MW00835212

To Harriett

with love +

Kisses.

Jules

Learning Disabilities and Psychic Conflict

Learning Disabilities and Psychic Conflict: A Psychoanalytic Casebook

Arden Aibel Rothstein, Ph.D.
and
Jules Glenn, M.D.

with case contributions by
Denia Barrett, Karen Gilmore, Roberta Green,
Jill Miller, Morris Peltz, Sherwood Waldron,
Antoinette Ambrosino Wyszynski, and Judith Yanof

INTERNATIONAL UNIVERSITIES PRESS, INC.
Madison   Connecticut

Library of Congress Cataloging-in-Publication Data

Rothstein, Arden.
    Learning disabilities and psychic conflict : a psychoanalytic casebook / Arden Aibel Rothstein and Jules Glenn.
       p.   cm.
    Includes bibliographical references and index.
    ISBN 0-8236-2952-X
    1. Learning disabilities—Psychological aspects—Case studies.
    2. Child analysis—Case studies. 3. Psychoanalysis—Case studies.
    I. Glenn, Jules. II. Title.
RJ506.L4R65   1998
616.85'889—dc21   98-51468
                                               CIP

Manufactured in the United States of America

Table of Contents

v

Authors

Jules Glenn, M.D., is Clinical Professor of Psychiatry, New York University Medical Center; Training and Supervising Analyst Emeritus, NYU Psychoanalytic Institute.

Arden Aibel Rothstein, Ph.D., is on the Faculty, NYU Psychoanalytic Institute; Clinical Associate Professor of Psychiatry, New York University Medical Center; private practice in New York City as an adult psychoanalyst, and child, adolescent, and adult psychotherapist and diagnostic tester.

Case Contributors

Denia G. Barrett, M.S.W., is Clinic Associate and Faculty Member, Cleveland Center for Research in Child Development; private practice as a child and adolescent analyst in Cleveland, Ohio.

Karen Gilmore, M.D., is Training and Supervising Analyst in Child, Adolescent, and Adult Psychoanalysis; Chair, Child Psychoanalysis Program, Columbia University Center for Psychoanalytic Training and Research; Training and Supervising Analyst, New York Psychoanalytic Institute; Associate Clinical Professor of Psychiatry, Columbia University.

Roberta Green, M.D., is a pseudonym used in this volume by an analyst in private practice.

Jill M. Miller, Ph.D., is on the Faculty, Denver Institute of Psychoanalysis and the Colorado Center for Psychoanalytic

Studies; private practice as a child, adolescent, and adult analyst, Denver, Colorado.

Morris L. Peltz, M.D., Training and Supervising Analyst, San Francisco Psychoanalytic Institute and Society; Assistant Clinical Professor of Psychiatry, University of California at San Francisco.

Sherwood Waldron, Jr., M.D., is a graduate in child and adult psychoanalysis, New York Psychoanalytic Institute; Director, Psychoanalytic Research Consortium.

Antoinette Ambrosino Wyszynski, M.D., Clinical Associate Professor of Psychiatry, New York University Medical Center; Faculty, NYU Psychoanalytic Institute.

Judith Yanof, M.D., is Training and Supervising Analyst and Child Supervisor, Boston Psychoanalytic Society and Institute; private practice as an analyst, Newton, Massachusetts.

PART I

Theoretical and Clinical Framework

Introduction

Although present in 5 to 10 percent of the population (Interagency Committee on Learning Disabilities, 1987), the psychoanalytic literature pays scant attention to patients suffering from learning problems with a clear neuropsychological underpinning. There are few in-depth studies of the clinical process of discovering the existence of learning disabilities in the course of an analysis. Nor has much appeared on several other related subjects: technical considerations in working with such patients, and clarification and exploration of the meanings of their particular learning disabilities in the context of the patient's complex of compromise formations, as they unfold in an analysis.

In our experience, the same is true in the clinical situation. Learning disabilities of patients in analysis or psychoanalytically oriented psychotherapy have often been overlooked entirely, or are not approached in a balanced fashion. Their contribution to the development of the patient's personality, and their implications for the analytic process, may either fail to receive careful consideration or, alternatively, be overemphasized. Rarely does the therapist direct his attention to specific details of the learning difficulty as discovered by the psychologist who has tested the patient. Instead, learning disabilities are typically considered in a more global manner.

A major purpose of this book is to alert clinicians to these and other issues in working analytically with patients who have learning disabilities, and thus help to prevent these kinds of oversights in the future. In our view, neuropsychologically based abnormalities contributory to learning disabilities, like any physical illness, do not derive from conflict and may need to be treated in their own right. However, when psychoanalytic work is undertaken with such patients, their neuropsychological difficulties cannot be considered apart from psychic conflict. Inevitably, the dysfunction and the fantasies which accrue

3

to it contribute to the shaping of psychic structure, psychodynamic conflicts, and the compromise formations which result (Hartmann, 1950; Weil, 1978; Rothstein, 1992, 1998). In this context isolating the dysfunction may be used for purposes of resistance by the patient or may reflect countertransference problems on the part of the analyst.

To prevent confusion, we will clarify our usage of a number of terms in this volume. *Neuropsychological* implies the existence of neurocortical abnormalities or so-called "developmental lags."[1] We use the term *neurophysiological* as a synonym for *neuropsychological*; it emphasizes the fact that the neurocortical anomalies are functional in nature, i.e., no anatomical findings have been discovered. Neuropsychological disturbances may be of many types. Some examples are disorders in memory, visual discrimination, regulation of attention, visual–motor coordination and sequencing. In turn, deficits in such neuropsychologically based skills may (but do not inevitably) contribute to problems in diverse aspects of learning, resulting in "learning disabilities." Similarly, another condition of neuropsychological etiology, Attention Deficit/Hyperactivity Disorder, applies to patients without known cerebral pathology, not all of whom display "learning disabilities," although most do. We further distinguish between *learning disabilities* and more general terms such as *learning problems, learning disorders*[2] and *learning difficulties* which do not imply a specific etiology but rather are

---

[1]In our view the term *developmental lag* may be misleading, since it is often taken to mean that, with time, a normal developmental course will be resumed. This is not always the case. In addition, it is not possible to differentiate, in advance, those instances in which a "lag" will abate and those in which it will persist.

[2]The diagnosis "Learning Disorder" in DSM-IV (APA, 1994), refers to problems in achievement of a quantitative nature, without specifying etiology. To quote, "Learning Disorders are diagnosed when the individual's achievement on individually administered, standardized tests in reading, mathematics, or written expression is substantially below that expected for age, schooling, and level of intelligence. The learning problems significantly interfere with academic achievement or activities of daily living that require reading, mathematical, or writing skills. A variety of statistical approaches can be used to establish that a discrepancy is significant. *Substantially below* is usually defined as a discrepancy of more than 2 standard deviations between achievement and IQ. A smaller discrepancy between achievement and IQ (i.e., between 1 and 2 standard deviations) is sometimes used, especially in cases where an individual's performance on an IQ test may have been compromised by an associated disorder in cognitive processing, a comorbid mental disorder or general medical condition, or the individual's ethnic or cultural background. If a sensory deficit is present, the learning difficulties must be in excess of those usually associated with the deficit.

descriptive in nature. When we refer to a learning problem as "neuropsychologically based," this does not imply that we dismiss the significance of psychological factors. It simply means that we assume a significant neuropsychological contribution.

Looked at historically, in the 1940s patients with learning disabilities were frequently diagnosed as having "minimal brain damage" (see Shaywitz, Fletcher, and Shaywitz [1994] for an excellent and more detailed historical survey). Indeed in many instances a history of actual illness (such as encephalitis, otitis media, or head injury) accompanied by positive neurological findings on examination, or "soft" neurological signs,[3] pointed in that direction. Often children with no history of physical disorder but with "soft" neurological signs were placed in the same category, giving rise to the diagnosis of "minimal brain dysfunction" rather than "minimal brain damage" (see Silver's [1992] introduction for an extensive review of the history of terminology in this field).

Because learning disabilities involve many types of dysfunction, we cannot expect to find a simple localized structural area of defect. We differentiate the vast number of learning disabilities which are functional (i.e., in which no structural lesion is known to exist, and thus the alterations of functions are neuropsychological in nature), from those which involve actual brain lesions (as in cases of aphasia).[4] Although we are concentrating on functional disorders of memory, perception, attention, sequencing, and the like, we have included one case (that of Dr. Miller) which involves known damage to the brain.

The methodology we used in assembling this volume is in keeping with Freud's view of psychoanalysis as a technique of treatment, a research method, and a theory. He believed that

---

Learning Disorders may persist into adulthood" (pp. 46–47). The disorder is specifically delineated as Reading Disorder, Mathematics Disorder, Disorder of Written Expression, and Learning Disorder Not Otherwise Specified.

[3]"Soft" signs are different from definite neurological findings such as reflex changes or a positive Babinski sign. Examples of "soft" signs are the finding that when a child is asked to extend his arms before him, one arm drifts downward, or the presence of an "equivocal Babinski" (Kennard, 1960).

[4]Ideally, one should differentiate patients whose poor functioning (such as a learning disability or hyperactivity) was caused by neurological lesions from those where no lesion is discovered. However, in practice that distinction cannot always be made.

the therapeutic procedure allows us to collect detailed observations of patients which can be used to build theory, while at the same time aiding them therapeutically. In this book we use detailed information from nine psychoanalyses to help delineate and understand the interweaving of psychodynamic and experiential issues in patients with learning disabilities from a clinical theoretical point of view, as well as issues pertinent to technique.

With this purpose in mind, we asked analysts to send us rather detailed summaries of analyses of patients with learning disabilities. To find suitable cases we placed notices of our intended volume in several psychoanalytic newsletters and directly contacted analysts to whom our colleagues referred us. After screening the papers we received, we chose cases we regarded as suitable, and asked the authors to elaborate their case reports, according to guidelines we supplied. In some instances we interviewed the analyst to get additional information.

The resulting approximately twenty- to forty-page writeups are comprehensive but not exhaustive. A full description of an analysis would fill a large book and overwhelm the reader. We asked the authors to condense their work, and at the same time present sufficiently detailed material for us to reach convincing conclusions. The contributing analysts provided subtle information, such as the development of the psychoanalytic process, the nature of transferences and countertransferences, the past and present environmental influences, and the character of defenses and the affects and wishes they defended against. And of course case reports revealed how individual patients coped with their learning disabilities before and during the analysis.

In addition, our contributors presented some extra-analytic information. Each patient had one or more diagnostic psychological testing evaluations, affording information about the presence and specific configuration of the learning disability. The nature of these evaluations varied from case to case; some were more detailed and elaborate and others were relatively cursory. In some instances this reflected the type of testing generally employed at the time the analyses were undertaken. Test findings were integrated into the analytic work to varying degrees. Some analysts also provided data about their patients' tutoring or other treatment modalities supplementary to the analysis.

This study is retrospective in the sense that it involves case material that was already gathered. Most of the analyses we examined were already completed, and the others were well under way. We did not change the technique of information gathering; nor did we request tests different from those already administered or alter the analysts' interventions by suggesting new interpretations or questions about which we were curious. We could, of course, reinterpret the data for scientific purposes, and note possible technical changes, but we could not change the course of an actual analysis.

The limitations of our method are intertwined with its strengths. The authors did not have preconceived ideas about how learning disabilities affect the personality and psychopathology of their patients. Psychoanalysis, involving four or five sessions a week for years, provides a tremendous amount of data, even about questions not considered prior to the treatment. With only one exception (Dr. Miller's case of Julia),[5] no patient was treated less than four times per week; even in that case much of the treatment was conducted four times a week. Much of the literature on patients with learning disabilities derives from less intensive treatment, which does not yield the in-depth data of the psychoanalytic situation or the greater degree of conviction about conclusions which these data permit.

Cohen (1998) has suggested that a methodology needs to be developed for verifying psychoanalytic findings regarding patients with neuropsychological disorders. We believe our method does just that. We examined the data on learning disabilities gathered from nine analyses, most reported from start to finish.

Others have tried to verify psychoanalytic constructs regarding matters other than biological–psychological interactions through the study of multiple cases. Breuer and Freud (1893–1895), describing patients treated before psychoanalysis

---

[5]In addition, Dr. Wyszynski's patient was seen at a reduced frequency for a brief period of time.

was developed, reached important conclusions regarding hysteria and its treatment. Later Freud stated or implied that conclusions he reached were based on a number of similar cases, but he did not specify how many or detail the analytic work (see Freud, 1919, for instance).

Others have relied on vignettes and details of analyses examined in study groups, records of analyses and information gathered from other analysts to reach conclusions, but have reported only a few such treatments (E. Furman, 1974; Sandler, Kennedy, and Tyson, 1980; Abend, Porder, and Willick, 1983; Schmukler, 1991; Fonagy and Target, 1996). Cohen and Cohler (in preparation) have described analyses of children who have been reanalyzed as adults. A number of chapters in Geleerd's (1967) and Harley's (1974) volumes on child and adolescent analysis cover much of the course of the analyses, as does another case book by Sholevar and Glenn (1991) which contains several more or less full analyses; in the overview Rangell offers in this volume, he used the four analyses presented to compare past and present technique.

In closing, we would like to describe the organization of this volume. In chapter 1 we present general clinical theoretical and technical issues of significance in analyzing patients with learning disabilities. In chapter 2 we critique recent contributions to this subject and briefly review older contributions. (See Rothstein, Benjamin, Crosby, and Eisenstadt [1988] for a more comprehensive review of the literature prior to this period.) In chapters 3 through 20 detailed accounts of the analyses of patients over a spectrum of ages are elaborated, followed by discussions we have written to highlight salient issues particular to each patient. The first five cases are children, from preschool to schoolage; the next one is an adolescent; and the final three cases are adults. These can be read in light of the controversies presented in chapters 1 and 2. Finally, we summarize our findings in the Conclusion.

Chapter 1

Clinical, Theoretical, and Technical Issues in the Analysis of Patients with Learning Disabilities

INTRODUCTION

This book consists of detailed studies by eight psychoanalysts of the treatment of their nine patients, each of whom had learning disabilities (one analyst described two cases). These reports are followed by our discussions of the patients and their treatments. We have explored these cases carefully from the perspective of the mutual influences of the patients' neuropsychological and psychodynamic contributions to their personality structures. In addition, we have studied the in-depth clinical material provided by the contributing analysts from the vantage point of previous contributions to this subject. In some instances this has led us to refine existing ideas or to comment on misconceptions.

It has been our experience that, despite the present climate of sophistication about learning disabilities, in practice a number of common myths, misunderstandings, and overgeneralizations persist. Many analysts manifest at least a tendency to overlook or subtly deemphasize the possible contribution of neuropsychological dysfunction to patients' difficulties in learning, achievement, and other presenting problems. Related to this, they may isolate psychodynamic from neuropsychological contributions to a patient's clinical picture, failing to fully consider the possibility, or indeed the inevitability, of coexisting and/or intertwining psychodynamic and neuropsychological contributions.

The analyst then feels an unnecessary pressure to determine whether a symptom or other type of surface presentation is due to psychic conflict *or* neuropsychological dysfunction, or at least to come to a conclusion about which one is more significant. This is especially common when patients are bright, verbal, and evidence compellingly relevant psychodynamic constellations which appear to sufficiently explain their presenting complaints. Much of the psychoanalytic and nonpsychoanalytic literature on this subject reflects a similar perspective (see Rothstein, Benjamin, Crosby, and Eisenstadt [1988], as well as the updated review of the literature in chapter 2 of this volume).

When a neuropsychological contribution is considered, and if a proper diagnostic assessment reveals the existence of circumscribed cognitive problems of this etiology, we believe that it is actually more useful to think about *how* (rather than *whether*) the neuropsychological dysfunction (one manifestation of which may be a learning disability) affects development and current functioning, and *how* it is incorporated in the patient's compromise formations.[1]

Toward this end, there is enormous value in knowing the details of the dysfunction, and exploring and conceptualizing the *specific* ways in which they are elaborated in fantasy and interwoven in the patient's psychodynamic constellations. This

---

[1]In our view it is valid to reach a neuropsychological diagnosis when, after a very careful diagnostic study, the patterning of findings is such that problems in cognitive functions correspond with what we know about the organization of the brain. That is, every time a particular function is required in a complex task, the patient has difficulty with it. For example, this would be the case when a diagnostic evaluation reveals problems with visual sequential memory (evident in a patient's performance on mazes, spelling, tests of visual sequential memory per se, and visual sequential portions of the standard IQ test) and sound blending, in the presence of strength in auditory sequential memory and constructional abilities. This pattern would not be explainable on the basis of the invasion of ego functions of integration by psychic conflict since, by this reasoning, the latter areas of strength should be affected as well. Conversely, one can have variability that does not correspond to the patterning of the brain, but which reflects such psychological phenomena as depression, anxiety about working alone, or anxiety about knowing.

perspective is contrasted with a tendency to rest solely with more *general* formulations and interpretations which, while crucial, are incomplete (Rothstein, 1992, 1998). Two examples of such general ideas are the learning disabled patient's experience of himself as damaged, and the recruitment of this sense of damage for defensive purposes, as in the unconscious thought, "I have no aspirations as an oedipal rival. I'm defective and helpless."

Since this volume is primarily addressed to psychoanalysts and psychoanalytically oriented clinicians, we emphasize several aspects of psychoanalytic work with patients who have difficulties in learning and achievement. One is the importance of transcending a tendency to make clinical assumptions which are not followed up with a combined psychological, educational, and neuropsychological diagnostic evaluation. Rather than competing with an analytic perspective, such diagnostic study ought to facilitate the richness of the analytic exploration. From the perspective of compromise formation theory, neuropsychological dysfunction inevitably has a shaping influence on the development of unconscious fantasies, which are composed of drive derivatives, affects, and defenses. In the absence of a detailed evaluation, a great deal may be lost to analytic understanding.

A number of additional issues will be discussed. The scope of an adequate diagnostic evaluation is presented, as are considerations in making a referral and reporting the findings of this evaluation when this is done during the analysis. We describe the multiple ways in which an analyst may become aware of the possibility of a neuropsychological contribution to a patient's clinical presentation, including a problem in learning. Finally, questions of analyzability and the patient's and analyst's fantasies of cure and experience of termination are elaborated.

In order to address these issues, our contributors have typically described their patients' analyses from beginning to end. The reports they have provided include passages that demonstrate the analytic processes essential to understanding their analysands, some of which appear to have little to do with their learning disabilities. In a given case, the patient's associations

may continue for many pages and many months without manifest discussion of cognitive issues. Although eventually the interaction of neuropsychological and conflictual aspects can
often be seen, this is not always the case. While some authors
tend to emphasize aspects of the analyses involving learning
disabilities (indeed we invited them to elaborate on these aspects of their analytic work), our aim is to present a balanced
picture of the roles of neuropsychological dysfunction (including learning disabilities) and psychic conflict.

NEUROPSYCHOLOGICAL DYSFUNCTION AND
COMPROMISE FORMATION

Even when careful diagnostic study documents the existence
of irregularities (or immaturities) in the functioning of the
brain, there is no less reason to consider their involvement in
the patient's psychological makeup. To say a particular type of
learning disability could not have taken shape without certain
types of neuropsychological dysfunction is not to say that it fails
to become embroiled in conflict or can be considered apart
from conflict.

Therefore, we feel that the efforts of an analyst to differentiate between what is "dysfunction" (or "damage," "deficit,"
or "defect") and what is a manifestation of psychic conflict,
may result in an impossible quagmire, and is of little clinical
value. The potential limitations in the scope of an analyst's
interventions which may result from a tendency to isolate
"deficit" from "conflict" were emphasized by Willick (1991)
who noted, "the importance of maintaining a dynamic point
of view in the face of what might appear to be an ego deficit. . . .
The danger in conceptualizing this impairment as a defect is
that it may lead to the therapist's reluctance to make interpretations of conflict . . . " (p. 83).

Some of the contributing analysts (Mrs. Barrett in chapter
3, Dr. Miller in chapter 5, Dr. Yanof in chapter 11, and Dr.
Wyszynski in chapter 19) subtly expressed wishes to distinguish
between "defect" and "conflict"; at the same time it was clear

that they intuitively appreciated and clinically worked with the multiple facets of their patients' conflicts. Of course for practical reasons that differentiation sometimes has to be made, even as one recognizes the intimate interactions. This is seen in Dr. Miller's case of Julia (chapter 5), the one most dramatic in terms of disordered brain functioning. The analyst attempted to help her patient differentiate between a sense of loss in the context of absences due to epilepsy and feeling lost due to conflict. However, from the perspective of our book we would emphasize the importance of exploring with the patient the multiple meanings of her physical symptoms as expressions of psychic conflict.

In one sense there is nothing unique about treating patients with documented neuropsychological dysfunction, often manifested in learning disabilities. In another sense there are common potential pitfalls in working with such patients if the analyst does not carefully attend to the specific and complex ways in which the patient's neuropsychological dysfunction influences the development of his conflicts, best understood as complexes of compromise formations. Brenner (1976), following Freud (1923, 1926), delineated the elements of compromise formations as follows:

When defenses are used to counter a dangerous instinctual wish or superego demand in order to avoid anxiety, it is the resulting compromise formation that appears in an individual's mental life and behavior as an observable phenomenon. It is the compromise that one hears and perceives as one listens to and observes a patient. *Wish, anxiety, guilt, and defense* all enter into the final result—the compromise—in every case, though the relative importance of each varies from one instance to another. The compromise is invariably the result of the interaction of them all. . . . It may be added, for the sake of completeness, that a compromise formation is often influenced by *current environmental circumstances* as well [pp. 10–11; emphasis added].

As with "current environmental circumstances," numerous features of the patient's ego also contribute to the shaping of the patient's compromise formations.

Where neuropsychological dysfunction exists, it likely shapes every component of a patient's constellation of compromise formations. Elsewhere one of us (Rothstein et al., 1988) has delineated the multiple neuropsychological developments, the intactness of which is assumed in the normal development of object relations. To cite a few, language and fine and gross motor coordination contribute to self-object differentiation, just as memory, perceptual processing, and the capacity to integrate these processes, contribute to the development of object constancy. Particular types of dysfunction may be especially suited for incorporation in unconscious fantasies, in that there is a convergence between the content of the dysfunction and the fantasy. An illustration would be problems with ocular control or visual processing in a child in the throes of the oedipal phase. Neuropsychological dysfunction will also become intertwined in superego functioning; for example, in fantasies that so-called "deficits" are punishments for unacceptable wishes. Superego formation may be affected in another sense; patients with certain types of cognitive dysfunction (e.g., a disability in expressive or receptive language) may be more likely to misunderstand parental prohibitions or statements of standards and develop a superego which differs from what the parents intended to advocate. Also, the parents may misunderstand a child whose communication is poor; their reactions to verbal behavior which they misconstrue may have a severity appropriate to a child with different intentions and capacities.

While broad statements about the vulnerabilities, dynamics, problems in analyzability, and transference configurations of learning disabled patients are of interest, in actual analytic work particular types of neuropsychological dysfunction contribute to development in complex and highly individual ways. The degree to which a specific type of neuropsychological dysfunction shapes development will depend upon a "complemental series" (Freud, 1937); for example, the degree of severity and/or pervasiveness of the dysfunction and the extent to which it "fits" with the psychodynamic constellations of the patient and of his or her parents. Thinking of "learning disabilities" as if they are entities with universal implications is of limited value in capturing the realities of the clinical situation, in which knowledge of the individual analytic patient's cognitive disabilities is more helpful.

When this perspective informs the initial diagnostic work (including testing and/or clinical interviewing) with a potential analytic patient, as well as the ongoing psychoanalytic exploration, the reward is the richness and complexity of the analytic understanding gained. An appreciation of the combination of strengths and weaknesses with which a particular individual presents obviates the need to rely upon generalities. Instead one can maximally explore the individual interweavings of the particular features of a patient's neuropsychological dysfunction (e.g., disturbances in ego functions such as perception, learning, and memory) with his wishes, defenses, superego elements, anxiety, depressive affect, and current environmental circumstances.

The analysts who have contributed their cases for this volume vary in the degree to which they had access to the kind of detailed diagnostic data which would equip them optimally to explore such interrelationships. For some of them, the growing awareness of additional perspectives on their patients' clinical presentation (behavior, style of communication) in the analytic hours led them to revise and augment their understandings of these clinical phenomena. For example, Dr. Green expanded her conceptualization of what she had previously regarded solely as Ms. Ames' obsessional symptomatology (chapter 15). She also came to view these characteristics of her patient as an effort to anchor her sense of disorientation and confusion in dealing with space, sequence, and numbers—her areas of neuropsychological dysfunction.

Although the psychologists who performed the multiple evaluations of Dr. Waldron's patient Frank (over the course of many years) did not integrate their cognitive findings (problems with language, memory, and written expression) with the nature of Frank's psychological structure and functioning, Dr. Waldron came to appreciate and address this in the analytic work (chapter 9). He gradually understood how Frank's "woodenness," immaturity, phobic distortions of reality, omnipotent fantasies, and confusion of pronouns were amalgamated in complex ways.

Dr. Miller (chapter 5) beautifully describes how her patient Julia used her frank brain pathology, including the experience of seizures, as a defense against overwhelming affects as the analysis proceeded. In so doing Dr. Miller attempted to differentiate between moments when such clinical phenomena were used primarily in the service of defense. More specifically, she tried to help Julia identify inner experiences that were primarily reflective of her neurological disease, in contrast to similar experiences which were basically a result of psychic conflict. It is worth considering whether this can actually be done, and what the clinical advantages of attempting to do so would be. Dr. Miller also does a masterful job of elaborating the interweaving of aspects of her patient's organicity in the formation of her unconscious fantasies.

Drs. Gilmore (chapter 13) and Yanof (chapter 11) richly explore the way in which their patients' problems in sustaining attention, distractibility, impulsivity, and other associated aspects of cognitive dysfunction both shaped their experience of self and others, and became involved in the development of compromise formations.

Dr. Gilmore believed that many characteristics of her patient Rebecca were related to an Attention Deficit/Hyperactivity Disorder which had been diagnosed years before the analysis began. This significantly informed Dr. Gilmore's clinical work as she explored with Rebecca her use of activity to reduce her awareness of painful insights and internal conflicts, and her recruiting of a sense of herself as vulnerable in the service of denying her aggressive wishes. She also explored Rebecca's experience of her cognitive functioning and the way in which her limitations had become caught up with feelings of being defective as a girl.

Dr. Yanof (chapter 11) was not certain that her patient Eric had an Attention Deficit/Hyperactivity Disorder (she used the term *Attention Deficit Disorder,* the one employed before DSM-IV). Nevertheless, she portrays with richness and vividness how her patient's impulsivity and distractibility contributed to his experience of himself and his surround as fleeting and lacking in continuity. She also elaborated the ways in which these experiences and behaviors came to be used defensively, as well as how they were incorporated in central unconscious fantasies.

An awareness of their patients' specific cognitive disabilities (e.g., deficits in language, memory, visual–spatial concepts, sequencing, conceptualization) led some of the contributing analysts to technical modifications. To illustrate, as he came to appreciate that his patient Frank had significant problems in expressive and receptive language, Dr. Waldron (chapter 9) altered the form and/or content of his interventions. He became more forthcoming in explaining actual facts or events to Frank, preliminary to further clarifying which feelings and thought processes led to his (Frank's) confusion. Dr. Waldron also increasingly grasped and interpreted the contribution of Frank's language problems to his compromise formations, as seen, for example, in his tendencies to clown, to avoid, and to engage in dishonest behavior. However, Dr. Waldron did not seem to explicitly take into account diagnostic findings of Frank's deficits in memory in making his interpretations.

THE DIAGNOSTIC TESTING EVALUATION

Many common kinds of misdiagnosis result from the tendency to emphasize psychodynamic *or* neuropsychological factors. Some reflect the imposition of preconceived notions of "deficit" on the data, while others result from insufficiently evaluating the range of possible etiological routes to the presenting problems. One broad group of misdiagnoses derives from the supposition of cognitive "deficits" of varying types by specialists in learning problems who are not also general clinicians. For example, a diagnostic tester may overdiagnose "language processing disorders" when, in reality, a patient has a case of what might be called "averageitis" (average intelligence when higher potential is presumed), or a major inhibition in functioning related to oedipal conflicts. Or a diagnostic evaluator may mistakenly conclude that the patient possesses limited intelligence, without adequately considering the effects of constriction resulting from anxiety associated with the fantasied consequences of aggressive and erotic wishes.

Similarly, patients of psychoanalysts or psychoanalytically oriented clinicians are sometimes erroneously assumed to have problems of a purely psychological nature (e.g., inhibitions in learning due to psychological conflict or failures to function due to lack of mirroring by self objects [Kohut, 1977]), especially when these patients are of superior intelligence. This reflects a belief that a patient cannot be bright and successful academically and nevertheless have a learning disability. A tendency to overlook the possibility of a neuropsychological contribution also frequently occurs when psychodynamic explanations seem sufficient to account for the psychological phenomena presented. Common examples are the failure to recognize Attention-Deficit/Hyperactivity Disorders or specific types of cognitive dysfunction (e.g., problems in visual sequential memory, sound blending, or visual discrimination) which contribute to problems in reading.

An opposite type of misdiagnosis occurs when the clinician concludes that patients suffering from disabling anxiety have Attention Deficit/Hyperactivity Disorders because they conform to the list of behavioral traits characterizing such conditions (see Silver, 1989, 1992; Weinberg and Brumback, 1992). *The Diagnostic and Statistical Manual,* 4th edition (DSM-IV; APA, 1994), as well as previous DSM's provide such lists[2] with the

---

[2]An "Attention Deficit/Hyperactivity Disorder" is diagnosed if four conditions are met. One is "a persistent pattern of inattention and/or hyperactivity-impulsivity" more frequent and severe than is typical for the patient's age. A second is that some of the symptoms must have been present before age 7. Third, the symptoms must be observed in at least two settings, such as at home and at school or work. Finally, clear evidence is required of compromised social, academic, or occupational functioning. A choice can be made between three types of Attention Deficit/Hyperactivity Disorders. To qualify for the diagnosis "Attention-Deficit/Hyperactivity Disorder, Combined Type" the patient has to have six or more symptoms of inattention and six or more symptoms of hyperactivity-impulsivity which have persisted for at least six months. The diagnosis "Attention-Deficit/Hyperactivity Disorder, Predominantly Inattentive Type" (comparable to the former diagnosis "Attention Deficit Disorder") is made if the patient has six or more symptoms of inattention but fewer than six symptoms of hyperactivity-impulsivity which have persisted for at least six months. "Attention-Deficit/Hyperactivity Disorder, Predominantly Hyperactive-Impulsive Type" is diagnosed if the patient has six or more symptoms of hyperactivity-impulsivity but fewer than six symptoms of inattention (although inattention may still be a significant clinical feature) which have persisted for at least six months. The nine possible behavioral manifestations of "Inattention" are: failure to give close attention to details or making careless mistakes, difficulty sustaining attention in tasks or play, apparently

expectation that the clinician will make the diagnosis mechanically. The fact that there is overlap among items in the lists used to diagnose other disorders (such as Conduct Disorders and Anxiety Disorders) increases the likelihood that the diagnostician will rely upon arbitrary decisions or conclude that a dual diagnosis applies. From a psychoanalytic perspective reliance upon such behavioral descriptions is frequently of little value in our effort to understand the patient's constellation of psychodynamic conflicts.

Furthermore, an assumption is sometimes made that a patient with ADHD necessarily has a learning disability, and that this does not need to be independently and specifically evaluated. In fact, while there is a significant correlation between the two, it is not inevitable (Silver, 1992). Furthermore, when there is an associated learning disability, its particular configuration can have unlimited variations.[3]

To minimize clinical errors, the scope and the specific nature of the learning disability should be determined. Conclusions about the existence of neuropsychological dysfunction can only reliably derive from a careful diagnostic evaluation of patients who usually present with problems in learning. This is

---

not listening when spoken to directly, failure to follow through on instructions and to finish schoolwork, chores, or duties in the workplace, difficulty organizing tasks and activities, avoidance, dislike or reluctance to engage in tasks which require sustained mental effort, a tendency to lose things necessary to tasks or activities, distractibility by extraneous stimuli, forgetfulness in daily activities. The nine behavioral characteristics involved in "Hyperactivity-Impulsivity" are: fidgeting with hands or feet or squirming in seat, leaving one's seat in the classroom or in other situations, running about or climbing excessively in situations in which this is inappropriate, difficulty playing or engaging in leisure activities quietly, being "on the go" or acting as if "driven by a motor," talking excessively, blurting out answers before questions are completed, difficulty awaiting turn, and interrupting or intruding upon others.

[3]As Shaywitz et al. (1994) noted, "although attention deficit-hyperactivity disorder (ADHD) and learning disabilities frequently co-occur in the same child, each (ADHD and LD) is a separate problem. Diagnosis of ADHD is established on the basis of a history of symptoms representing the cardinal constructs of ADHD—inattention, impulsivity, and sometimes hyperactivity (American Psychiatric Association, 1980, 1987, 1991). In contrast, the diagnosis of learning disability is established on the basis of performance on tests of ability and achievement" (p. 108). Shaywitz et al.'s (1994) review of the literature showed that, the prevalence of learning disabilities in the ADHD population is substantial (Keogh, 1971; Wender, 1971). Results of studies to date support this belief, with estimates of learning disabilities in a hyperactive population ranging between 9% (Halperin, Gittelman, Klein, and Ruddel, 1984) and 80% (McGee and Share, 1988) to 92% (Silver, 1981)" (pp. 110–111).

contrasted with a reliance upon clinical preconceptions which shape what one will find. General diagnostic impressions, such as that a patient's problems are "organic" or that a patient has a "learning disability," are only a starting point. The particular features of learning that are affected can and should be delineated; for example, overall intelligence, conceptualization, expressive and receptive language, reading, mathematical calculation, writing, attentional processes, sequential concepts, visual–motor coordination, and the array of memory functions.[4]

A comprehensive evaluation includes the intelligence test appropriate to the patient's age, achievement tests (including a full examination of academic skills which are not explicitly mentioned among the presenting problems, for example, math should be examined, even when only reading is reported to be a problem), more specialized tests of the individual building blocks for these more complex functions (e.g., an array of auditory and visual memory functions, sequencing, motor coordination, various types of sensory processing) and projective tests. This is a extensive procedure, which typically involves four sessions of $1^{1}/_{2}$ to 2 hours each (see Rothstein et al. [1988, pp. 129–163] for a more in-depth discussion of an optimally comprehensive test battery).

In our experience, diagnostic testing evaluations are all too often of insufficient scope, leading to overly general conclusions about learning disabled patients, and sometimes false negative or false positive findings. Typical examples are the conclusion of "organicity" without delineation of the particular aspects of functioning involved. The administration of an intelligence test alone, and the omission of achievement tests which permit careful study of the specific components of the learning disability, is surprisingly common. We have found that this may occur even when central presenting problems relate

---

[4]One published example of attention to specific cognitive disabilities in the clinical situation is Athey's (1986) fine-grained delineation of different types of disorders in memory functions, with their implications for clinical interventions. Squire (1987, 1995) has also described a multitude of memory functions and dysfunctions which he has used to clarify psychoanalytic findings regarding repression and other aspects of remembering and forgetting.

to school performance. So too is the practice of simply administering an achievement test in the absence of an intelligence test and/or specialized tests of the specific neuropsychological building blocks for academic tasks.

Furthermore, many diagnosticians have a misconception that there is a "typical organic pattern," such as a large discrepancy between the patient's Verbal and Performance IQ scores.[5] In this volume, this tendency is exemplified by the diagnostic workup in Dr. Wyszynski's case (chapter 19). In fact, there are multiple etiological routes to such a discrepancy, a learning disability being only one of them. In addition, a patient may have a neuropsychologically based learning disability in the absence of such a discrepancy.

Such practices are particularly common in a number of settings. Evaluations performed within schools are necessarily brief (for example, see the evaluation of Mrs. Barrett's patient Leah, chapter 3); given the limitations of resources more than a screening can rarely be provided. The approximately eight hours necessary to administer a comprehensive battery alone (not taking into account the time for scoring, interpreting and reporting of findings) make such evaluations unfeasible within the school.

More generally, clinicians who carry out optimally comprehensive evaluations are sometimes difficult to find, especially outside of areas with sophisticated training settings in which the necessary tests and their value is taught. We have found that the ability to find properly trained clinicians is not to be

---

[5]The concept of specific types of disability, rather than "typical organic patterns," is one which has been generally accepted for a long time. More than two decades ago, Denckla (1972), a behavioral neurologist and expert in the field of learning disabilities, advocated that the field had moved beyond "lumping" children into single diagnostic categories. Arguing for the value of syndrome analysis, she proposed three categories of learning disability: specific language disabilities, specific visuospatial disabilities, and dyscontrol syndromes. In her seminal paper she called for continued investigation of subtypes. In this spirit, Mattis, French, and Rapin (1975) described three independent forms of dyslexia. Studies of types of learning disturbances continue. Two excellent recent examples are the contributions of Pennington (1991a, b) who offers five subtypes (dyslexia and other developmental language disorders, Attention Deficit/Hyperactivity Disorder, right hemisphere learning disorders, autism spectrum disorder, and acquired memory disorders) and Hooper and Swartz (1994) who review all previous contributions regarding subtypes.

taken for granted even in major cities with first-rate teaching hospitals and graduate programs.

Paradoxically, in some of these settings another problem may develop. The frequent proliferation of subspecialists can result in the practice of having professionals of different disciplines, each of whom carries out only a portion of the type of evaluation we recommend, without fully integrating their findings. For example, a clinical psychologist may administer the intelligence test and projective tests, while an educational psychologist administers achievement tests, and a neuropsychologist or learning specialist assesses specific aspects of cognitive functions such as memory, perceptual processing, and the like. When these findings are apparently inconsistent, or even in conflict with each other, a single clinician does not provide an overview of the array of subtle clinical possibilities which can account for this. As a consequence, both false positive and false negative conclusions may result.

The cases we have selected for this volume exemplify the gamut of approaches to diagnostic testing evaluation. The one which best approximates the comprehensiveness we believe to be optimal is Dr. Green's case of Ms. Ames (chapter 15). A detailed study of the nature of Ms. Ames' cognitive (including academic) functioning was undertaken, along with an in-depth examination of her psychodynamic constellation as conveyed in projective testing. This permitted an appreciation of the interplay of her specific weaknesses in visuospatial reasoning, sequencing, and other cognitive functions, with her personality configuration.

The diagnostic evaluations of other patients in our volume fall short in a variety of ways. In several cases (see the evaluations reported by Dr. Peltz in chapter 7, Dr. Green in chapter 17, and Dr. Wyszynski in chapter 19), despite the analyst's and/ or psychologist's suspicion that a learning disability affected academic work, achievement testing was omitted. This made it impossible to reach a definite conclusion.

In those instances when some type of achievement test was included and the patient's performance *was* below expectations based upon his or her overall level of intelligence (see Mrs. Barrett's case of Leah in chapter 3, Dr. Waldron's case of

Frank in chapter 9, and Dr. Yanof's case of Eric in chapter 11), there was often a less than optimally detailed analysis of the specific reasons for this. For example, when reading levels are well below expectations, the possibility of weaknesses in particular cognitive functions (e.g., visual sequencing, visual processing, visual memory, auditory discrimination, and sound blending) should be explored. When such evaluation is not undertaken, findings are left more inconclusive than need be.

Although most often a neuropsychological contribution to a learning problem can be ruled in or out and its nature specified, there *are* critical situations when it is not possible to reach definitive conclusions. One example is work with children of preschool age (e.g., Dr. Yanof's patient Eric in chapter 11), with whom a comprehensive evaluation of academic skills cannot be carried out. However, it is often eminently possible to gauge whether a child is at risk for a learning disability because of unevenness on other tests. Since this *can* be further evaluated in the early school grades, it is wise to recommend a reevaluation. In addition, when questions remain, it is useful to retest a child at regular intervals (for example, in 1st and then again in 3rd grade), to determine whether additional vulnerabilities will appear in the context of new academic demands.

The cases in this volume also illustrate clinicians' widely varying practices with regard to including complete projective testing (the Rorschach, Thematic Apperception Test, and Figure Drawings at a minimum) in batteries of patients being evaluated for problems in learning. One possible result of the omission of such tests is minimization of the contribution of psychic conflict. This was evident in Dr. Gilmore's report of the diagnostic testing evaluation done with her patient Rebecca (chapter 13) years before they met. Another is a failure to fully appreciate and delineate the interrelationships between specific aspects of cognitive and psychic functioning. This was evident in the multiple partial evaluations performed with Dr. Waldron's patient Frank (chapter 9) in which the interplay between Frank's expressive and receptive language disorder and his "flights of ideas" and "loosening of secondary process," his immaturity, omnipotent fantasies, and phobic distortions of reality seemed to have been overlooked. In contrast, the psychologist who evaluated Dr. Green's patient Ms. Ames (chapter 15) engaged in a rich integration of the patient's problems in visuospatial organization and visual memory with her conflicts over seeing and knowing, her difficulty in retrieval of visually encoded memories, her obsessional symptomatology, and her struggles at work.

Technical Issues in Preparing a Patient for Testing and Using the Test Findings

Testing may occur as part of the initial evaluation, or take place once the analysis is under way. It may be initiated by the analyst, by another professional involved with the patient, or by the patient himself (or his parents). Some child analysts routinely arrange to have patients tested, while others may do so only in selected cases, such as when they suspect a learning disability. The adult patient or parents (and sometimes the child patient) will want to know the reasons for undertaking a diagnostic evaluation, and the analyst will inform them of his particular rationale.

The patient's fantasies about the meanings of this procedure are likely to be expressed in the analytic material. When the analyst initiates the referral for testing, some preparatory work (much of which involves analysis of these fantasies) may be involved as well. When testing takes places after the analysis is under way, it is often an outgrowth of the treatment process. Preparation similarly becomes a part of the analysis in which patient and analyst discuss and try to understand the significance of this evaluation for their understanding of the patient. Only rarely does the analyst have to help the patient master the testing procedure because it is experienced as traumatic, as was the case in Dr. Miller's work with Julia (chapter 5).

Three of the cases in this volume fruitfully explore issues around preparing a patient for diagnostic evaluation. In her work with her two patients (chapters 15 and 17) Dr. Green was sensitive to the psychodynamic meanings of pursuing a detailed diagnostic study of areas of their functioning which were intensely affect laden. These issues were also highlighted in the analysis of Julia reported by Dr. Miller (chapter 5); in fact, Dr. Miller felt that one goal of the initial months of analysis with Julia was to help her stabilize sufficiently to be able to weather a proper diagnostic evaluation. This was necessary because Julia, in fantasy, equated the benign psychological testing situation with the dangerous traumatizing surgical procedures she had suffered. The preparation was compatible with the analytic goal of helping the patient understand the determinants of the anxiety that testing elicited in her. In fantasy Julia equated the benign psychological testing situation with the dangerous traumatizing surgical procedures she had suffered.

When testing is completed, the analyst has to evaluate the advisability of sharing the results with his patient. The determination of how much and what to tell the patient is a complex decision. If too great an emphasis is placed on cognitive dysfunction, the patient may use this knowledge defensively to avoid recognizing conflictual neurotic determinants of his personality. Furthermore, the patient may experience the information he is given as a deep narcissistic injury. He may feel, with a conviction that makes analysis difficult, that the analyst has inflicted a sadistic blow.

Although of course each case has to be considered individually, it is probably best to let most patients participate in some way in the gradual assimilation of knowledge about their cognitive dysfunction, and its role in the development of their personalities. In part, this is because if insufficient data are supplied, the patient may not be able to decide on what the best treatment would be. In addition, it is not possible to engage in the valuable exploration of the diagnosed neuropsychological dysfunction's contribution to and interweaving with the patient's psychodynamic constellation unless diagnostic findings are available to the patient. Moreover, the analyst's concealing of knowledge derived from a psychological evaluation he has recommended is generally antithetical to psychoanalytic aims and practice. Furthermore, not discussing this material may be experienced as a repetition of relationships with parents who were unaware, or otherwise avoidant, of the patient's cognitive difficulties. These questions are explored in depth in the cases reported by Dr. Green (chapters 15 and 17) and Dr. Miller (chapter 5). In contrast, although testing was performed during or just prior to the beginning of the analyses reported by Drs. Peltz (chapter 7) and Waldron (chapter 9) and Mrs. Barrett (chapter 3), the exploration of findings with their patients was not detailed.

ROUTES TO DISCOVERY OF A LEARNING DISABILITY

The cases in this volume exemplify variations in the processes by which analysts come to consider the existence of a patient's neuropsychological dysfunction, including a learning disability. In some instances, problems in learning and/or behavior in school or at work are central to the initial referral to the analyst. In others the patient (and/or his or her parents, in the case of children) is unaware that neuropsychological difficulties are contributory to the clinical picture, since it does not explicitly involve academic or work functioning.

Referral to the analyst may precede or follow diagnostic evaluation by another professional. In the cases reported by Drs. Wyszynski (chapter 19) and Yanof (chapter 11) the patient had psychological testing just prior to referral to the analyst. In these instances, psychotherapy or psychoanalysis was either the sole, or one of several, resulting recommendations. In some cases (such as Dr. Peltz's) the diagnostician did not seem to feel the learning difficulties significantly involved neuropsychological problems. In Dr. Wyszynski's case of an adult (chapter 19), the diagnostician believed that Mr. G evidenced residua of a childhood learning disability, the psychological consequences of which required psychotherapeutic attention, along with his other broader psychological problems. In Dr. Yanof's case of Eric (chapter 11), the referring psychologist thought the young boy had an Attention Deficit Disorder (the term used at that time) which should be treated with stimulant medication; in addition, she believed that he was at risk for a learning disability and required psychotherapy. She also thought that he would profit from repeating kindergarten to have an extra year to benefit from these interventions, prior to undertaking more rigorous academic work. Mrs. Barrett's patient

Leah (chapter 3) was tested as a preschooler coincident with the beginning of the analysis, as part of the school's routine screening process. Although Leah was noted to have difficulty with many aspects of learning and performance, this seems to have been attributed predominantly to intrapsychic conflict, and the question of a neuropsychological contribution was de-emphasized.

In several of the cases, diagnostic evaluation had been undertaken years before the patient was seen by the analyst. However, the clinician at that time did not fully appreciate the interweaving of neuropsychological and psychodynamic considerations necessary to understand the patient's clinical picture. Nor did the clinician consider or recognize the suitability of the case for analysis. Dr. Gilmore's patient Rebecca (chapter 13) was diagnosed three years prior to consultation with her as having an Attention Deficit Disorder (again the term at that time) which, according to the consultant, needed to be treated with stimulant medication, tutoring, and only brief supportive psychotherapy. She did not grasp Rebecca's need for more intensive psychotherapeutic treatment to explore her conflicts over sexual and aggressive wishes (which were interfering with her social and academic functioning), or the contribution of Rebecca's ADD to this clinical picture. Dr. Waldron's patient Frank (chapter 9) had been tested two years before referral to the analyst, when he was in preschool. The referral problems did not concern school performance, but rather nightmares and other fears. At the completion of the earlier evaluation, prompted by Frank's mother's distress that her son was not accepted by the school of her first choice, the diagnostician did not recommend any type of intervention at that time, but suggested reevaluation a year later. Thus she neither ruled in, nor ruled out, the existence of a learning disability, or the possibility of being at risk for one.

Two of the contributing analysts (Drs. Peltz and Waldron) recommended diagnostic testing, as part of their initial consultation, to better determine the contribution of neuropsychological dysfunction to the patient's presenting problems. Dr. Peltz' patient Andy (chapter 7) was referred for diagnostic testing to assist in understanding the reasons for his difficulties in school (persistently poor reading, weakness in other academic skills, and daydreaming) and the state of his psychological integration. Dr. Waldron (chapter 9) requested diagnostic testing to further assess his patient's potential and resources, both to consider the advisability of analysis and to better understand the nature of Frank's academic functioning.

Dr. Miller's report of her work with her patient Julia (chapter 5) exemplifies yet another clinical possibility. With the knowledge of Julia's frank cerebral pathology, Dr. Miller assumed there would be consequences for her learning. She believed that a careful diagnostic testing evaluation would be crucial as her patient approached school entry. She also anticipated that the evaluation itself could potentially be traumatic, and thus required preparatory work in the analysis. Further, independent of Dr. Miller, and even prior to her involvement, other diagnostic procedures such as neurological examinations, X rays, lumbar punctures, and EEG's had been performed.

The clinical processes of discovery of the learning disabilities were quite different in Dr. Green's analysis of her patients, Ms. Ames (chapter 15) and Mr. Young (chapter 17). On the basis of observations in the psychoanalytic situation, corroborated by emerging facets of her history, Dr. Green began to consider the possibility that Ms. Ames had undiagnosed learning disabilities. In Mr. Young's case, Dr. Green initially suggested testing to help her patient with his unremitting investment in seeing himself as defective; she did not expect to find that he indeed had some areas of significant cognitive difficulty, but rather thought the tests would rule out this possibility.

NEUROPSYCHOLOGICAL DYSFUNCTION AND ANALYZABILITY

Some psychoanalysts subtly (or not so subtly) convey a belief that patients with learning disabilities are not analyzable, or need not be analyzed. This may reflect a number of factors.

Some clinicians may experience the needs of such patients for additional interventions (such as tutoring or stimulant medication to treat Attention Deficit/Hyperactivity Disorders) as competing endeavors. This may reflect a failure to consider that analysis may improve a patient's ability to make use of educational, tutorial, and psychopharmacological interventions as his capacity for relationships improves (see for example the cases by Mrs. Barrett in chapter 3 and Drs. Peltz, Waldron, Yanof, and Gilmore in chapters 7, 9, 11, and 13).

Unfortunately the analyses reported in this volume do not include in-depth studies of the patients' relationships with teachers and tutors since the contributing analysts did not specifically attend to this subject as they worked with their patients. Even if they had, it might not be possible to understand in detail how changes in the patient's personality affected his or her ability to learn. Hence we may sometimes assume that a patient's growing capacity to deal with his learning problems resulted from an improved adaptive relationship with teachers and tutors, without being able to demonstrate exactly how that occurred.

The fact that so few cases of psychoanalytic patients with learning disabilities have been reported may also reflect the existence of analysts' blind spots in regard to suggestions of learning disabilities and their psychological consequences. No doubt this has many sources. A tendency to ignore external realities, as one concentrates on psychodynamics or the transference, may unconsciously result in minimizing the role of learning disabilities. A desire to treat all conditions psychoanalytically, an expression of the idealization of analysis, may have similar effects. Denial of the existence of neuropsychological dysfunction in general, and learning disabilities in particular, may also result from a therapist's hidden anxiety about his own personal cerebral functioning. The brain, after all, serves as an extremely important organ in persons such as analysts who spend their professional lives engaged in thinking. They may avoid recognition of the brain's vulnerability, since the idea of cerebral dysfunction causes narcissistic distress or castration anxiety, through a brain–genital equation.

A more specific case of potential clinical oversight is the tendency to exclude from psychoanalytic consideration patients with language disabilities. As analysts, we are heavily invested in the significance of language and conceptualization, which are so central to our work. This may predispose us prematurely to assume that a person disabled in this sphere is unsuitable for analysis. Such a leaning was evident in the initial misgivings of Dr. Waldron and his supervisor about recommending analysis for Frank (chapter 9). Even though Dr. Waldron was not fully aware of his patient's language disability, which had not been clearly diagnosed, he was sensitive to Frank's "limited capacity to grasp or respond productively to my comments." This made him and his supervisor initially hesitant to think that the boy could make use of analysis. As Dr. Waldron proceeded nevertheless, and the necessity of taking language problems into consideration in making and formulating interpretations was grasped, a fruitful and rich analysis unfolded.

PATIENTS' AND ANALYSTS' FANTASIES OF CURE AND THE EXPERIENCE OF TERMINATION

Like many analysands, those with neuropsychological dysfunction frequently harbor fantasies (conscious or unconscious) that they will emerge from the analysis repaired, in a state of perfection; in addition, they wish to have been perfectly understood. In contrast to other patients, the specific content of their ideas about this will, at least in part, incorporate the fact that they have learning disabilities or other manifestations of neuropsychological difficulties.

Fantasies of this sort were evident in all the cases reported in this volume, although they were more pronounced in some than in others. Dr. Green described her patient Ms. Ames' (chapter 15) wish that the analyst would remove the "deficit," rather than merely help her to adapt, compensate for, and accept its existence and its meanings. Dr. Miller's patient Julia (chapter 5) similarly expressed such a wish in her associations to the Heidi story in which Clara, Heidi's crippled friend, was cured of her long-standing disability merely through her relationship with Heidi. Dr. Waldron's significantly learning disabled patient, Frank (chapter 9), and Dr. Green's patient, Mr. Young (chapter 17), expressed their fantasies that just coming to analysis would repair them, without their having to put in the hard work necessary to achieve a better (and yet imperfect) result. Similarly, Dr. Yanof's patient Eric (chapter 11) conveyed his unconscious fantasy that his analyst would declare (and make) him "okay," and Mrs. Barrett's patient Leah (chapter 3) repeatedly appealed to her analyst to help her rid herself of the "I-can't-read feelings."

Rage is common in the analysis of learning disabled patients who have had repeated experiences of frustration in attempting to achieve their goals or live up to their ideals. So too may fury arise because parental intentions have been misunderstood and because parents have failed to provide appropriate empathy for their disabled children. Furthermore, rage derived from these and other sources can accentuate oedipal rage.

These features of patients with learning disabilities are frequently highlighted during termination, when it is ultimately necessary for patients to analyze and mourn their fantasies of perfection in conjunction with the loss of their analyst. Aware that their wish to rid themselves of all deficiencies has not come true, they may become angry at the analyst for not accomplishing this, and then erect defenses against their antagonism and disappointment. Their fury at this failure can be immense, the analyst often being the object of feelings such as hatred. To make things worse, not only will their learning disabilities remain, but so too will remnants of their limitations. In some instances, these may, in turn, interfere with the patient's ability to engage in a more complete analytic understanding of themselves. This was seen, for example, in the analysis of Dr. Wyszynski's patient (chapter 19) whose problems with abstract reasoning sometimes compromised his ability to grasp the complexity (especially the overdetermination) of his conflicts. These specific sources of anger may combine with the analysand's typical experience of fury, anxiety, and depressive affect more generally associated with the impending loss of the analyst in termination.

This set of feelings is in some respects a repetition of the rage children with learning disabilities often experience because they believe, rightly or wrongly, that the adults important to them have not recognized their condition and helped them. Even when parents recognize, and do their best to correct, their child's learning disability, the fact that they do not achieve a conclusive success frequently evokes rage and depressive affect.

A dramatic example of this syndrome is Dr. Wyszynski's patient Mr. G (chapter 19). His growing recognition that he would not overcome his pathology or be reborn or perfect, combined with his intense anxiety over erotic transference feelings, and possible cognitive limitations in grasping analytic meaning; this culminated in his growing need to end the analysis.

The analyst too may find it difficult to resign himself to an imperfect analysis as he tries to decide whether as much as possible has been accomplished. These deliberations are also exemplified by Dr. Wyszynski's reflections about the advisability of her patient's decision to terminate the analysis earlier than she would have liked. The analyst will search his soul, as he seeks evidence that he has carried out the analysis optimally for this patient. He may chastise himself when he notices the errors and failures of empathy which so frequently occur in treating a patient with a cognitive disability.

DRIVES, DEFENSES, CONFLICT, AND THE ROLE OF PARENTS IN PATIENTS WITH LEARNING DISABILITIES

We have seen that the presence of a learning disability can increase the intensity of patients' aggression and have detailed some of the sources of that intensification. The nature of the patient's libidinal attachment can also be intensified. The patient may need to rely to a greater than usual degree upon his parents in order to obtain realistic help with his difficulties in learning. When parents tutor their own children (as, for example, in the case of Dr. Gilmore's patient Rebecca, chapter 13, whose father also gave her medication), this is likely to shape the child's sense of dependency as well as his oedipal experience. Furthermore, the fantasy of cure through borrowing or stealing the power of others (which is particularly clear in Dr. Waldron's patient Frank [chapter 9]) may involve clinging to wishes for union with potent grown-ups. In addition, increased love for parents may result from a defensive need to counter rage. Such intensification of aggressive and libidinal drives contributes to the likelihood of heightened conflict, as superego strictures clash with drive demands, to which the patient responds with an array of defensive maneuvers.

As in psychoanalytic work with any patient, the nature of the resulting compromise formations will require exploration and delineation on a case by case basis. Nevertheless in studying the analyses in this volume, we have observed a number of trends. While they are by no means invariant or inevitable, we feel it is worth highlighting them for consideration by analysts working with patients who evidence learning disabilities and other manifestations of neuropsychological dysfunction.

In most of the cases denial was conspicuous as a defensive response. We account for this in a variety of ways. First, in some instances, the existence of the patient's particular cognitive disturbances results in compromised perception of the outer world. This potentiates the development of denial, which (among other things) involves poor or distorted perception or evaluation of the environment. Second, the parents of children with learning disabilities often experience pain in relation to their child's difficulties. Failure of the child to gratify their narcissistic desires for perfection may cause parents to suffer and become angry at their offspring. They may be ashamed of their child's defects, which they attempt to hide. It is common for many parents of children with learning disabilities (and other manifestations of neuropsychological dysfunction) to have themselves had a similar cognitive difficulty, whether diagnosed or undiagnosed. When this is the case, the parents' distress about their children's trouble may be accentuated. Parents' denial may stem from other types of personal experiences as well. Denial in these children is also promoted by the likelihood that they will identify with their parents' proclivity for this type of defensive activity. This was seen, for example, in the case of Dr. Green's patient Mr. Young (chapter 17) whose mother, finding both her son's learning difficulties and short stature distressing, insisted he had no failings in either area. Mr. Young identified with his mother in this regard and, at times, also denied the existence of these limitations.

We have also observed that the nature of defenses and drive derivatives produced a sadomasochistic picture in quite a few of the cases. We suspect that parents frequently became angry and depressed at indications that their children were deficient; poor functioning, such as difficulty tying shoelaces (again seen in Dr. Green's patient Mr. Young) upset and irritated them. The children may have responded with an amalgam of craving for acceptance, a depressive sense of hopelessness to bring this about, feelings of entitlement to repair these (as well as cognitive) injuries, anger that was libidinized, hatred for their attackers, and a pleasure in being attacked. Once such sadomasochistic relationships were established, the children could seek further pleasure in the form of provocative cognitive failures, for instance, exaggerating their faults in a vexing way. To illustrate, Mr. Young's (chapter 17) practice of seeking driving lessons from teachers with whom he could only poorly communicate, not only made it likely he would fail; it also created a situation in which his instructors could become angry at him and he with them.

Finally, related to this, it was common for these patients to employ their disabilities for defensive purposes. As Brenner (1982) wrote, "the ego can use for defense anything that comes under the heading of normal ego functioning or development" (p. 75); we elaborate this perspective by emphasizing that this is also true of anything that comes under the heading of *abnormal* ego functioning or development. Thus neuropsychologically based difficulties came to be used simultaneously for defensive purposes, as well as in the service of seeking drive gratification, promoting and opposing superego standards, and facilitating adaptation to the environment.

This introduction will help prepare the reader for his journey through the nine analyses in this book, each of which is followed by our discussions. The next chapter, a review of the psychoanalytic literature on learning disabilities, will serve as further preparation. A final chapter will briefly summarize many of the conclusions we have reached.

Chapter 2

Review of the Literature

INTRODUCTION

Although the field of learning disorders has burgeoned into public awareness in the last three decades, relevant psychoanalytic contributions had appeared as early as the 1920s and 1930s by such prominent authors as Abraham (1924), Glover (1925), Bornstein (1930), Strachey (1930), M. Klein (1931), and Fenichel (1937). Early interest most probably reflected the excitement sparked by Freud's (1923, 1926) introduction of the structural hypothesis and subsequent advances in ego psychology. This fueled exploration of the impact of the drives and the superego on various functions of the ego. Publications reflective of psychoanalytic attention to the psychodynamic aspects of problems in learning continued at full strength into the 1940s, 1950s, and mid-1960s, until they all but ceased in the late 1960s and early 1970s (with some notable exceptions). They were then renewed to some extent in the late 1980s and 1990s.

The period of diminished psychoanalytic interest was precisely at a time when papers on the neuropsychological etiology of "learning disabilities" and "minimal brain dysfunction" proliferated (Black, 1974). These became household phrases as heated controversy about etiology and treatment was brought to public attention. The existing psychoanalytic literature of that period had given little consideration to neuropsychological contributions to learning problems. This was despite

Hartmann's (1950) fundamental paper calling for investigation
of the impact of the child's ego equipment upon his intrapsychic and ego development. He wrote:

> We come to see ego development as a result of three sets of
> factors: inherited ego characteristics (and their interaction), in-
> fluences of the instinctual drives, and influences of outer reality.
> Concerning the development and the growth of the autono-
> mous characteristics of the ego we may make the assumption
> that they take place as a result of experience (learning) but
> partly also of maturation . . . [pp. 120–121].

> We have to assume that differences in the timing or intensity
> of their growth enter into the picture of ego development as a
> partly independent variable; e.g., the timing of the appearance
> of grasping, of walking, of the motor aspect of speech. *Neither
> does it seem unlikely that the congenital motor equipment is among
> the factors which right from birth on tend to modify certain attitudes
> of the developing ego* (Fries and Lewi, 1938). *The presence of such
> factors in all aspects of the child's behavior makes them also an essen-
> tial element in the development of his self-experience* [p. 121; empha-
> sis added].

> So far we have in analysis mainly been dealing with the interven-
> tion of conflict in [the autonomous ego apparatus's] develop-
> ment. *But it is of considerable interest not only for developmental
> psychology but also for clinical problems to study the converse influ-
> ence too: that is, the influences which a child's intelligence, his percep-
> tual and motor equipment, his special gifts, and the development of
> all these factors have on the timing, intensity and mode of expression
> of these conflicts.* We know infinitely more, in a systematic way,
> about the other aspect, the ego's development in consequence
> of its conflicts with the instinctual drives and with reality [p.
> 123; emphasis added].

Most analysts working on the subject of learning disorders
believed them to be of exclusively psychogenic etiology, without
sufficiently ruling out neuropsychological contributions. In so
doing they frequently addressed themselves to a limited spectrum of learning disordered patients, without making this explicit. Furthermore, when a neuropsychological etiology was

evident, they often relegated such patients to a group they considered unanalyzable. The major exception was Weil (1961, 1970, 1971, 1977, 1978) who published a number of masterful psychoanalytic contributions to our understanding of how the neuropsychologically based deviations that affect learning simultaneously interact with the psychological sphere in the development of a neurotic personality organization.

In recent years there has been a renewed and broader interest in this subject. However, authors of more modern contributions still vary in the degree to which they appreciate that learning disabilities and neuropsychological dysfunction are general terms, the specific nature of which requires careful diagnosis. Concomitantly, some analysts grasp that these difficulties contribute to development in complex, intertwining, and highly individual ways, shaping every component of a patient's constellation of compromise formations. In contrast, others assume that there are universal psychological derivatives of neuropsychological dysfunction or learning disabilities.

Among these recent contributions, several clusters may be identified. There have been many papers on neuropsychology. Some authors have undertaken theoretical integrations of neuropsychology and psychoanalysis. In part these contributors based their ideas on the growing experimental literature documenting abnormalities in neuropsychologically based conditions such as learning disabilities and ADHD.

There have also been a handful of recent clinical contributions pertinent to the interweaving of neuropsychological dysfunction with other aspects of the patient's personality: its impact upon ego development and its psychodynamic elaboration. A number of authors describe in some detail the place of a learning disability in an individual patient's overall development and in the analysis or psychoanalytically oriented psychotherapy. In contrast to this individual case approach, a small group of analysts offers more general perspectives on how learning disabilities (and neuropsychological dysfunction in a broader sense) may affect, and be affected by, psychological development. The relationship between conflict and "deficit" is examined. Several authors explore the complexities of specific neuropsychological syndromes, such as Attention Deficit/

Hyperactivity Disorders. Other related contributions reflect a self psychological orientation; their authors focus upon the narcissistic difficulties they assume to be the central characteristic of patients with learning disabilities.

Finally, there is also a small, but growing, literature on technique, including diagnosis and treatment. Some analysts demonstrate that patients with neuropsychological dysfunction are analyzable or treatable by other psychoanalytically oriented methods. Several emphasize the need for multiple interventions, one essential component of which is psychoanalysis or psychotherapy.

We will review each of these clusters of psychoanalytic (and psychoanalytically oriented) contributions in sequence. Pertinent studies from other fields will also be briefly presented.

NEUROPSYCHOLOGY

Integration of Neuropsychology and Psychoanalysis

The application of neuroscience to a psychoanalytic understanding of the mind, although promising, has not produced definitive findings. Nor have investigators discovered a clear anatomical or physiological basis for what we call neuropsychologically based learning disabilities.

However, a number of interesting contributions have appeared in the literature in recent years, all of which refer to Freud's pioneering work in his monograph *On Aphasia* (1891). Freud, while recognizing that different aphasias were associated with lesions in different areas of the brain, challenged the narrow approach to localization then postulated by his contemporaries. Freud's interest in aphasia adumbrated his later more ambitious attempts to explain psychoanalytic findings on the basis of the functioning of the brain. He himself never published his "Project for a Scientific Psychology" (1895), which appeared posthumously in the Standard Edition in 1964. Because he thought he failed in his endeavor, Freud decided to abandon his attempts to integrate psychoanalytic findings and brain functioning. Rather, he asserted, the mind must be understood on the basis of observations in psychoanalytic treatment. Psychoanalytic theory must stand on its own feet, and not depend on neurological hypotheses. However, the shadow of the "Project" can be seen in the metaphors and concepts of many of his later metapsychological formulations. In addition, he thought a biological basis for mental illness existed and that one day we would use medication to treat mental disorders.

Prior to abandoning his efforts, Freud arrived at several important ideas. He recognized that the notion of a specific connection of the area of damage and the type of pathology was misleading. He asserted that "a mental phenomenon corresponds to each part of the chain [of events], or to several parts" (p. 55), an approach that Levin (1995a) regards as a "general systems perspective" (p. 542). Jones (1953) called Freud's a "functional explanation" (p. 214). Subsequent studies of aphasia have borne out Freud's misgivings about precise localization. It has become clear that information is not stored in specific areas of the brain. Nor is mental functioning located in specific neurons or groups of neurons; rather, it involves many parts of the brain, although certain areas have crucial nodes. For example, it was (and is) known that motor aphasia is generally associated with damage to Broca's area, which is located in the left frontal lobe adjacent to the motor areas, and that sensory aphasia is generally associated with lesions in the temporal lobe abutting the somatic sensory area. (The injury occurs on the left side of the brain of right-handed people and the right side in persons who are left-handed.) However, the exact location of the lesion can vary from patient to patient (Benson, 1993), sometimes surprising the clinician who is too confident in his ability to establish the cite of the lesion.

L. Miller (1991, 1993), a major contributor to this field, sees himself as continuing Freud's tradition of integrating clinical neuropsychology and psychoanalysis. He is one of a number of recent writers within psychoanalysis who study the relevance of data derived from clinical neuropsychology to broader questions of consciousness, psychodynamics, and personality (see also Levin and Vuckovich, 1983; Reiser, 1984; Watt, 1990; Levin,

1991, 1995a,b; Schore, 1994; Levin and Kent, 1995). He has coined the term *neuropsychodynamic* to describe his model of brain and psyche. Miller cautions against the pitfalls of premature "reification and oversimplification of neuropsychological models" (1993, p. 184), in which particular psychological features are assigned to specific locations in the brain. Instead, to be effective, models of the brain must rely upon the dynamic notions of functioning Freud (1891) emphasized in *On Aphasia*. In Miller's words:

> According to this view, the different lobes, loci, and hemispheres contribute interactively to determine the various forms of expression of thought, feeling, and consciousness. Thus, the effect of a brain lesion is not to leave a "hole" in the psychological apparatus, but to *cause a neuropsychodynamic reconfiguration* in which the resultant clinical presentation—the person after brain damage—represents the residual pattern of strengths and deficits, the efforts of the remaining neuropsychological system to come to grips with itself and the world . . . [p. 184; emphasis added].

Miller also emphasizes that neuropsychology should not be used to substantiate or refute psychoanalytic metapsychology. Indeed he believes that basic questions within psychoanalysis also exist within the domain of neuropsychology, for example, "the nature of consciousness, fantasy versus reality, the role of thoughts and passions in personality structure . . . " (p. 185).

Miller focuses upon three subjects of major interest to Freud: hysteria, dreams, and parapraxes. He discusses these in light of the findings and concepts of modern neuropsychology, summarizing its perspective on the functions of the brain and their implications for human psychology. The brain systems which control sensation, movement, language, memory, thought, emotion and consciousness are elaborated. Miller explains that the left hemisphere is the seat of the capacity to articulate to oneself, with the guidance of the frontal lobe. In this way we control behavior and assess feedback about the impact of this behavior on others and on the physical world. Knowledge of the self is gradually attained, and personal identity derives from such daily experiences involving emotion, perception and activity. As volitional control of the ability to verbalize grows, the developing person can more directly communicate his feelings, desires and perspectives to others in a more refined manner; correspondingly, self-communication develops in this manner. A growing appreciation of the self as agent facilitates "ego-autonomous action" (p. 246). With the use of many case histories, Miller documents:

> [T]he brain damage-produced dissociation of such neurocognitive functions as language, memory, perception, and movement from active, conscious, volitional control. The argument has been made that these severe, frankly "organic," cases are merely the boldly instantiated exemplars of more common everyday neuropsychodynamic events that continually determine and shape our fears and wishes, goals and aspirations, personalities and pathologies [p. 246].

In recognition of Freud's view that man is neither "functional" nor "organic," but rather "functional" *and* "organic," Miller presents his "neuropsychodynamic" model. This is an effort to weave disparate observations and findings into a coherent conceptualization which can be utilized for further clinical work and research.

Covering much of the same ground (including a review of much of the same clinical neuropsychological literature), Watt (1990) also attempts to bridge neuropsychological and psychoanalytic ideas. In his view, psychoanalytic concepts about the organization and structure of affect, thought, behavior, and their interrelationships must be built upon basic brain mechanisms; he explores concepts central to both disciplines in light of each other. He, like Miller, explicitly rejects the practice of "locating" psychoanalytic concepts in particular areas of the brain. Having said this, Watt makes clear his belief that Freud's most basic ideas about the ego as a structure mediating inside and outside are paralleled by the mediation between biological needs relating to both individual and species survival; this is the function of the limbic regions, paralimbic cortex and heteromodal cortex (see also Schore, 1994).

Watt reviews the now plentiful literature on hemispheric specialization, both in "split-brain" research and in the newer

concept of "alterations in interhemispheric relations" or
"functional commisurotomies" (Hoppe, 1977). The right and
left hemispheres of the brain encode data in modes partially
incompatible with each other. The left hemisphere encodes in
terms of language, time, sequence, and categories, while the
right hemisphere encodes in terms of visual imagery and gestalt. When these cannot be communicated, and therefore
smoothly interrelated, there are likely to be consequences for
defensive, cognitive and characterological styles (see also Shapiro, 1965; J. Levy, 1974; Hoppe, 1977; Galin, 1977; Smokler
and Shevrin, 1979; Levin and Vuckovich, 1983; Schore, 1994).
Some of these contributors have also noted similarities between
these findings and Freud's descriptions of primary and secondary process. As Watt (1990) wrote:

> The equation is not the simplistic left hemisphere=conscious
> and right hemisphere=unconscious but a more complex one.
> Conscious may imply that representations in each hemisphere
> can be transposed, whereas the unconscious may involve a type
> of relationship between the hemispheres that prevents such
> transposition. Psychoanalytic notions about the unconscious
> have always stressed the individual's blindness to various aspects
> of experience related to drive and affect [p. 497].

In addition, Watt commented that psychoanalysis has
taken little note of the now extensive empirical literature on the
relationship between lateralization and emotion. Most studies
suggest that the right hemisphere is dominant for the processing of emotional events and affective stimuli. However, others point up different roles for the two hemispheres, depending
upon the valence of the affect; the left hemisphere may mediate
more positive affects and the right hemisphere more negative
affects. Watt places special emphasis upon the implications of
neuropsychology for the psychoanalytic concepts of self and
object representations and their linkages with pleasurable and
unpleasurable affects. In this regard Watt also takes up the
subject of right hemisphere processing in the transference:

> Given that the right hemisphere is able to operate with visual,
> kinesthetic, somatosensory, and auditory data very much in a

nonlinear and nontemporal fashion, it would have major advantages over the more literal and sequential left hemisphere in the construction of such condensations of multiple experiences [pp. 510–511].

Watt also reviews the studies which serve as evidence that the psychoanalytic concept of "the executive functions" of the ego are supported by the prefrontal cortices.

He discusses the implications of the dialogue between the cerebral hemispheres for psychotherapy and for adaptation:

> It is in the analysis of the transference (and related phenomena) that the image-based units of primary representation from the right hemisphere are forced to enter into dialogue with the lexical units of primary representation from the left hemisphere. Put more conventionally, the patient's affect is gradually put into words, understood in terms of primary and highly ambivalent self- and object representations, and connected to primary traumatic experience [p. 519].

From this perspective characterological, and more broadly structural (in the psychoanalytic sense), change must at some level reflect neurological change.

Watt closes with a call for further work and a cautionary note about analysts' tendency not to concern themselves with the integration of biological and psychic processes:

> [N]euroscience must resist reductionism, and not ignore issues that currently defy easy neurological quantification, such as character or defense, while psychoanalysis must resist passivity and defensive isolationism. Those who respect the great contributions psychoanalysis has made to understanding human experience must actively participate in building a more integrated theory of mind-body. *Psychoanalysis can ill afford to take the challenges posed by biological psychiatry lightly, or leave the work of bridge building solely to those who distrust, fear, or misunderstand analytic perspectives, or who mistakenly regard psychoanalysis as a stop-gap language that will eventually be replaced by a "true" neurobiological language.* . . . Although the neurosciences will have much to contribute to an understanding of how our internal meaning making and organizing processes become biologically

disordered (and therefore reveal their neurobiological foundations and deeper structure), there will always be a need for a
science and language of personal meaning(s), a language of
personal love and hate that attempts to understand the unique
and deeply personal organization of our images of pain and
pleasure [p. 524; emphasis added].

Levin (Levin and Vuckovich, 1983; Levin, 1991, 1995a,b;
Levin and Kent, 1995), a psychoanalyst, has published many
studies with the goal of making "novel, specific, and detailed
correlations between psychological/psychoanalytic variables,
on one hand, and neuroanatomical/neurophysiological considerations on the other" (1991, p. xxi). He offers a tentative
set of formulations and speculations reflective of his belief in
the importance of developmental models in understanding the
relationship between psychological development and the
changing organization of the brain.

With the use of material from psychoanalyses he has conducted, Levin discusses the implications of these models for a
range of clinical subjects. These include the management of
the transference, nonverbal communication, and the power of
interpretations including their employment of metaphor.
Levin believes that there is much of value in studying "hemispheric collaboration and the significance of blocks between
the hemispheres" (1991, p. 17):

> [I]t is possible to take what psychoanalysts call defense and what
> neuroscientists call interhemispheric communication and relate
> these to each other in some interesting ways. My theory (testable
> with modern noninvasive techniques for brain visualization) is
> that what we call repression (forgetting, especially of highly per-
> sonal experience) and disavowal (downplaying the emotional
> significance of experience) are left to right and right to left
> blocks, respectively, of the flow of information between the cere-
> bral hemispheres [p. 17].

Levin gives special emphasis to the evolution of language
and its impact, when there is adequate exposure to language
in infancy and childhood, upon brain organization. He believes

it is possible that acquired (native) language is a later development of "a language originally used by the brain for internal
communications" (1991, p. 221).

Levin feels that neuroscience can help psychoanalysts better appreciate the "basic design features of the brain" (1991,
p. 220), while psychoanalysis can highlight the significance of
biological data. He elaborates, "Most simply stated, what we
see determines what we want, but what we want, know, and are
capable of conceptualizing also impacts upon what we look
for, see, and appreciate." To illustrate, "the prefrontal cortex
selectively utilizes from the rest of the brain a system for the
pursuit of its goals and further directs the selective attention
that guides the sensory system so that principally 'desired'
(meaning appropriate and useful) sensory input is obtained"
(1991, p. 220).

In his discussion of learning disabilities per se, Levin concentrates on the biological as he attempts to keep a balanced
view. He recommends the use of detailed diagnostic testing,

> to keep an open mind since in some instances, the frequency
> of which is difficult to determine at present, the self-pathology
> may not be the cause, but rather the result of learning block
> (e.g., stemming from a processing problem within any of the
> brain systems for eye tracking). There appear to be situations
> in which the boundary between 'organic' and 'psychological'
> disappears . . . [1991, p. 64].

Levin speculates about disruptions occurring at many levels within the brain: the reticular activating system or midbrain
level when there is an attention deficit disorder, at the neocorti-
cal level with late myelinization of the parietal lobe, "at the
level of specific perceptual systems controlled by the brain stem
and vestibulocerebellar mechanisms" (p. 63) and the like.

Lewis (1992) is another contributor to the subject of correlations between neurological models of mental functioning and
psychological phenomena. She particularly focuses upon their
implications for psychotherapy. Like Miller and Watt, she ac-
knowledges the danger of reductionism, which she intentionally eschews. For purposes of exposition Lewis treats separately

two neuropsychological models of normal brain functioning: cerebral laterality and hierarchical brain organization. With regard to the former, she reviews much of the same split-brain and functional disconnection research, in the service of making two points.

One is the similarities between the functional capacities of the right hemisphere and the psychoanalytic concept of primary process, and those of the left hemisphere and secondary process. Empirical research suggests two ways in which mental activity of the right hemisphere can be dissociated from that of the left hemisphere. Early experiences may be represented in the right hemisphere alone, due to the functional immaturity of the corpus callosum. Second, callosal inhibition may render right hemisphere activity and memories unavailable to language representation of the left hemisphere.

Lewis' second point concerns the therapeutic implications of these findings. She suggests that psychotherapy may be viewed as a way of facilitating communication between the left and right hemispheres. She describes the hierarchical organization model, which regards the brain as an archaeological site involving three systems of special intelligence: memory, sense of time and space, and motor functions. In her view these may make a special contribution to treating patients with psychosomatic and anxiety disorders. Times of conflict may highlight differences in how these three different brains perceive and react to the world. Lewis views psychosomatic and anxiety-disordered patients as lacking the ability to express emotion verbally. Thus verbal approaches at the beginning of treatment would be unlikely to be effective. Instead she proposes the greater efficacy of "disalarming" (p. 30) the visceral brain of these patients, for example, through the use of tone of voice, tempo, and manner of gestures. As calming is achieved and the therapist–patient relationship is strengthened, verbal methods of insight may more effectively permit verbal, rather than somatic, mediation of affects and drives.

Several other contributors to this area (Fisher, 1954; Dement and Kleitman, 1957; Reiser, 1984, 1991; Solms, 1995, 1997) have considered the possibility of correlating changes in the brain during dreaming and the psychological phenomena of dreaming, alerted by the observation that dreams occur during REM sleep (when rapid eye movements appear). Solms (1997) has studied the effects of pathological anatomical lesions on dreaming. He has especially described nonvisual dreaming and cessation or restriction of visual dream imagery, and recurring nightmares. Reiser and Solms have each offered cogent hypotheses regrading the pathways utilized during dreaming. Reiser implicates the prefrontal, sensory, temporal, and occipital cortex, the diencephalon, amygdalin, hippocampus, and basal forebrain, and Solms describes similar brain activity. In a series of discussions at the New York Psychoanalytic Institute, Solms and the analysts who participated have tried to determine further correlates between brain structure and function and psychoanalytic findings and theory.

Experimental Studies on Abnormalities in Neuropsychologically Based Specific Learning Disabilities and Attentional Problems

Some mounting evidence for a biological basis for Attention Deficit/Hyperactivity Disorders (ADHD) and specific learning disabilities comes from electroencephalogram (EEG) and positron emission tomograph (PET) studies. Mann, Lubar, Zimmerman, Miller, and Muenchen (1992) and Janzen, Graap, Stephanson, Marshall, and Fitzsimmons (1995) reported that the EEGs of children with the inattentive type of ADHD displayed excessively slow wave (theta band) activity. Kuperman, Johnson, Arndt, Lindgren, and Wolraich (1996) revealed that ADHD children have less delta band relative percent power and more beta wave relative percent power. Satterfield, Schell, Backs, and Hidaka (1984) demonstrated increased alpha and beta band power in boys over $8^1/_2$ with ADD.

Zametkin, Liebenauer, Fitzgerald, King, Minkunas, Herscovitch, Yamada, and Cohen (1990), using PET scans to determine brain glucose uptake, found that children with ADD metabolized glucose at a lower rate than controls. Overall the rate of glucose metabolism was 8 percent lower than the control group, but frontal lobe metabolism was even less than that in other parts of the brain. Similarly, Lou, Henricksen, and Bruhn (1984) found decreased blood flow in the frontal lobes, especially in the right hemisphere of children with ADD. On the basis of these and other studies, Chelune, Ferguson, Koon, and Dickey (1986), Hallowell and Ratey (1994), and Casey, Rourke, and Picard (1991) suggest that poor frontal lobe functioning results in failure of inhibition with consequent hyperactivity.

EEG, PET scan, MRI, and brain blood flow deviations from the norm have also been found in patients with learning disabilities, indicating neurophysiological disturbances (Harris, 1995). In these conditions evaluation is more difficult because there are so many variations in the nature of learning difficulties, many of which have not been investigated. The MRI studies of Rumsey, Dorwart, Vermes, Denckla, Krues, and Rapoport (1986) revealed greater symmetry of the planum temporale in children with severe reading disabilities than in normal children or those with ADHD alone. Rumsey, Andreason, Aquino, Hamburger, Picus, Rapaport, and Cohen (1992) discovered abnormalities in cerebral blood flow to the left temporoparietal area, which is involved in language, in boys with severe reading disorders. Standard electroencephalography had limited value in distinguishing or classifying learning disabilities (Shapiro, 1994). However, difficulties in visual perception, delayed speech and motor development, as well as disorders of higher cognitive functions, have been related to EEG abnormalities (Hughes, 1985). Also event-related brain potentials (ERPs) indicate that physiological differences exist between children with reading disorders and children with normal reading, in terms of their cognitive processing, including linguistic categories (Landwehrmeyer, Gerling, and Wallesch, 1990). PET studies have demonstrated prefrontal cortex and inferior occipital lobe differences between some dyslexics as compared with normal children (Gross-Glenn, Duara, Barker, et al., 1991).

Recently Beitchman and Young (1997) reviewed the literature on reading disabilities and the brain. They note that "while none of these findings can be considered conclusive, they seem to support the view that at a neurofunctional and neuroanatomical level, at least some reading-disabled individuals differ from the non-reading disabled" (p. 1024). However, they caution that "until the results of more definitive studies are known, the findings . . . should be considered tentative" (p. 1024).

Controversy has arisen as to whether ADHD and learning disabilities are discrete conditions, or ones which lie on a continuum. Levy, Hay, McStephen, Wood, and Waldman (1997) state that their study of 1938 families with twins and siblings "suggest that ADHD is best viewed as the extreme of a behavior that varies genetically throughout the entire population rather than a disorder with discrete determinants" (p. 737). Similarly, Shaywitz, Fletcher, and Shaywitz (1994) conclude that "[r]eading difficulties occur along a continuum that blends imperceptibly with normal reading ability" (p. 10).

Nonetheless these authors regard ADHD and learning disabilities as biologically based conditions. Levy et al. (1997) assert that their "results indicate that ADHD has an exceptionally high hereditability compared with other behavior disorders" (p. 741). Shaywitz et al. (1994) insist that the etiology of dyslexia is "indisputably biological in nature" (p. 10). Another more recent article by Shaywitz, Shaywitz, Pugh, Fulbright, Constable, Mencl, Shankweiler, Lieberman, Skudlarski, Fletcher, Katz, Marchione, Lacadie, Gatenby, and Gore (1998) has greatly fortified the evidence for a biological basis for one type of learning disorder, which they label "dyslexia." They examined the functional Magnetic Resonance Imaging system (MRI) findings in twenty-nine dyslexics and thirty-two nonimpaired individuals while the subjects were performing tasks involving reading, in particular phonological processing. The subjects ranged from 16 to 63 years of age. Only one of them met the DSM-IV (APA, 1994) criteria for Attention Deficit/Hyperactivity Disorder.

Shaywitz et al. found that during the tasks nonimpaired subjects displayed greater activation of Wernicke's area, the angular gyrus, and the striate cortex. In contrast, the posterior areas of the dyslexic population manifested greater inferior frontal gyrus activation. The more difficult the phonologic tasks, the greater was the degree of activation. The authors concluded that "the impairment in dyslexia is phonologic in nature and that these brain activation patterns may provide a neural signature for this impairment" (p. 2636).

Evidence for the inheritance of types of dyslexia has varied with the type of disability. Studies of families and of twins reveal that "genetic factors are of major etiological significance in the development of *some* forms of dyslexia" (Grigorenko, Wood, Meyer, Hart, Speed, Shuster, and Pauls, 1997; emphasis added). Attempts to link learning disabilities and defects of specific chromosomes have been only partially successful. The Fragile X Syndrome, a rather rare subtype of learning disability (appearing in less than one person for every thousand births) associated with a nonverbal learning disorder as well as with social and emotional impairment, is caused by an X-linked chromosome mutation. A permutation within the FMR-1 gene results in less severe dysfunction, while a mutation of the gene produces more serious conditions like autism and mental deficiency (Baumgardner and Reiss, 1994).

In another condition, Familial Dyslexia, the patterns of occurrences within families strongly suggest inheritance, but a proposed specific linkage with chromosome 15 has not been confirmed (Lubs, Gross-Glenn, Duara, Feldman, Stottun, Jallad, Kushch and Rabin, 1994). However, Grigorenko et al. (1997) have provided significant evidence of a linkage between specific types of dyslexia and Chromosomes 6 and 15. They studied six extended families with dyslexia and correlated particular cognitive defects with markers on these chromosomes.

Studies of Language Development and Its Evolution

Levin (1991) attempts to trace the evolution of language. His hypotheses are based on archaeological findings regarding the evolution of primates. In accordance with recent discoveries, he traces hominoids from Australopithecus (which appeared 4 million years ago) to homo habilis (starting 1.75 million years ago), to homo erectus (which spread out from Africa 1 million years ago), to homo sapiens which evolved into the form of modern man 100,000 years ago.

Australopithecus walked and used simple tools. The structure of his arms suggests a capacity to gesture. Homo erectus used fire and constructed symmetrical tools. Homo sapiens not only hunted and used tools; early man painted beautiful cave paintings and carved sculpture, indicating an aesthetic capacity as well as symbolization and abstract thinking. Levin suggests that examination of tools used by hominoids and the art of homo sapiens indicate that gestures were used for communication before vocalization and that early on nonstandardized utterances were employed in conjunction with gestures. He adds that about 40,000 years ago hominoids' intonation apparatus became sufficiently developed so that vocalization became more standardized and the naming of objects became possible. Syntactic language and then the naming of abstract entities became possible.

A further advance occurred with the development of writing and, associated with that, reading (Coulmas, 1989; Chernow and Valassi, 1993). Writing is the visual recording of language, while reading is the recognition of the meanings of what has been written. Homo sapiens is the only species to develop writing and hence reading. However, chimpanzees have been taught by humans to recognize, react to, and, many believe, to interpret written words.

Scholars estimate that writing first appeared at about 4,000 B.C.E. It developed independently in Egypt, Mesopotamia, China, and Central America. Writing takes many forms, among them pictograms or ideograms (which symbolize ideas, things, or letters), cuneiform and the use of patterns of written letters to convey the sound of individual consonants or vowels which indicate words. Because a particular letter does not always refer to a specific sound (especially in English), the resulting confusion puts writers and readers in jeopardy, and compounds the difficulties of people with learning disabilities.

A number of other types of research involving the biology of learning have not been integrated into the study of learning disabilities. The work of Chomsky (1965) and his followers (Pinker, 1994) has not been incorporated into psychoanalytic knowledge of language development. Chomsky maintains that the ability to know and use grammatical structure is innate, not learned, although societies do influence the details of grammar in particular languages. Piaget's findings (1923) have been incorporated into psychoanalytic thinking (Wolff, 1960; Silverman, 1971) to some degree, but have not been applied to the subject of learning disabilities.

CLINICAL CONTRIBUTIONS TO A PSYCHODYNAMIC UNDERSTANDING OF LEARNING DISABLED PATIENTS

Individual Psychoanalytic and Psychoanalytically Oriented Case Studies

A number of authors have published accounts of their clinical work with learning disabled patients. In some instances the existence of the learning disability was known at the time of consultation; in other cases aspects of the patient's presentation in the analysis and/or history led to its discovery. These papers also differ in the degree to which the treating analyst gives balanced consideration to the role of the learning disability in the individual patient's overall development and analytic treatment.

Some case reports are intended to prove the point that certain types of problems invariably accompany the existence of a learning disability. In these instances, the particulars of a specific patient's neuropsychological difficulties are generally not discussed. This is contrasted with an open-minded exploration of what is found in an individual patient, without preconceptions as to the nature of the neuropsychological dysfunction, or the ways in which it may be psychologically elaborated. Such open-mindedness also permits the richest process of discovery in psychoanalytic work. Several examples of this type of work will be presented, followed by examples of contributions involving preconceived notions.

The most detailed and comprehensive case report in the psychoanalytic literature is that of Rubovits-Seitz (1988) who illustrated that "analyzability does not depend upon general intelligence" (p. 213). Having reviewed the literature on intelligence, psychological mindedness, and analyzability, he cautions against the assumption that patients without high intelligence and advanced education are less analyzable. He also demonstrated that "brain damage" did not impair his patient's integrative and synthetic functions in a way which seriously compromised his ability to profit from an analytic approach. Toward this end, Rubovits-Seitz presented his experience analyzing a man with a Full Scale IQ of 107 (in the "Average" range) who, in addition, had documented neuropsychological dysfunction. He had been a very slow learner who had had difficulty with most of his classes in childhood.

This case report is unique in two ways. One is Rubovits-Seitz's careful study of the place of the patient's level of intelligence and specific neuropsychological difficulties in his overall constellation of compromise formations. Another is the use of diagnostic test material, along with analytic process data, to do so. Rubovits-Seitz referred his patient for a diagnostic evaluation in the course of his treatment as an adult. In addition the analyst reviewed an evaluation which had been performed many years before he met his patient.

A partial testing evaluation had been undertaken when the patient was 17. At this time he had a Verbal IQ of 102 and a Performance IQ of 100, giving him a Full Scale IQ of 102. Despite some individual subtest scores (general factual information, forming verbal concepts) in the "Bright Normal" (i.e., above average) range, the patient's academic functioning was well below average. Projective testing showed him to be prone to isolation, avoidant of active engagement in meaningful relationships, and very concerned about the adequacy of his attempts to conduct his life.

About one year into the analysis Rubovits-Seitz referred his patient for another evaluation in the context of the patient's having lost his job. This very comprehensive psychological and neuropsychological study revealed a comparable Verbal IQ of 107 and Performance IQ of 106, giving him a Full Scale IQ of 107, all in the average range. He had an adequate fund of factual information, vocabulary, arithmetic, and comprehension of social norms and nuances. In contrast, several areas of weakness were identified. In the verbal sphere, he had difficulty forming verbal concepts and retaining auditory stimuli. Furthermore, his spelling was impaired and he had a mild developmental language disorder characterized by paraphasic errors (the substitution of one word for another similar in sound or meaning, e.g., "public" for "pubic"). He also evidenced weakness in visuospatial constructional tasks in which the gestalt was preserved and in executing a rote graphomotor task. Projective testing highlighted the patient's sense of intellectual inferiority which was "overdetermined, having roots both in his actual neuropsychological problems and in castration anxiety" (p. 191).

In presenting detailed analytic process material, Rubovits-Seitz made it clear that neither its form, nor its content, was specifically or irreparably shaped or compromised by the existence of average intelligence and neuropsychological dysfunction. He felt his patient's thoughts and fantasies during free association seemed at least average in amount and rate. Although perhaps less complex and rich than those of an intellectually gifted patient, they were by no means impoverished or unimaginative. Furthermore, over time his ability to think abstractly and to be self-reflective emerged as a previously latent talent, his low scores on a test of verbal abstraction notwithstanding. Conflicts at all levels of psychosexual development were evident in the analytic material, and were interwoven with the patient's experience of his cognitive characteristics, including his areas of disability.

Kafka (1984) contributed another individual case study. He reported his process of discovery of the neuropsychological dysfunction of his adult analytic patient, Mr. R, and discussed its possible implications for analytic technique and character development. Kafka stated that such "cognitive difficulties, whether or not recognized in childhood, play a significant part in adult analyses and therapy. This is both through their effects on development and, if they persist, through their continuing effects in adulthood" (p. 533). Mr. R presented for analysis after consulting with his internist for a potency disturbance which the internist could not explain. This was a more extreme version of his chronic complaint of anxiety about performing sexually. In general, Mr. R considered himself a "faker" who "pretended" sexually, as well as in other areas of his life.

A series of symptomatic acts, about which Mr. R felt intensely humiliated and was reluctant to explore, prompted the analyst to become more curious about the forms these parapraxes took. Kafka did not feel that his patient's cognitive idiosyncrasies could be explained solely on psychodynamic grounds. Hints of a cognitive disability arose in this context, leading to childhood memories of right–left confusion, impulsiveness, reading problems, clumsiness and difficulty with abstraction. Kafka then considered these observations in light of some of his earlier thoughts about the patient. He had noted Mr. R's intense underlying anxiety and defensiveness, rigidity of character, and constriction of dream and fantasy life, along with the pronounced degree of his bisexual conflicts, the severity of his separation problems, and his repeated use of imagery involving location, especially when this involved right–left discrimination.

Using this case as a centerpiece, Kafka raised several general questions about working with patients with neuropsychological dysfunction. How may we take note in analysis of the residua of unrecognized cognitive problems from childhood which may persist into adulthood? What are the consequences for development of these difficulties? How do they affect analysands? Do they necessitate alterations of technique or of emphasis? Is there more for us to learn about the sources of such cognitive problems, or must we be confined to their individual manifestations in relation to individual patients? He also wondered why analysts so rarely address these issues.

Kafka offered several tentative answers to these questions. He cited Wender's (1971) description of characteristics of children with "minimal brain dysfunction": impaired coordination, clumsiness, short attention span, impulsivity, and an obsessive quality. He felt Mr. R suffered from these difficulties. Kafka believed that Mr. R's sense of defect contributed to his vulnerability to separation and to castration anxiety, as well as to his sense of loss, depressive ideas of incompetence, and his susceptibility to humiliation. Kafka did not feel he had to make major technical modifications in his work with Mr. R. However, he sometimes needed to repeat or rephrase interpretations (in different words and/or with the addition of examples) and to do so with more tact and patience than with other patients.

In Kafka's view, his patient's cognitive symptoms could not be entirely attributed to psychic conflict. At the same time he believed the case of Mr. R exemplified the uses to which neuropsychological problems may be put for purposes of defense and wish gratification, both consciously and unconsciously. In this sense these problems become shaping elements of compromise formation. Had Kafka referred his patient for a neuropsychological diagnostic assessment, it may have been possible to elaborate upon these issues even more informatively, or at least in a manner more specifically tailored to discussion of Mr. R's individual psychological picture. In closing, Kafka commented that when such cognitive problems in adults are subtle, they may go unrecognized. By the same token, he thought, when they are sufficiently severe to be noted, such patients may frequently be considered unanalyzable—an opinion with which he did not agree.

Myers (1989, 1994) has very briefly described two pertinent cases; in neither one was a diagnostic evaluation performed. In one (1989), the analyst was alerted to the possibility that his 30-year-old patient had a learning disability when he reported two dreams in which he reversed the sequence of the letters of several words: "stug" for "guts" and "DM" for "MD." This prompted the analyst to inquire whether the patient had suffered from dyslexia or another kind of learning disability as a child. The man replied with surprise that he had; indeed he was unaware that he had not previously disclosed this to his analyst. Myers, who had interpreted many aspects of his patient's prominent sense of humiliation (including his sense of himself as "stupid," "a dummy," and "a dunce"), now was able to identify another highly significant source. Myers (1994) regarded the "addictive sexual behavior" of another patient as an expression of, and an attempt to gain relief from, her sense of inner turmoil related to an Attention Deficit Disorder which had been diagnosed in adolescence. He added, "It would not be surprising to learn that a number of adults exhibiting addictive sexual behavior had earlier in their lives suffered from attention deficit disorders" (p. 1181).

Schwaber (1992) presented the analysis of a patient, Mr. I, who was an intelligent man with "considerable dyslexic difficulties which had been quite burdensome to him throughout his life" (p. 349). (The existence of a diagnostic evaluation, or the possibility of referring Mr. I for such an evaluation, to delineate the nature and scope of the dyslexia was not mentioned.) While the subject of the patient's reading disability was not central to Schwaber's purposes, several thoughts pertinent to this subject are stimulated by a reading of her account. In the course of the analysis Mr. I became aware that "the dyslexia also served as a defensive shield, protecting him from having to grapple with painful or conflictual issues" (pp. 340–350), in part related to his sexual identity. The patient, who was not satisfied with his work life, wished to continue his education beyond the college level. However, the prospect of applying to graduate school was a source of intense anxiety. Schwaber encouraged Mr. I to apply, with the view that this might shed more light on a sexual difficulty which was coming up in the analysis at that time. However, when he became extremely disorganized and confused in the context of doing so, Schwaber inquired why he felt under such pressure to apply at this time. He replied, "I feel damned if I do and damned if I don't. . . . I feel you're giving me mixed messages."

Emphasizing the issue of countertransference, Schwaber felt her patient was correct. From her perspective, she *had* engaged in a familiar reenactment with him because the predicament about school and sexuality he presented stirred something in *her*. She did *not* seem to consider the possibility that she was responding to Mr. I in a way that his parents had. Perhaps, like a parent, she wanted him to apply and subtly urged him to do so. But when he had trouble with his desire to face and overcome his learning disability, when he panicked at the possibility, she reneged. Schwaber then implicitly indicated to Mr. I that he need not confront his problem and the anxiety it evoked at that time. It is possible that she, like some parents of learning disabled children, tried to calm him by suggesting avoidance. Receiving a double message, Mr. I felt guilty and unable to please his parents (or analyst in the transference) whatever he did; he was damned if he did or did not. Thus Schwaber did not seem to take into account the specific link between Mr. I's dealings with his conflicts over his learning disability. Instead she emphasized her patient's conflict between "his essence" and "society" and between analyst and patient which, in her view, led to a loss of sexual identity and loneliness.

Garber (1991) published an account of the $3^1/_2$-year analysis of an 11-year-old learning disabled boy to demonstrate that the emotional sequelae of a learning disability can be addressed in a psychoanalytic setting. His other thesis was that the fantasy of being defective and damaged was most fundamental to this patient, although sexuality and sexual acting out were an important component of the boy's conflicts. In this paper, as in several others (1988, 1989, 1992), Garber emphasizes the centrality of problems in self-esteem regulation, to which he believes sexual issues are secondary. In his view they are often used to fill the patient's emptiness. (For more in-depth discussion of these ideas, see the section below entitled "Recent Contributions on General Characteristics of Patients with Learning Disabilities," pages 68–71.)

Garber's patient had been diagnosed as learning disabled and as having ADHD since the age of 8. Treatment with Cylert was inconclusive. Weekly psychotherapy with another therapist for one and one-half years, starting when he was 9, was stopped since there was no apparent progress. At this earlier age testing indicated a Verbal IQ of 98 and a Performance IQ of 89. The patient scored relatively high on measures of abstract reasoning, practical judgment, vocabulary, and fund of information. Alertness to the environment and nonverbal reasoning were also relative strengths. There were serious weaknesses in symbolic reasoning and short-term auditory memory. Performance tests were particularly uneven. On tests of visuomotor integration, weaknesses were noted in spatial organization and integration and in psychomotor speed. In addition, poor attention and concentration may have lowered the patient's scores on these subtests.

In light of his initial contacts with this boy, Garber regarded these test scores as underestimates of his patient's potential. Clinically, he had an extensive fund ot knowledge and
was keenly observant. Garber acknowledged that, at the outset
of treatment, he questioned what he had to offer to a boy with
these problems, since he (unlike an analyst such as Rubovits-
Seitz) assumed there would be serious limitations in the boy's
ability to be self-observant and introspective based on his IQ
scores. Nonetheless he agreed to work with the boy in a three
times per week analytically informed treatment, with parental
contacts as well. Garber ultimately concluded that the "emotional sequelae" of a learning disability are best addressed in
such a setting.

Indeed he came to believe that there are "recurrent dynamic configurations" unique to such children who "are vulnerable to the development of narcissistic psychopathology"
(p. 149). Garber felt that his patient left treatment with a more
stabilized sense of self and better self-esteem regulation. He
attributed this to the provision through analysis of consistent,
predictable, and reliable mirroring responses. In Garber's view
the fantasy of being defective and damaged is central to these
patients. Learning disabled children build on the notion that
something has gone awry in their brains or minds. They nurture a sense of defect in excess of the reality of their limitations
and beyond the time when these limitations exert an effect.
This fantasy has to be explored, worked through, understood,
and integrated.

This emphasis was so dominant in Garber's approach that
there seemed to be no consideration of further testing, remediation, or medication. In addition, Garber apparently did not
discuss with his patient the specific nature of his neuropsychological difficulties. Nor did he directly address the fact that, at
the end of the analysis, his patient's cognitive deficits remained. The reasons for these clinical decisions were not discussed.

Bucholz (1987) briefly presented the analysis of a man
who had a learning disability in childhood. This case was used
to illustrate her developmental model, which is also heavily
reliant upon self psychological ideas. These include the need

for parental attunement and mirroring and the establishment of object constancy, all of which may have been compromised in the learning disabled patient. Bucholz explored the impact of neuropsychological dysfunction upon the establishment of object constancy in particular, and on the attainment of satisfying object relations in general. In her analytic work with adult patients of at least average intelligence with learning disabilities, she views their difficulties from the perspective of what has gone awry in their "object relations and self systems." From this perspective, these patients, who are often insecure about their strengths and deficits, are likely to accept that they need help, without, however, grasping the nature of the help they require. Instead they are prone to feel "everything is out of kilter." Bucholz often finds that neither patient nor analyst recognizes the centrality of the patient's learning difficulties in this picture. She did not specifically comment, in this regard, on the contribution of a detailed diagnostic evaluation.

Palombo (1995) has described the case of a 10-year-old boy to illustrate his thesis, reflective of a self psychological perspective, about patients with "nonverbal learning disabilities." Palombo has identified what he regards as a constellation of associated psychological sequelae (delineated in the section below entitled "Recent Contributions on General Psychological Characteristics of Patients with Learning Disabilities"). When his patient did not understand the rules of a game other children had just taught him at camp, he insisted that the rules he created were the correct ones. This produced a chaotic situation in which he, enraged when the others disagreed with him, assaulted another child. Avoiding a simple cognitive explanation, Palombo points out the importance of additional factors in this episode such as fear of rejection.

Silbar and Palombo (1991) reported the twice weekly psychoanalytically informed psychotherapy of M, a 19-year-old man, which lasted only 13 months. M sought help because of school and social difficulty and a fear he was gay. He turned to drugs such as marijuana and LSD to sooth himself, but did not succeed in this effort. The authors conceptualized M's problems largely as a result of a lack of cohesion of the self due to his parents' failure to be available as supportive figures. However, when he was discovered through testing to have a learning disability, these findings were incorporated into the explanations of his pathology. M's subjective experience of lacking cohesion, furthered by his failure to achieve significant goals, was thought to be an essential part of his disturbance. It was not clear whether recommendations for tutoring or any other type of educational intervention were made. Despite the fact that M was often late to sessions and his father terminated the treatment prematurely, M's father reported improvement five months after the therapy ended.

Moore (1995), in an article on narcissism, described the psychoanalytically oriented psychotherapy of a physician who probably had a learning disability. This man had learned by listening because he had difficulty reading, as well as with mathematics and abstract concepts. Although psychological testing results were equivocal, Moore believed his patient had an Attention Deficit Disorder for which Ritalin was helpful. In his report of the skillful psychotherapeutic work he did with his patient, Moore described certain narcissistic traits, including rage when he was narcissistically deprived, and a strong desire to blend with others which manifested itself in fears of homosexuality and of closeness with women. Although these characteristics might well have been related to his learning disability, an attempt at integration of the patient's cognitive and conflictual aspects in the analytic work was not mentioned.

Gensler (1993) presented brief reports of four cases of adults with documented learning disabilities. Two he treated in psychotherapy; the other two were treated by other professionals who referred their patients to Gensler to carry out diagnostic testing evaluations. In none of these cases did the patient begin psychotherapy with an awareness of having neuropsychologically based difficulties, or a focus on a history of learning problems. These cases were intended to demonstrate the value of defining the patient's specific disabilities. For example, it was only after years of work that Gensler came to consider this possibility with Mr. A, who sought treatment for depression, a troubled relationship with his girl friend, and disturbing dreams. Gensler reports that the psychotherapeutic work was greatly deepened by his alertness to his patient's problems with verbal expression (grammar and word finding). He could better appreciate the complex interweaving of these cognitive limitations with Mr. A's anxiety about making phone calls, his inhibition in seeking appropriate levels of employment, and his sadomasochistic relationship with his girl friend. These repeated his childhood dependency upon his mother, his conflicts over having a severely disabled younger brother, and his identification with a narcissistic and self-preoccupied father. The wishful, defensive, and self-punitive aspects of his psychic elaboration were also explored; in Gensler's terms, he examined the effects on "adult character, defensive style, and relationship patterns" (p. 673).

In treating an adult borderline patient with a learning disability Migden (1990) discussed with him how it felt to be "intelligent yet illiterate; how it felt to see so many of life's opportunities pass him by; and how it felt now to see he could use remediation" (p. 112). This 33-year-old man was "essentially a non-reader" (p. 108). He "was given a full psychoeducational evaluation which found him to be functioning only at the second grade level in reading, spelling, and math; he exhibited specific deficits in visual recall, visual-motor integration, and auditory recall" (p. 109). Migden helped Mr. S recognize that his temper outbursts were not meaningless explosions, but rather results of his low self-esteem, failures of compensatory grandiosity, and his self-defeating behavior. As Mr. S learned to read, with the help of tutoring, he developed a new capacity to sublimate which provided outlets for his drives, and helped him control his outbursts. Migden points to a similar accomplishment in normal latency age children who sublimate through reading.

Because of the less detailed data available in less intensive treatments, the interesting suggestions made in these papers (i.e., those reviewed immediately above) are difficult to verify. Their authors make clinical observations which are worthy of further exploration in the psychoanalytic situation.

Contemporary Psychoanalytic Perspectives on Conflict and "Deficit"

In recent years there have been a number of attempts at conceptualizing the intertwining of neuropsychological dysfunction and psychological functioning. Many of the resulting contributions take up the interrelationships between "deficit" and "conflict," and rely upon the notion of compromise formation (Freud, 1926; Brenner, 1976). As early as 1926, Freud realized that, "The presence of a symptom may entail a certain impairment of capacity, and this can be exploited to appease some demand on the part of the super-ego or to refuse some claim from the external world. In this way the symptom gradually comes to be the representative of important interests . . . " (p. 99). He thus viewed symptoms as "a compromise between the need for satisfaction and the need for punishment" (p. 98). At the same time Freud cautioned against a misuse of this concept: "There is a danger, too, of exaggerating the importance of a secondary adaptation of this kind to a symptom, and of saying that the ego has created the symptom merely in order to enjoy its advantages. It would be equally true to say that a man who had lost his leg in the war had got it shot away so that he might thenceforward live on his pension without having to do any more work" (p. 99).

In recent contributions there is general agreement that when neuropsychological dysfunction is present, it does not derive from conflict but inevitably becomes incorporated in fantasy (Cohen, 1985, 1993; Coen, 1986; Allen, Lewis, Peebles, and Pruyser, 1986; Rothstein, Benjamin, Crosby, and Eisenstadt, 1988; Pine, 1991, 1994; Rothstein, 1992, 1998). These authors refrain from specifying particular types of associated fantasies, in contrast to other contributors (Palombo and Feigon, 1984; Shane, 1984; Palombo, 1985a,b, 1987, 1991, 1994, 1995; Bucholz, 1987; Garber, 1988, 1989, 1991, 1992; Palombo and Berenberg, 1997), who emphasize psychological configurations they believe to be universal in patients with learning disabilities.

Weil (1961, 1970, 1971, 1977, 1978) was the first analyst to systematically pursue Hartmann's (1950) call for an in-depth examination of the ways in which the neuropsychologically based deviations which affect learning simultaneously interact with the psychological sphere. More specifically she explored how the maturation of the ego apparatuses (including the rate, timing, and other qualitative and quantitative factors) influences a number of aspects of psychic development. These include the establishment of concepts of the object and of the self, psychic structure formation in general, and the emergence of structural conflicts. In her last paper on this subject, Weil gave particular emphasis to differences in perception, motility, and language. In her view, variations which occur very early in life are most likely to affect ego structuring and the potential for anxiety and aggression. She believed such variations would, in addition, find later expression. Those which occur subsequent to the development of speech, symbolic thinking, and self-awareness, she posited, would primarily be elaborated neurotically.

In several previous papers one of us (Rothstein et al., 1988; Rothstein, 1992, 1998) has written about the impossibility of considering neuropsychological difficulties apart from psychic conflict. The importance of investigating how particular types of neuropsychological dysfunction contribute to development in complex and highly individual ways was emphasized. This exploration encompasses unconscious fantasies, including wishes, defenses, and superego manifestations. An illustrative case analyzed from this point of view was detailed (1998).

Coen (1986) has demonstrated that, both in cases in which there is an actual problem of a physical (and, we might add, a neuropsychological) nature, and those in which there is not, the experience of "defect" represents a compromise formation. He contrasts this with an actual defect existing somewhere in the body, or in a psychological structure. Such a compromise formation must be analyzed in its complexity, rather than reduced to a "real" limitation or abnormality, since "it becomes the nidus around which much is crystallized" (p. 47).

Similarly, Willick (1991) has emphasized the importance of preserving "a dynamic point of view in the face of what might appear to be an ego deficit." He comments that the notion of "defect" may well contribute to a reluctance on the part of the analyst to interpret the conflicts which have become associated with the limitation. Arlow (1969) called attention to "how the symptoms of organic disturbances affect the fantasy life of the patient and how they facilitate the emergence of pathogenic fantasies" (p. 18). Beres and Brenner (1950) maintained that neurological symptoms become psychologically traumatic because of their association with a preexisting unconscious conflict.

By contrast with these authors, Pine (1994) has found it useful to distinguish between "conflict," "deficit" (which he defines as "an insufficiency of appropriate input from the surround—ordinarily from the primary caretakers" [p. 223], and "defect" (which he regards as aspects of faulty ego functioning). In his view, "deficit" can stem from biological conditions (for example, the effects of blindness, or a neuropsychologically based learning disability, upon some aspects of ego development) or from a "deficit" (e.g., the impact of unreliable care on the development of a capacity for delay). From Pine's perspective there is a dual relationship between conflict and "defect" or "deficit." In agreement with the above-mentioned analysts, he believes that "defects" and "deficits" inevitably become caught up in conflict and are psychologically elaborated. At the same time, he finds it useful to consider that "defects and deficits have an existence of their own as well . . . though conflict may be everywhere in mental life, it is not everything" (p. 237). In Pine's opinion it is possible to distinguish between "what is primary and what is secondary" (p. 235). Thus he maintains a distinction between so-called "conflict pathology" and "developmental pathology." Interestingly, despite the differentiation he suggests, his vision of its clinical implications is unclear; Pine recommends that therapeutically, not only a corrective relationship, but also interpretive work is necessary in the developmentally troubled areas of "deficit" and "defect."

Allen et al. (1986), writing from a slightly different vantage point, concern themselves with the ideal neuropsychological evaluation in a psychoanalytic setting (the Menninger Clinic). They argue against the polarization of neuropsychological and psychodynamic explanations for a patient's pathology; instead they favor an integrated conceptual framework in which neuropsychological and psychological considerations are intertwined. Only in this manner, they believe, can respect be paid to complexity, and ambiguity and reductionism avoided.

Recent Contributions on General
Characteristics of Patients with
Learning Disabilities

Some contributors find it useful to identify general characteristics of patients with learning disabilities. Typically these are clinicians who regard learning disabilities as a whole, rather than considering the particularities of the neuropsychological problems of individual patients. Many of their observations and clinical speculations may be exceedingly useful in selected cases. However, it is very important to bear in mind the tentative nature of such hypotheses, rather than assuming they will invariably apply. In addition, these ideas generally do not derive from the data of an intensive psychoanalytic treatment conducted on a four or five times weekly basis which, in our view, provides the best opportunity for discovery, clarification, and verification.

Broadly speaking, three types of general statements appear in the literature with some frequency. Learning disabled patients are said to evidence limitations in their capacity for empathy (Garber, 1988, 1989, 1991, 1992), in the accuracy with which they interpret nonverbal communications (Palombo, 1995), and in the appropriateness of their social relatedness (Gabbard, 1990). The compromising of their ability to achieve object constancy and a stable sense of self has also been noted by a host of analysts and other clinicians (Bucholz, 1987; Gabbard, 1990), as have their problems with separation-individuation (Herman and Lane, 1995), self-esteem regulation, and the development of a sense of competence (Garber, 1988, 1989, 1991, 1992; Aleksandrowicz and Aleksandrowicz, 1987; Lewis, 1986; Shane, 1984; Heisler, 1983; Burka, 1983).

A major contributor to this subject is Garber who writes from a self psychological perspective, emphasizing the narcissistic problems of patients with learning disabilities. He, along with Shane (1984), also addresses the narcissistic difficulties experienced by the parents of such children: "The damaged child may be experienced as a disappointing selfobject for the parents, thus seriously interfering with the transformation of narcissism normally and expectably an outcome of parent-hood" (1984, p. 121). In keeping with the review of the psycho-analytic literature published by Rothstein et al. (1988), Garber (1988) noted the "dropping out" of psychoanalytic contributions beginning in the 1970s. He critiqued what he views as the excessive emphasis of these authors upon ego psychology, at the expense of other considerations, most notably narcissistic development from the perspective of self psychology. Garber regards his papers as attempts to "redress" the neglect of psychoanalytic perspectives in treating patients with learning disabilities.

He believes that the excessive preoccupation of learning disabled children with how they are seen renders them less available to be concerned about the feelings and perspectives of others. This, combined with limitations in cognitive equipment, compromises their empathy as well. Thus such patients are prone to be insensitive and selfish vis-à-vis their peers.

Garber has also highlighted the significance of a sense of defect in learning disabled children; indeed he feels this is central to their pathology in self-esteem regulation. Aleksandrowicz and Aleksandrowicz (1987) have found that self-esteem problems persist well beyond other manifestations of neuropsychological dysfunction, such as academic underachievement or hyperactivity. In the case of adolescents (1992), Garber stresses their sense of loneliness and lack of acceptance by peers. Problems in accurately perceiving social signals from others, and therefore in appropriately and successfully relating to them, were also noted by Gabbard (1990) and Palombo (see below). Writing specifically about children with ADHD, Nathan (1992) points out the "long-term, entrenched, primitive view of the self and others born of long-standing, conflictual interaction produced by primary, core ADHD symptomatology" (p. 305).

Also writing from a self psychological perspective, Palombo (1985, a, b, 1987, 1991, 1994) has given special consideration to what he terms "nonverbal learning disabilities" (NVLD) and their relationship to disorders of the self and relational problems as well as borderline conditions. He defines these as "the disabilities related to visuospatial processing of information and disorders associated with the reception, expression, and processing of affective communications" (Palombo, 1995, p. 147). In Palombo's view children with such disorders have difficulty interpreting a range of nonverbal communications, leaving them with an incomplete, and to some degree distorted, understanding of their interpersonal relationships.

These patients nonetheless attempt to create meaning, constructing a self-narrative and view of reality which may not be shared with others. When there is a lack of concordance, their relationships with others, including their caretakers, is compromised. More specifically, the child's capacity to obtain sustenance from parental objects or to make use of them as "selfobjects" is affected, leading to narcissistic vulnerability. Palombo believes that the resulting relational problems have significant consequences for the child's sense of self as well. He has also linked neurocognitive deficits and borderline personality development, asserting that "a borderline condition represents an inpairment in a child's sense of self cohesion that is the result of a neurocognitive delay, distortion or deficit, for which the milieu of selfobjects has found it impossible to compensate" (1987, p. 326).

For the most part Palombo makes general statements about his patient population, or presents brief illustrative clinical vignettes. He does not, however, report in-depth clinical material to illustrate or validate his conclusions. (The exceptions are Palombo [1995] and Palombo and Berenberg [1997], described above.) A vignette from the psychotherapy of a boy who was 6 at the beginning of his treatment exemplifies the type of child he discusses and the type of evidence Palombo accumulates. Larry was a "chaotic, disorganized child who attacked his environment in a most disruptive way" (Palombo, 1994, p. 145). After observing him clinically and with the help of psychological testing, Palombo concludes that he was a "classically borderline child with marked neurological problems which were never clearly diagnosed" (p. 145). Because there was a significant discrepancy between verbal and performance scores, the author suggests the child has a nonverbal learning disability. In our view, since these findings can have many causes and consequences, it would have been enhancing to have access to more detail about the psychological test results of Palombo's patient.

Gabbard (1990) has written about the adverse impact upon the development of object constancy of "defects" in visual and auditory perception and memory. Also contributory, he believes, is the learning disabled child's difficulty in self-soothing; this he relates to an inability to internalize and maintain images of comforting maternal figures.

Migden (1996), in an unpublished article, makes a number of important suggestions about the effects of learning disabilities on several aspects of psychological functioning. He states that the language-based learning disabilities of many ADHD children contribute to their hyperactivity and inattentiveness. Because their linguistic ability is limited, these children are unable to adequately use speech and language to express and organize their ideas and emotions; they use action instead. Unable to use language (and, we may add, in many cases motor skills) to control and organize their drives, they become impulse-ridden.

Herman and Lane (1995) have accentuated the role of separation-individuation in learning disabilities. After criticizing early psychoanalytic authors for "overextending their somewhat simplistic, narrow, id-defense theory" (p. 15), the authors attempt "to show how the capacity for academic learning is founded on the earliest phases of cognitive/affective ego development" (p. 18), including the progress from autism "toward object constancy" that Mahler, Pine, and Bergman (1975) described. Herman and Lane discuss related cognitive aspects and later developmental stages as well. They attempt to place patients into groups based largely, but not entirely, on their developmental stages. The treatment they outline appears to pertain to the most mature group, and pays little attention to separation-individuation. Their examples are extremely brief vignettes which do not clarify the frequency of their patients' treatment or the nature of the learning disabilities they consider. Thus it is difficult to evaluate the accuracy of their clinical concepts.

Early Psychoanalytic Contributions to Problems in Learning

An infinite number of fantasies may accrue as a result of neuro-psychological dysfunction and learning disabilities, whether diagnosed or undiagnosed. There are also limitless psychodynamic purposes for which the existence of such dysfunction may be employed. Contemporary analysts may find much of value in the earliest psychoanalytic contributions on learning disorders in which the myriad of fantasies associated with learning problems is richly explicated. This is so, even though these papers are dated in some respects, and most of the analysts who wrote them failed to consider the existence of neuropsychological factors in the patients they analyzed; at the same time, some accurately identified the population who suffer from learning disabilities on a purely psychogenic basis.

All contributions are elaborations of the fountainhead, *Inhibitions, Symptoms and Anxiety* (Freud, 1926):

> [T]he ego function of an organ is impaired if its erotogenicity—its sexual significance—is increased. . . . The ego renounces these functions, which are within its sphere, in order not to have to undertake fresh measures of repression—in order to avoid a conflict with the id.
>
> There are clearly also inhibitions which serve the purpose of self-punishment. . . . The ego is not allowed to carry on those activities, because they would bring success and gain, and these are things which the severe super-ego has forbidden. . . .
>
> The more generalized inhibitions of the ego obey a different mechanism of a simple kind. When the ego is involved in a particularly difficult psychical task . . . when a continual flood of sexual phantasies has to be kept down, it loses so much of the energy at its disposal that it has to cut down the expenditure of it at many points at once [pp. 89–90].

In this spirit, the early psychoanalytic authors explored an array of disorders with differential emphasis upon one or more of the following factors: dynamic, genetic, structural, representational, and environmental. Conflicts—whether predominantly oral, anal, or oedipal—were shown to result in a great variety of manifestations: general disruption of the learning activity itself, specific kinds of errors (e.g., misinterpretations of words based on drive-determined distortions), or particular conditions under which the activity finds interference (e.g., in the presence of special dynamically laden contents).

Other analysts consider the relative involvement of the three psychic structures, ego, id, and superego, in a particular learning pattern (Pearson, 1952). This approach highlights the fact that the psychodynamic meanings of learning may fuel a disruptive breakthrough of impulses or, conversely, a special investment and high level of proficiency (Plank and Plank, 1954). Disorders may arise when there is (1) failure to achieve sublimation in a child who has not experienced optimal frustration or gratification (E. Klein, 1949; Plank and Plank, 1954; Rubenstein, Falick, Levitt, and Eckstein, 1959; Vereecken, 1965); or (2) deneutralization of drives (E. Klein, 1949; Plank and Plank, 1954; Newman, Dember, and Krug, 1973). The latter may be due to the ego's impoverishment with respect to energy available for learning by virtue of its absorption in other tasks, or in response to an unconscious need to fail.

Psychodynamic formulations of both extensive and delimited learning disorders differ in their relative emphasis upon preoedipal and oedipal factors. Theories of unconscious oral conflicts find especially great currency in the literature on reading problems, although they are also called upon to explain general problems in learning. Reading has been viewed as a derivative and symbolic expression of the following oral activities: when done in bed, a nightcap or good kiss (Glover, 1925), "eating" another's words (Strachey, 1930), or incorporation by way of the eye (Fenichel, 1937). Oral conflicts and consequent reading disorders may include fear of destroying the object through incorporation (Pearson, 1952), reluctance to relinquish oral passivity as seen in difficulties in shifting from the passivity of being read to, to the activity and initial frustration of being the reader (E. Klein, 1949). Plank and Plank (1954) offered a similar formulation for arithmetic disabilities. The persons whose autobiographical statements they reviewed could not give up the desire for maternal oral gratification necessary to move into a world of symbols. Conversely, those who excelled in arithmetic evidenced special maternal deprivation.

Learning impairment in general has been noted to reflect an equation with having food shoved down the throat (Pearson, 1952), given the association between imbibing knowledge and eating (Abraham, 1924; E. Klein, 1949), or a disorder of frustration tolerance (Pearson, 1952). Narcissistic issues are also thought to contribute to stunted learning, as when the child cannot bear to suffer comparison and possible competitive loss. He attempts to maintain a superior stance by virtue of apparently not needing to study, holding those who do in contempt (E. Klein, 1949; Newman et al., 1973). A somewhat different emphasis is given by Kaye (1982) who views the learning problem as a manifestation of the maintenance of "innocence in relation to the self-system" (p. 92).

Anal issues and conflicts which are said to contribute to or interfere with learning include the special appeal of particular subjects (e.g., arithmetic) because of their demands for precision, the possible use of knowledge to express anal sadistic and exhibitionistic impulses (Pearson, 1952), and the negativity of hostility manifested in a specific symptom, for example, writing words backwards or not learning at all (Blanchard, 1946).

Oedipal determinants of learning disorders have been much discussed. Intellectual inhibition as a whole or in a particular subject with sexual associations (e.g., biology) may be a symbolic derivative of the suppression of sexual curiosity (Mahler, 1942; Blanchard, 1946; E. Klein, 1949; Pearson, 1952; Jarvis, 1958; Vereecken, 1965). Pseudoimbecility, for example, permits the child to do, see, and say things otherwise not permissible. Inhibition may also reflect associations between learning and femininity, creating a conflict for boys, or masculine strivings with resulting conflicts for girls (E. Klein, 1949; Pearson, 1952; Plank and Plank, 1954; Jarvis, 1958). Castration anxiety elicited by the prospect of excelling over parents or older siblings is another commonly noted contributor to learning problems (E. Klein, 1949; Pearson, 1952; Jarvis, 1958; Buxbaum, 1964; Vereecken, 1965) and other kinds of success neuroses (Buxbaum, 1964).

Arithmetic disorders have been attributed to unconscious

hostile fantasies associated with the processes of manipulating numbers: breaking them up, taking parts away, and the like. Such concerns over aggression and integrity of the object may be orally colored as well. Jarvis (1958) discusses reading disorders which result in a situation of being read to, rather than reading oneself, as a regressive solution to oedipal dangers. This general idea is further elaborated by some to explain fear of use, but not acquisition, of knowledge which is equated with use of the penis, often beginning in early adolescence (Pearson, 1952). The sense of having a damaged head is construed as an upward displacement of castration anxiety. Fears of humiliation in examination of one's learning are symbolically related to the boy's humiliation in the course of having his genitals compared with those of his father.

Several authors (Hellman, 1954; Rubenstein et al., 1959; Buxbaum, 1964; Newman et al., 1973; Berger and Kennedy, 1975) place greater emphasis upon environmental factors, although their clinical illustrations suggest that, when prolonged, environmental stress will result in internalized conflicts and maladaptive identifications. Children reared in terribly poverty-stricken neighborhoods where crime (including murder) is rampant and primal scene traumata are repeatedly experienced because of cramped, overcrowded quarters, often have difficulty learning (Meers, 1970, 1973; Burland, 1984, 1986). Denial, a defense necessary to tolerate such a perilous world, interferes with learning. Paradoxically, in these ghettos, overstimulation is often complemented by the understimulation of parents who fail to engage their children's academic interests and stir their curiosity. When schools, instead of being havens in which learning is fostered, become dangerous places in which the teachers must be more concerned with discipline than teaching, learning becomes difficult if not impossible.

Overstimulation and understimulation need not be neighborhood matters. They can also characterize particular families with devastating effects. Various constellations of parental psychopathology shape the child's development at particular stages. In some cases, the mother's unconscious need to externalize her own sense of inadequacy, which finds embodiment in her child, is highlighted (Blanchard, 1946; Buxbaum, 1964;

Berger and Kennedy, 1975). In their patients, Berger and Kennedy note the mother's early expectation of defectiveness and consequent failure to nurture development. Faulty maternal resolution of separation–individuation processes is emphasized in others. The child's ability to learn threatens an especially intimate tie between mother and child. Preoedipal encouragement of oral fixation was suggested by histories of excessive stimulation or inconsistent patterns of excessive indulgence and frustration. In these cases, general stupidity or a particular disorder represented an unconscious collusion with mother in order to preserve her love by remaining in a partially symbiotic relationship. This precluded independent functioning or recognition of ability. Later oedipal elaboration sometimes occurred in the form of an impairment of ego function, inhibition of curiosity, and scoptophilia as a defense against knowing forbidden family secrets, especially when they were sexual (Mahler, 1942; Staver, 1953; Hellman, 1954; Buxbaum, 1964; Sprince, 1967). Pseudoimbecility permits looking without being thought to be able to see. Hellman (1954) describes a special situation in which the mothers' distortion of reality made it impossible for their children to see realistically without compromising closeness.

A predominantly preoedipal constellation which incorporates some of the above elements is elaborated by Newman et al. (1973) to account for poor academic performance in boys with exceptionally high IQs. Uneven development, a strong command of language, accompanied by poor conceptualization, attention, and motor functions, is attributed to the mother's excessive valuation of verbal production without concomitant encouragement of motor activity, since the latter signals the child's ability to separate. This early imbalance interferes with the normal intertwining of such functions necessary for the formation of sensorimotor schemata, lending a shallowness to later language and other higher cortical functions. Maternal attitudes are noted to reflect their depression and devaluation of spouses in the child's early years, rendering them excessively needy of the child for companionship. The child's precocious speech leads mother to believe he is a genius, without need for ongoing stimulation. Lack of activity and autonomy, not regarded as problem areas by mother, are identified as such only at school age.

This preoedipal substratum sets the stage for a difficult oedipal phase. Having earlier gained a sense of omnipotence associated with talking, the child has exaggerated expectations that talking alone will help him negotiate. In school, where this is not the case, he experiences intense narcissistic injury at the prospect of having to struggle and not know immediately. This leads him to avoid less developed areas, resulting in a further disequilibrium of functions. Conflicts with father are significant as well. In some respects the child has already won an oedipal victory, which makes the ultimate oedipal defeat more humiliating, and simultaneously fuels fears of retaliation by the father he defeated. The learning disorder is conceptualized as an expression of ambivalence toward mother—verbal facility expresses love, and failure in performance expresses hostility—as well as a means of maintaining closeness with mother through verbalization; both provocatively defy father by physical inadequacy and school failure, and placate him by not being more successful academically.

Other environmental contributions to learning disorders of a current, rather than chronic, nature are noted by Pearson (1952): unpleasant conflictual experiences with teachers, ongoing family traumata (e.g., parental fighting) which absorb ego energies, and pressure from or identification with peers who discourage learning.

CONTRIBUTIONS ON TECHNIQUE WITH LEARNING DISABLED PATIENTS

Diagnosis and Analyzability

With rare exceptions, contributors to the psychoanalytic literature prior to the 1980s gave inadequate consideration to the careful assessment of the specific nature of the learning disability. This was despite Pearson's (1952) cautionary remarks long ago:

[E]very child who shows any form of steeple-like or valley-like learning patterns requires an evaluation by a psychoanalyst. It is important that those psychoanalysts who specialize in the psychoanalysis of children have *a broad knowledge of the factors which may produce such problems and of how they may be cured* ... [p. 322]. Most of this data [neuropsychological bases for learning problems] is well known to physicians and educators but I have felt it necessary to re-emphasize because *at the present time when there is so much emphasis on the importance of intrapsychic processes in all phases of medicine and education, psychiatrists tend to become overenthusiastic about dynamic intrapsychic processes to the complete neglect of physiological and organic processes, for which they seem to have a psychic blind spot* [p. 328; emphasis added].

Several other excellent, relatively early exceptions are papers by Heinicke (1972), Silverman (1976), and Pine (1980), in which the multiple etiologies of these disorders and their varied clinical manifestations were carefully delineated. McDevitt (1975) discussed the many causes of learning disabilities in a sophisticated way but without offering clinical illustrations or recommending a comprehensive diagnostic evaluation.

More common were the countless cases reported which did not reflect the degree of sophistication, specificity, and comprehensiveness with which such diagnostic studies can be performed. In many instances this was an expression of the author's specific view of learning disabilities—a preconception that they consisted of invariant features, when they are actually highly individual in nature. To illustrate, Weil's (1961, 1971) discussion and clinical examples emphasize one type of learning disabled child (the neuropsychologically impaired child who presents with hyperactivity and attention deficits) for whom *these* behavioral indicators, coupled with an IQ test, may be sufficiently diagnostic. However, even in the case of such children an IQ assessment alone would be inadequate for remedial purposes. Therefore, what many clinicians construe as a complete assessment is in fact only a partial evaluation.

Newman et al.'s (1973) study of 15 "underachievers"—boys with IQs 130 and above and grades of C and below—is one of many psychoanalytic papers which exemplifies the pitfalls of a partial diagnostic evaluation. It will be discussed in some detail to serve as an illustration. The uneven development of these children was also evident in their strong command of language accompanied by poor conceptualization, attention, and motor functions. This was attributed by the authors to the mother's excessive valuation of verbal production without concomitant encouragement of motor activity which signals the child's ability to separate. This early imbalance was hypothesized to interfere with the normal intertwining of such functions necessary to the formation of sensorimotor schemata, lending a shallowness to later language and other higher cortical functions.

In detailing the contrasts between hypertrophied verbal capacities and impaired motor functioning, Newman et al. note their patients' sloppiness, restlessness, sluggishness, and poor handwriting, which they do not regard as evidence of motor incoordination: "on their psychological tests *they did not show even slight signs of any actual motor incoordination, and their total test performance was in no way suggestive of the presence of minimal brain damage*" (p. 92; emphasis added). However, just preceding this statement is another: "Their scores on the coding subtest of the WISC, the only subtest that requires use of pencil, were the only scores that were almost uniformly low" (p. 92).

These two assertions are contradictory: if visuomotor coordination problems are present, this is precisely where they are likely to be in evidence. A footnote to the first quotation cited is intended to further discount the possibility of neuropsychological dysfunction by equating an average IQ with intact ego equipment: "While their Performance IQ's were typically somewhat lower than their Verbal IQ's they were nevertheless well above average, in the superior range" (p. 92). Since the WISC is the only tool used to assess cognitive functioning, and since there *is* a single finding suggestive of dysfunction, it is not possible to rule out a neuropsychological contribution to the constellation described.

While modern contributors are far less likely to fundamentally overlook the neuropsychological etiology of a learning disability, most nevertheless fail to appreciate the value (and often even the possibility) of a detailed diagnostic assessment of the nature of the neuropsychological involvement.

An example of the degree of specificity with which one may assess even a single cognitive function, memory, was conveyed by Squire (Panel, 1995), who identified many types. "Declarative memory" involves retention of facts and recalling of events. "Non-declarative memory" includes "procedural memory" in which particular actions can be repeated. Remembering how to drive a car or ride a bicycle or writing are examples. Another subtype, "priming," occurs when the subject responds to a second identical stimulus more quickly after the stimulus was previously introduced. A subject may be asked to identify a number of pictures of objects; he will do so more rapidly if he has previously been shown a particular picture. Another subtype, "classical conditioning" is contrasted with nonassociative memory. "Evocative memory" is differentiated from "recognition memory," and "long-term memory" is distinct from "short-term memory."

The failure to sufficiently integrate the knowledge neuroscientists are accumulating into the study of learning disabilities has to do with the fact that "[o]nly a beginning has been made at understanding the complex problem of how the brain accomplishes learning and memory" (Squire, 1987, p. 241). There are a number of achievements of knowledge of which parts of the brain are involved in different types of memory. For instance, to name just a few of the many connections, declarative memory is said to be localized in the median temporal lobe and diencephalon; procedural memory involves the stria, priming is associated with the neocortex, and conditioning involves the cerebellum.

It is apparent that since memory is so complicated and involves so many interconnected parts of the brain, we cannot expect that there is but a single type of learning disability with a simple structure that applies to all patients with problems in memory. Nevertheless it is common for analysts and other clinicians to lump such learning disabilities together, rather than attending to particular details of the learning difficulty as discovered by the psychologist who has tested the patient.

One noteworthy exception is a paper by Aleksandrowicz and Aleksandrowicz (1987) who herald the great value of accurate diagnosis of subtle cognitive or integrative impairments in enhancing a patient's self-esteem. They refer to the frequent statements of these patients such as: "You are the first person who ever understood and told me what is wrong with me." They add, "Proper diagnosis is also a powerful tool to relieve the parents' guilt and shame, to inspire them with hope, and to motivate them to embark on a treatment program" (p. 585). These authors strongly advise that an accurate and detailed diagnostic picture be shared with both patient and family as does Silver (1989). Rubovits-Seitz's (1988) above-described case report also exemplifies the value of such specific diagnostic evaluation.

More typical, however, is the work of Garber (1992). On the one hand he underlines the failure of learning disabled adolescents to understand the precise nature of their cognitive disability and/or how it impacts upon their social interactions and learning:

> *It is difficult to differentiate the actual effect of the disability from the meaning that they have given to it.* As a result, learning disabled adolescents believe that there is something seriously damaged in their heads. This is a pivotal fantasy around which psychology crystallizes. The adolescent will use and embellish the fantasy beyond the point that is reasonable and appropriate [p. 342; emphasis added].

Therefore, it is surprising that in none of his general clinical papers or case studies does Garber specify the nature of the learning disability he discusses; nor does he seem to clarify this via detailed diagnostic testing or in the course of the clinical work. Indeed he (1992) indicated his belief that learning disabilities are overdiagnosed in adolescents, conveying a subtly skeptical tone about the value of diagnostic evaluation.

In their recent review article about the state of psychiatric diagnosis and treatment of children with learning disabilities, Beitchman and Young (1997) note "tremendous advances within the field over the last ten years" (p. 1029). However, in our view, their characterization of current assessment practices in working with patients who are possibly learning disabled is generally too circumscribed—often far more so than is true of the evaluations of many of the patients in our volume. The authors state that the most basic assessment is an intelligence test (most often the WISC-III) along with an "assessment of academic content areas including reading, mathematics and spelling through achievement tests" (p. 1022). Focusing particularly upon children with reading disabilities, they comment that, in addition to standardized tests of cognitive ability (they do not specify which tests), a thorough examination should include "measures of a child's ability to read words both in isolation and in text, ability to sound out unfamiliar words, knowledge of word sounds and corresponding letters and letter patterns, and reading comprehension skills" (p. 1023). The necessity of more specialized tests (such as those measuring sequencing and visual and auditory memory) (Rothstein et al., 1988) and projective testing is not emphasized. Although evaluation of aspects of the child's personality, and family and societal demands is mentioned, the value of a thorough psychoanalytically based study is not. Nor are neurological examinations (or the need to evaluate "soft" or gross neurological findings) included as part of the current workup. A contribution such as Silver's (1992) monograph on ADHD is a model of the comprehensiveness with which a diagnostic evaluation can be performed.

Treatment

While many of the early psychoanalytic contributors on learning disorders claimed that their psychodynamic formulations accounted for the learning problems of a broader range of patients than was accurate, their views regarding the applicability of their clinical methods were typically too narrow. With several exceptions (Sarvis, 1960; Rappaport, 1961; Hartocollis, 1968; Weil, 1971, 1977; De Hirsch, 1975; Silverman, 1976; Pine, 1980) these contributors did not sufficiently appreciate the value of psychoanalytic concepts and techniques in treatment planning for patients with neuropsychological dysfunction. The growth of diagnostic techniques did not contribute to a "widening scope" (Stone, 1954) of patients considered treatable by psychoanalysis. Instead patients without intact "equipment" were frequently dismissed as unsuitable. This was particularly true when the aspects of functioning involved were of central importance to psychoanalytic work, for example, expressive language and conceptualization (Waldhorn, 1960; Doris and Solnit, 1963). There may also have been concerns about the effect of other needed interventions upon the transference and analytic process.

In contrast, many of the above-described recent case studies (Kafka, 1984; Bucholz, 1987; Rubovits-Seitz, 1988; Garber, 1991; Palombo, 1995; Palombo and Berenberg, 1997) were written with the intent of demonstrating the usefulness (and indeed the necessity) of treating learning disabled patients in psychoanalysis or psychoanalytically oriented treatment. Several papers report the importance of psychodynamic psychotherapy of patients with frank brain damage due to traumatic injury (Lewis, 1986; Buskirk, 1992; Leichtman, 1992). Buskirk explicitly counters the view that psychodynamic approaches are contraindicated; he notes that such assumptions are based upon the common view that treatment relies upon highly developed verbal skills, reflectiveness, tolerance of frustration, and the capacity for abstract thinking and generalization.

All of these authors maintain that, precisely because even subtle neuropsychological dysfunction may affect important psychological processes, psychodynamic approaches are crucial. Several contributors specifically address the treatment of ADHD from this perspective, emphasizing the need for long-term psychotherapy in conjunction with stimulant medication (Smith, 1986; Nathan, 1992; Cohen, 1993). Emphasizing the characterological effects of this neuropsychological experience, with which we agree, Nathan elaborates on the rationale for psychotherapeutic treatment, albeit in a passionate (if not hyperbolic) style:

> *I am speaking here about changing the long-term, entrenched, primitive view of the self and others born of long-standing, conflictual interaction produced by primary, core ADHD symptomatology.* These core symptoms are identical to the "nonspecific ego weakness"

described in the histories of patients with borderline character pathology (Kernberg, 1975). The evolution of such character pathology is undoubtedly the reason for the devastating findings in outcome studies on ADHD youngsters. . . . Because such individuals represent a large proportion of the approximately 3–9% of youngsters who had ADHD . . . the coordinated treatment of this disorder should be viewed as nothing less than an assault on a major psychiatric public health problem [p. 305; emphasis added].

Although the effectiveness of Ritalin and other stimulants in controlling ADHD has suggested that a biological etiology of that condition is primary, Richters, Arnold, Jensen, et al. (1995) state, after an extensive study of the literature, that matters are more complex. They conclude that "there is a substantial body of evidence demonstrating the *short-term* effectiveness of stimulant medication in normalizing many of the core clinical symptoms of ADHD" (p. 993; emphasis added). However,

[S]timulants appear less reliable in producing *long-term* benefit, although this has not been adequately studied. . . . Also stimulants seem to have weak and/or unreliable therapeutic effects on many secondary or comorbid and academic deficits of children with ADHD. . . . Stimulants may be most effective in normalizing and stabilizing the primary functioning characteristics of some hyperactive children, *whose behavior and learning problems must then be addressed directly and strategically through a range of psychosocial treatments* . . . [p. 993; emphasis added].

A number of the studies they reviewed show that drug treatment alone is not as effective as multimodal treatment which includes stimulant treatment and psychosocial treatment. These authors do not, however, refer to psychoanalysis or psychoanalytically oriented psychotherapy.

Beitchman and Young (1997) reported a similar finding in their examination of the literature on the effects of medication on reading disabled children. They concluded that "evidence of *long-term* academic benefits of stimulant medication is lacking" (p. 1027; emphasis added). This is true despite the fact that medication may have the immediate effect of increasing attention and concentration and improving behavior, thus enabling patients to participate in the learning situation at home and at school. The sole article indicating the long-term effects of a stimulant medication (Dexedrine) revealed improvement over a fifteen-month period (Gilberg, Melander, von Knorring, et al., 1997). Because this study was done in Europe where the criteria for the diagnosis and use of stimulants appear to be more restrictive than in the United States, one of the authors (Dr. Gilberg) warned against using this research to justify widespread use of medication for all hyperactive patients here (Gilbert, 1997).

R. A. Furman (1996) recently published a study of the comparative use of stimulant medication in the treatment of ADHD in the United States versus Europe. He cited the striking statistic that, taking England, France, Germany, and Italy as a whole (with an aggregate population comparable to that of the United States), the use of stimulant medication is less than one quarter of 1 percent that of the amount used in the United States. It is estimated that 1.3 million American school children between 5 and 17 are receiving stimulant medication for conditions diagnosed as ADHD. Furman highlighted two contributory factors: the contrasting bases for diagnosing ADHD (which lead to a higher incidence in the United States) and the more restrictive regulation of use of these substances in Europe.

Many contributions emphasize flexibility in treatment planning, including the frequent necessity of integrating multiple approaches (Abrams and Kaslow, 1976; Migden, 1983; Smith, 1986; Aleksandrowicz and Aleksandrowicz, 1987; Nathan, 1992; Leichtman, 1992). These may include psychoanalysis and/or psychoanalytically informed psychotherapy, remediation, psychopharmacological intervention, supportive psychotherapy (treatment in which the patient attempts to control his impulses and emotions), and parental counseling and/or individual treatment of parents.

PART II

Psychoanalytic Case Studies

Chapter 3

Leah's Analysis

Denia G. Barrett, M.S.W.

INTRODUCTION

The educational specialist who evaluates a child having problems learning in school uses a variety of diagnostic measures
to assess the difficulty. While the results of psychometric tests
help determine the intactness of the ego apparatus, the analyst
evaluating the child from a metapsychological perspective will
also consider the child's level of anxiety, his defenses, his progress along the developmental lines, the nature of his conflicts—both internal and internalized—in addition to assessing
his drives, superego, and object relations (A. Freud, 1962,
1963). A metapsychologically based evaluation can help determine whether or not an analytic treatment is indicated, but it
may not be until the end of such a treatment that one can
determine the relative contributions of psychopathology and
neuropsychological dysfunction in a particular child's learning problem.

This was true for Leah, whose analysis I will describe below.
Psychoanalysis helped uncover many of the sources of her
learning interferences. It allowed her to work through conflicts
that were expressed via her impaired learning, and it enabled
her to develop a capacity to use a relationship with another in

order to learn. It did not, however, eliminate her academic problems altogether. Although Leah needed ongoing remedial help after her treatment ended, her analytic material affords the opportunity to learn more about the complexities and rich individual meanings that attach to her particular disturbance in learning.

PRESENTING PROBLEMS

Leah was referred for an evaluation when she was 6 years old and in kindergarten at a private school where I was a consultant. Separations had always been hard for her. At the start of kindergarten Leah's distress showed in tears when she said goodbye to her mother at the start of the day and in withholding bowel movements and urine. She had episodes of both day and night wetting, demonstrating that she had not mastered toileting.

Leah's former preschool teacher described her as one of the most unhappy children she had ever met. Her kindergarten teacher observed that Leah often sat by herself, staring off into space. She was well-behaved at school and sought her teacher's attention by showing off her pretty clothes and asking for hugs after weekends at home. Leah did not, however, develop a more age-appropriate learning relationship with her teacher. She did not seem to grasp prereading concepts. Nor did she appear to have achieved secondary autonomy in either her self-care or her learning skills. She was able to tie her shoes and know letters and numbers one day, only to lose these abilities the next. Leah learned best on a one-to-one basis with her teacher, but seemed to become lost in a group. When she made a mistake or did not know how to do something, she berated herself as "too stupid" or "too little."

Leah's mother was embarrassed by her daughter and felt she was "weird." As an illustration she described a situation at the local library when Leah anxiously waved her hand to be recognized by the story teacher. When she was called upon, however, her answer had no apparent connection with the group discussion. Later, Leah could not complete a project related to the story because she had difficulty using the scissors. This, too, seemed "bizarre" to her mother.

PSYCHOLOGICAL TESTING

In addition to these observations from school and home, results of several tests administered by the school psychologist at the end of Leah's kindergarten year (Leah was a little over 6 years) indicated a problem with her learning. While Leah's overall intelligence was in the average range as measured by the Stanford-Binet, there were very significant differences between her performances on different portions of the test. In general, her vocabulary, comprehension of verbal material, and abstract visuospatial reasoning were considerably above expectations for a child her age. In contrast, she evidenced pronounced weaknesses in oral arithmetic skills and immediate memory for both visual and auditory stimuli. The achievement test administered at that time yielded similar and additional findings. Leah had a fund of general factual information which was well above age level but manifested weaknesses in basic aspects of spelling, mathematics, and reading; her scores spanned the 9th to 30th percentiles for her age. Her performance on these tests was also below expectations based upon her IQ.

In noting the unevenness between Leah's ability and her actual achievement, the psychologist observed that she had seemed anxious and confused by the testing situation. If she felt she did not know the right answer, she became upset and gave up. Though there were no other signs of problems with her motor skills, Leah had tripped and hurt herself slightly on her way to the office where the tests were to be administered.

CONSULTATION

Leah's parents initially sought parent guidance for help around her separation problems, obstinacy, and her enuresis. The child analyst with whom they worked recommended an evaluation for analysis when it became evident that these symptoms and the learning problems likely represented internalized conflicts which were not amenable to change through guidance alone. Although this analyst was unable to see Leah himself, he remained available throughout my evaluation to facilitate a transition that allowed the parents to express the disappointment and loss they felt as their work together ended.

Leah was a sturdy, pretty 6-year-old when her parents brought her for the evaluation with me. Although she was obviously worried and unhappy, there was nothing in her outward appearance that would cause others to describe her, as her mother did, as "weird."

Leah and I had two meetings prior to the start of her analysis. Her parents prepared her by telling her that the first analyst (whom Leah had met) thought it would help her to have someone to talk to herself. When they asked her if there were things she wanted help with, she said she wanted to be able to read as some of her classmates could.

Leah came to our first meeting wearing a brave smile. She let me know at the outset that she was going to be late to school because of our morning meeting. She was also worried that she would not be able to complete all her work. She spoke of the referring analyst, indicating that her mother would not be talking with him if she came to talk to me. When I acknowledged her concern to be losing school time and someone special, Leah's smile faded and she seemed to hold back tears. She told me she had not been allowed to see a movie because it had a lot of fighting. I said that her parents told me that there were lots of fights at home and they hoped talking with me might help with this. Leah said she and her brother fought, especially when he tried to take her doll. She went on to say that her mom and dad kissed, adding "They can do that in bed, but me and my brother don't like it when they do it in front of us so we try to get between them."

Between the first and second evaluation sessions, Leah told her mother she felt a wet spot when she sat down on my couch. She did not bring the problem of her enuresis directly to me. However, in the second meeting Leah spoke at length and critically about others who were either messy or out of control. She thought it would be hard to talk with someone she did not know. She wanted me to know how much she liked her mother, her teacher, and her school friends. Leah's worry about loyalty notwithstanding, she agreed to the idea of meeting before school every day.

Developmental History[1]

In providing a developmental history, Leah's mother indicated that she experienced Leah as somehow "different" from the very start. Her pregnancy had been normal, but the labor and delivery were complicated, and Leah suffered some temporary respiratory distress. However, she did not require any special attention after her birth.

She was an easily soothed infant who ate and slept well and adapted to her mother's household routines. The only remarkable aspect of the mother's report of the first six months was her exaggerated reluctance to let anyone else hold Leah. When pressed to explain what she found weird or different and when she began to experience this, she referred to times when Leah showed signs of readiness for increasing bodily separateness and independence—when she began to refuse the breast at 6 months and when she began to walk at 10 months.

It is difficult to sort out which partner in the mother–infant couple withdrew from the other first. Leah's mother became pregnant again when Leah was 6 months old. At this time, as Leah became more mobile and demanding, she began frequently to leave her in the care of babysitters. Leah reacted by beginning to awaken during the night. Her mother's response was to yell at her in helpless fury when her efforts to comfort her failed. Whereas initially each seemed to have gained pleasure and narcissistic supplies from their relationship, from the second half of the first year on, this favorable balance shifted

---

[1]The history has been disguised in several places in the service of maintaining confidentiality. In each instance where this is the case, care was taken to remain faithful to the psychological meaning and integrity of the analytic material.

toward a preponderance of sadomasochistic interplays and raw aggression.

Leah's brother Jacob was born when she was 15 months old. After Jacob's birth, Leah's mother was overwhelmed by the demands of an infant and toddler, the one nursing, the other still taking a bottle, and both in diapers. She yelled and hit Leah with increasing frequency. Her own early childhood experiences had left her ill-prepared for the tasks she faced in her maternal development. Leah's mother's capacity to gradually progress from a narcissistic investment in her children as extensions of her own body, to an object investment in them as separate persons, was impaired. Her aggression interfered with her assuming the role of educator of the drives and promoter of ego mastery. She was unable to help Leah with her ambivalence toward her and her jealousy toward her little brother.

Nor was she attuned to signs that Leah was ready for steps that could increase her sense of autonomy and self-esteem. By leaving Leah in diapers until she was 3, she failed to promote self-care and cleanliness, and the related reaction formations. She stated that she wanted to be the one to do things for Leah, and did not want to teach her to do for herself. She also wanted to avoid the mess and fight she anticipated. As Jacob's second birthday approached, she introduced the toilet to both children at about the same time. Jacob was compliant and gradually became clean and dry over a 6-month period that was developmentally on target. In contrast, the mother became locked in verbal and physical battles over messes with Leah. Eventually she acquiesced to her mother's demands, but Leah began to withhold urine and bowel movements frequently. She leaked and stained her pants during the day. She had some dry nights, but bedwetting occurred regularly.

The delay and failure to resolve anal conflicts at the developmentally appropriate time, and her mother's obvious preference for her brother, contaminated Leah's phallic phase. In addition, she experienced humiliating medical investigations and intrusions as a 4-year-old when her withholding resulted in recurrent urinary tract infections. All of these experiences contributed to Leah's sense of herself as an unlovable, out-of-control, dirty girl. Leah's father enjoyed her pretty looks and her interest in dolls and homemaking. He did not discourage her when she stated her intentions to marry him when she grew up. Despite her observations of nudity at home, neither parent could recall that Leah ever asked any questions about the sexual differences between boys and girls and adults and children, or about conception or birth. At the same time, both parents did relate doll play during which Leah was obviously delaying her use of the toilet, as she pretended she had babies growing inside her. Each was uncomfortable with the prospect of discussing or teaching Leah about these matters.

Recommendation for Analysis

Analysis was indicated as the treatment of choice for Leah because her toileting symptoms and her learning interferences posed significant threats to progressive development in latency. It appeared that her symptoms were interrelated and involved the consolidation of conflicts from every developmental phase. Leah provoked her parents to criticize or punish her and she berated herself cruelly, revealing the harshness of her early latency superego.

My recommendation for a five times weekly analysis was accepted and sessions continued at that frequency for the duration of the treatment. As the work got under way, I met with Leah's parents weekly. Over time, these meetings were reduced to biweekly and then monthly.

COURSE OF THE ANALYSIS

Leah brought a picture book to her first analytic hour. She pretended to read the title page and then went through the rest of the book, telling me the story page by page. It was a vividly illustrated version of Hans Christian Andersen's *The Little Mermaid* (1981). A voluptuous mermaid princess falls in love with a sailor prince and begs her father, the king, to allow her to follow him to land. In order to be transformed from a mermaid to a young woman, she must first take a dangerous journey to visit a witch. She is required to submit to a bloody rite of passage in which part of her tongue is cut off and her blood is added to the witch's cauldron. Pain and disappointment follow for the mermaid, as she discovers that to use her new feet feels like walking on sharp knives and that her beloved prince is to marry a real human princess. She sadly accepts this defeat and returns to the sea and her mermaid form.

After Leah told me that she really liked this book, I asked what it was that she liked so much. "The prince and the bride," she replied dreamily. She said her mom was going to buy her a bride outfit for playing dress up. After I reflected that it sounded hard to wait to be a bride, she added that she wanted to have three babies when she grew up. Before putting the book away, she pointed out that in the pictures the mermaids' "chests" showed. She went to unlock her supply cupboard but was unable to get it open, despite having done so without any problem earlier. She showed me a bad scrape from a bike fall and then said she had to go to the bathroom. She assured me she could go by herself.

When Leah returned, she confessed that she and a friend had taken off all their clothes while playing mermaid recently. She said this was not "appropriate" and her excitement seemed to grow. She told of fire drills at home, of boys playing with matches, and she asked about the fire exits in my office building. I addressed myself to Leah's worry about whether it was going to be safe to stay and try to understand her troubles through talking with me, or whether I, too, might join her in getting too excited and doing things her conscience considered inappropriate.

Leah then asked me to show her how to write "Exit." In her attempt to copy the word, she wrote the letters, E, X, and T correctly, but she did not place them in the right order and it was an effort for her to write them. She informed me that her mother gets furious when she is messy with markers. She wanted to know what time we would stop so she could leave for school. Since Leah did not yet know how to tell time, I offered to draw what the clock would look like when our time was up. She wanted to put in the numbers by herself, but reversed both the "7" and the "9." I commented that she seemed to want me to know about her wish to be able to learn to read and write letters and numbers. I went on to ask if she were showing me how it was for her at school sometimes, when something seems to get in her way as she works. "Yes," she said.

This account of the content and process of Leah's first analytic session suggested a classical example of a girl regressing from phallic–oedipal strivings to avoid the multiple threats and anxieties these arouse. Excitement and grown-up wishes lead to bloody injury and humiliating disappointment for the little mermaid. After sharing her own excited longings and guilty conscience, Leah retreated to the relative safety and familiarity of the bathroom and thoughts of struggles with her mother over messes. Along with this evidence of instinctual regression, furthermore, was the marked vulnerability of her ego functions. This showed in the loss of her former abilities to open the cubby or ride her two-wheeler safely and in the ease with which her newly acquired number and letter skills could be drawn into conflict.

Thus I also viewed these neurotic solutions as an overlay to an ego disturbance dating from the disturbance in her earlier relationship with her mother. The apparent "classical oedipal regression" was deceptive and an oversimplication. I will describe how this became evident during the first year of our work together when Leah's behavior and speech regressed to more primitive levels of bodily discharge, unlike work with a typical neurotic patient of this age.

After the initial hour, Leah's anxiety increased with each succeeding day. She was terrified by ordinary noises from other offices in the building. She let me know she was afraid of the scissors I supplied because she was worried she would not be able to stop herself from cutting her own hair. She could not use the stapler or the small pencil sharpener because she imagined she would hurt herself on the "sharp" staples and blade. I began to have a better appreciation for some of the examples her mother had brought, such as Leah's "bizarre" reaction to using the scissors at the library. When I asked her what was so worrisome for her, Leah replied simply, "I get angry."

Her projection of anger and aggression was pervasive. For example, when I wore a new pair of high-heeled shoes, Leah was afraid to walk down the hall to my office with me. At first she said she did not like the noise they made on the tile floor, but soon admitted that she thought I might stomp on her foot with the heels. As we talked about it more, she could let me know that she was really very jealous of my grown-up lady shoes and that she was the one who wanted to stomp on my foot.

Leah grew more and more unsafe, out-of-control, and attacking of me. I let her know I would stop her from being unsafe until she could find the 6-year-old part that could keep her own self safe. I had to restrain her sometimes, but she could also use my suggestion that she pick an area of the office to be a safe place where she could take herself. Throughout this time, Leah consistently managed to keep her out-of-control behavior out of school. The effort this cost her, understandably, left little neutral energy available for learning.

Over the course of Leah's first year of work, her sudden and very surprising attacks on me represented a passive-into-active defense whereby she attacked me as she had been surprised by her mother's yelling or hitting, both in the past and present. The attacks also demonstrated that while her libidinal development had proceeded more or less unimpeded to the oedipal level, her aggression remained at a primitive, oral sadistic level. She did not have reliably adequate signal anxiety, and introjection and projection remained prominent as defenses. Her conscience, which objected to her impulses, attacked her with raw aggression and cruel introjects. Verbalizing feelings did not always prevent Leah from discharging them motorically.

She began one hour telling me that she had something "sad and mad" to tell me. She reported a mean thing Jacob had done at home and then launched toward me saying, "And I want revenge." As I put my hand up to ward off her blows, she bit me. We were both surprised: I, because I thought she would stop herself and Leah, because she seemed to have no warning between the impulse and the bite. I said I was sorry that her mean mouth feelings can take over like that, surprising her and then getting the mean mouth yelling at herself.

Once I spoke of her mean, yelling conscience, Leah let me hear it more. She called herself lazy and stupid when she mixed up words or could not do something. When I expressed my hope that we would find words to help with the biting, yelling feelings, she added, "And the 'I can't read feelings.'" Her word confusions and her comparisons of herself with others in her class who were beginning to read wounded her narcissism, as did her mother's ongoing failure to keep her in mind.

These issues became available in the work around the first summer separation. After her mother forgot to tell her she would be waiting in a different location one day, Leah complained, "It feels mean when you forget me." The following day she brought a phonics book with short words she had previously learned. When Leah could not remember the sounds that went with the letters, I drew her attention to how she was forgetting words that she had known before. I reminded her of how angry she had felt about her mother forgetting her the day before. Leah ripped up her bookmark and yelled at me, "Shut up, you turkey. Forget it, just forget it!" She brought up the vacation then and I wondered with her whether she was worried that we would forget one another during the weeks we did not meet, as happens for her and her mother.

A few days later, Leah brought an alphabet game to her session. The card that matched with the letter V on the board had violins on it. She mispronounced the word and it came out "violence." She looked puzzled and ashamed and said, "I get words mixed up." Leah confessed that she had used a pacifier until she was almost 6. Without really considering why, I asked what she had called her pacifier. She blurted out "Some Fucker!" Worriedly, she tried to correct herself by saying "Some Thucker" and finally "Thumb Sucker." Her examples again demonstrated that language, like other ego functions, had not become autonomous. It could readily become instinctualized. Instead of using words to serve as a vehicle for neutral communication, Leah often repeated angry sarcastic comments or curses that she heard from others. At such times she did not sound like herself, leading me to feel the outbursts indicated the presence of unintegrated introjects rather than more selective identifications. The same difficulty was evident later when Leah's attempts to master written language were contaminated by instinctual breakthroughs.

At various points during the first year of work together, Leah alluded to her masturbation problem and said she had "secrets I'll never tell." Her excitement often intensified before a holiday or vacation and it seemed to help ward off the feelings of worthlessness and abandonment that the separations aroused. Initially, I addressed myself to this defensive function her excitement served.

This same mechanism was evident at the beginning of the next school year when she was worried about the work and her new teacher. Upon the recommendation of the private school she attended, Leah was enrolled in a transitional class designed for children who had already completed a year of kindergarten, but were not ready for first grade. When she returned to her analytic work in the fall, she was carrying a folder with a rock group on the cover, and she dressed and talked like her teenage babysitter. She thought the math book would be "too big" and that a primer she started would be "a real killer." As her anxiety was addressed, her excitement diminished.

Leah's curiosity about sexual matters and male–female differences gradually became more directly available in her analytic material. She began to ask about my husband and family. She asked if I had the "recipe" for girls. I said that she seemed to have lots of such questions about boys and girls, ladies and men, and how babies get made. She had an umbrella with her that hour and she stuck it between her legs and called it a magic stick. A few days later she bragged about having a new bathing suit. Almost immediately after telling me this, however, she turned on me and yelled, "I hate you, you're a zero." I noted that it sounded like something was making her feel like a zero. In addition to feeling unvalued by her mother, Leah also felt like a zero in response to her fantasies about anatomical differences. This problem showed in school when she could not correctly answer questions in her math group about which objects were bigger or smaller and which had more or fewer details. When I tried to explore this with her, she declared that she did not like differences.

One secret Leah closely guarded also contributed to her feeling like a zero—her enuresis and the leaking that dampened her pants when she postponed urinating. Shame and conflict over this symptom showed up in an interesting way, once her sessions had become less chaotic and words began to replace action. We had begun to notice her frequent use of reversals as a defense against her envy. For example, if I wore something she found pretty, she would berate it as ugly. If she liked something someone else had, she claimed she hated it. We had been working on this for a time, when Leah drew a picture during one of her hours. It showed a girl high atop many mattresses on a bed and she told me it went with the story *The Princess and the Bean.* As many children do, Leah often reversed the letters *p* and *b.* This was the first opportunity to interpret the conflictual meaning it had for her. I offered my idea that it was hard for her to know it was a story about a princess and a pea, not a bean, because of her own peeing in the bed problem. Not long afterwards, she reversed the number 9 in some work she was doing in my office. When I drew her attention to the mistake, she angrily retorted, "Are you saying it looks like a 'p'?" She then grudgingly let me know that she had wet the bed the night before.

In addition, Leah seemed to have unconscious knowledge about a forbidden secret of her mother's. In her first hour she had emphasized that she wanted to have three babies of her own. This fantasy reemerged in a game during the second year of her analysis, when Leah pretended to be a mother with three babies to look after. She switched roles at one point and became a policeman. She grew abusive of me and threatened to arrest me and take my children away because I was a neglectful mother.

Leah's mother soon told me of a secret that explained this play. At this point, her attitude toward Leah alternated between emotional unavailability and angry intrusiveness. In discussing this with me, Leah's mother recognized that she dreaded the sense of loss she anticipated when Leah moved on to first grade. She attempted to explain her feeling that there had been something "different" in her relationship to Leah from birth. I noted that it had been her first time to have a baby. She hesitated and then told me about an unmastered experience from her past. In college she had a brief relationship with a fellow student and she became pregnant. While not ready to become a mother, her decision to have an abortion was nevertheless an agonizing one for her. She recalled thinking when Leah was born, "No one's going to take this baby away from me." In this context, her possessiveness of Leah during the first months of her life, her subsequent resentment of her daughter's independent forays, and her current reactions became more understandable. This constellation of feelings had an impact not only on the relationship between Leah and her mother, but also on Leah's development of ego functions crucial to learning: perception, reality testing, and curiosity. Her identification with her mother's attitude that some things must not be known, such as the pregnancy and abortion, had the effect of inhibiting Leah's approach to learning in general.

The significance of this piece of Leah's mother's history could not be addressed at this point in Leah's treatment. However, Leah did begin to bring anxious fantasies and conflicts about pregnancy for us to explore. She was wild and out-of-control one hour, until she could tell me that she had to accompany her mother to her gynecologist's office later that day. She mentioned that on another occasion in this doctor's waiting room she had seen a video of a baby being born. Leah had some grapes with her during this session and as she talked about the video, she swallowed one whole. She went on to describe a giant swallowing a human being. She kicked at the desk violently and spoke of kicking inside of her mother, demonstrating her fantasy of oral conception involving babies being swallowed. In this fantasy the eaten-up babies inside are angry. Leah grew wild again, but at the end of the hour she secured her mother's promise that she would not be exposed to the video.

The following day Leah continued to kick and scuff the walls. "Oh, all right, punish me," she said. She complained that I blamed everything on her and that I wasn't a helper. However, she could not say what had happened inside her that turned me from a helper to a blamer. She announced that she could not use the cleanser I provided to repair the damage to the walls because it was poison. The next day Leah let me know that her reading had become involved in her regressive oral–sadistic fantasies. She was practicing for a play, but could not read the word *bad*. She guessed "Bite?" "Mad?" "Sad?" In the material that followed, Leah expressed directly a wish to kill Jacob. I offered a reconstruction of the bitter anger and sadness she experienced during her mother's pregnancy and after Jacob's birth.

Leah and I had also been working more directly on her masturbation conflicts. On a day she was scheduled to repeat her psychological testing, Leah touched her genitals during her analytic hour. I wondered if the touching helped keep away her worries about the testing. In response, she touched herself again and said, "Don't say that, you're so stupid." Though I spoke to her anxiety that she would feel stupid, she was beginning to reveal a fantasy that her masturbation was responsible for her learning problems.

On the second testing, after a year of analysis and at the end of her second kindergarten year, Leah's overall IQ score was 7 points higher. The spread between her verbal and quantitative reasoning scores was less pronounced. However, she still manifested a weakness in immediate memory for visual and auditory stimuli. Her percentile rankings on the achievement test administered had fallen, reflective of the fact that there was little improvement in her academic skills. The only exception was the elevation of her score on a test of general factual information.

We continued to address her learning interferences as they related to masturbatory conflicts as first grade approached. Leah brought a stuffed animal to her hour and showed me how she scratched and tickled it in bed at night. She wrote the first letter of her name backwards and turned the "L" into a "7." Leah then told me I had a stupid brain. I asked if it bothered her that she would be older than some of the other first graders, since she would be turning 8 during the year. In subsequent hours Leah's excitement continued. She flitted from touching one thing to the next, flicked the lights on and off and pointed out broken things. I interpreted that she was letting us know she thought her nighttime touching was what made her different from kids who were ready to start first grade when they were 6.

In anticipation of a routine doctor's appointment Leah excitedly performed an "examination" on the stapler to determine why the staples wouldn't come out. She told of doing things her mom says are bad for her, but which she likes to do anyway. I said that the liking was one thing, but the worry and feeling that she cannot stop doing something bad for her might be something we should try to understand more about. Leah excitedly put her finger in a hole in the plaster wall. At that point I interpreted the compulsive masturbation that followed the frightening excitement and shame she felt when she was younger and her urinary symptoms had led doctors to look at and touch private parts of her body.

Leah began to bring the sadomasochistic struggles that she and her mother had over her toileting into her analytic work and the transference. She again needed limits and grabbed at me or harmed something in my office and then warned, "Don't touch me." As Leah's hands got messy one hour, she said "My mother will kill me." When my stomach growled, she yelled at me. I said all of this must have come from the mean yelling that went on instead of loving teaching when Leah was trying to learn to use the bathroom. In the following hours, she began to leave to go to the bathroom frequently. She explained that she now used it when she needed to because she was tired of her mother nagging her about it. Leah also provoked nagging feelings in me by stubbornly refusing to talk in her hours.

Soon afterwards, Leah had a book report due. When she complained that her mother was nagging her about her homework, I remarked to each of them that it sounded like they were going back to the old ways. Leah's mother withdrew resentfully and Leah wet the bed on the morning she was to give the oral report. As she practiced in my office, she could not remember the author. When I commented that the old memories of fighting about the toilet seemed to get in her way as she tried to remember school things, Leah was able to recover the name and feel pleased with her own effort.

During the third year of Leah's analysis, she reintroduced the mermaid theme for us to work on directly. She began to draw mermaids in her hours and she told me sincerely, "Little girls love mermaids." When I asked why this was so, she said it was because of their tail. I commented that after seeing such a tail, girls might wish to have one too. Leah associated, "I dream of having a tail." I wondered how it felt when she awoke to find she did not really have one. While Leah did not answer directly, she told me about something she did better than Jacob. I pointed to this and to her recent experiments with fancy jewelry and hairstyles as signs she was not really feeling good enough. I expressed the idea that she had seen something boys and men have that made her feel no good about her own body. If we could talk about her body concerns, then she might be able to get the good feeling she had in the dream from being a girl who could do many things well, without having to pretend to have a tail.

Leah subsequently told me she had seen an adolescent boy leave my office. She began to cheat on the board game we were playing at the time. Leah was fiddling with one hand. I asked if she were again letting us know of things for hands to do which feel like rule-breaking and linked this to the work we had been doing on her observations of what males have on the outside. Leah named her own eyes and heart and said she could feel her heart inside of her. I said there are some parts she can see on the outside and some she can only know about by the way they feel inside (Kestenberg, 1975).

Leah held tenaciously to the fantasies that she had damaged herself and that she deserved to be punished for her masturbation. She found confirmation for this when a series of urinary tract infections again led to medical investigations. She acted out by engaging in excited observations with some girl friends following which she told me girls have "she weenies." Although she did not confirm this directly, Leah's drawings at this time suggested that her description of "she weenies" referred to her observations of her clitoris. When Leah was abusive toward me, I reflected what a hard time her conscience was giving her again. Demanding that I give her money and office supplies, she cajoled, "Please, please . . . just one teeny-peeny." I acknowledged how deeply she wished to have a penis instead of a "she-weeny" and hoped I would give it to her.

At the time, Leah had been trying unsuccessfully to read from the Shel Silverstein book, *The Missing Piece Meets the Big O* (1981). One day she threw the book in the trash after she could not decipher a word. I addressed how bad she thought she was when she could not read. I asked if we might try to solve the puzzle of what got in her way when she tried. I said sometimes kids were not able to read because the words were about something they had strong feelings about. I reminded her of her old trouble feeling like a zero in her mother's eyes and all the ways she was letting us know that she felt like she was a girl missing the piece she saw on boys.

Not long before her ninth birthday, Leah began one hour with play in which her Barbie doll was being cruelly tortured. Leah then left to go to the bathroom. She had been having trouble sleeping at night and had been going to her parents' room. We had begun to explore her sadomasochistic views of intercourse, based on her observations of her parents fighting, her own toileting battles with her mother, and the possibility that she had been exposed to the primal scene. I expected the material to lead us in that direction. Therefore, I was surprised when Leah forthrightly and genuinely said, "Mrs. Barrett, can I ask you a question . . . when your breasts started to grow, did they get purple?" She then pulled her t-shirt taut to show her nipples. This was the first time Leah had put into words her awareness of signs that her body was beginning to change. The relief with which she reported the next day that she had finally slept through the night revealed the intensity of the anxiety she had been experiencing about her body.

Any pleasure Leah took from this proof of her new feminine development was shortlived and soon outweighed again by anxiety and a sense of inadequacy. She wanted "boy lego" for her birthday because she felt "girl lego" was "too small." Provocative and unsafe in her hours, she picked at scabs and at her gums until they bled. I noticed aloud how unable she was to like herself or me, or to stop hurting herself, after telling me about the girl changes. Leah carelessly cut herself at home and had to have stitches. I asked her if she had questions about growing up and bleeding. Her reply showed her familiar defensive reversals: "I love blood, I don't care if it gets on my clothes."

Leah's mother's discomfort discussing sexual matters with her contributed to the difficulty in effectively preparing her for her pubertal development. One day Leah wanted me to look at her lips, which she said were blue and bleeding. I interpreted the displacement from her concerns about menstruation. She said her mother had told her about "shedding blood." A few days later, Leah was worried she had accidentally enlarged one of the holes in her recently pierced ears. I said her worry that she hurt herself by touching was like her concern that the bleeding which comes with growing up was also an injury, instead of something that indicated her body was healthy and doing the right thing.

Leah continued to work on trying to integrate her anxiety and her excitement, her fantasies and her inner genital sensations. She began to bring in her diary and talked about a teenage heart throb who was so "hot" he made her "sizzle." "One day he'll be mine, all mine," she said and added, "I know who you're hot for, your husband." I acknowledged her curiosity and said I hoped we could know about her sizzling feelings in words so that they did not cause her to make trouble for herself. Not long before her excitement with her father had led to a fight as he tried to help her with her homework.

The next day, Leah repeated her cruel play with Barbie and then pretended the doll was a mermaid. She folded her coat around herself in a clamlike shape. Commenting that it was a cave for the mermaid to sleep in, she settled in with a satisfied "Aaah!" I said that maybe she was beginning to like some of the good feelings a girl can get from the inside parts of herself. The following hour she wrote me a note thanking me for helping her.

However, the help also stirred Leah's homosexual conflicts and she soon called me a brat. I wondered aloud whether it had gotten too hard to talk about her romantic and excited feelings with me. Soon thereafter she told me a boy should have a girl friend and a girl should have a boyfriend. I asked if liking me and feeling friendly had turned into sizzling feelings that worried her. Following this, Leah became more contained. She asked if I noticed there were no more "fights" in the office. When I asked why she thought this was, she replied, "Because of the good feelings."

A regression was signaled when Leah brought hair gel to her hour and showed it to me with an admixture of excitement and disgust. She confirmed that she was beginning to notice similar discharge from her own body. She turned her Barbie into an acrobatic cheerleader who exclaimed, "Girls are best." At first this seemed to be another expression of Leah's compensatory phallic fantasies. However, later she said reflectively, "We're both girls, aren't we? Girls can do some things boys can't do."

After arriving late for one appointment, Leah (who was not quite $10^1/_2$ years old) shyly confided that she thought she had gotten her period. I asked what gave her the idea and she spelled B-L-O-O-D. She observed that she was starting "early," and worried the principal would find out. When Leah expressed her fantasy that she would get detention for a week, I noted she still seemed to view periods as punishment. The next day she brought a yo-yo to her hour. After explaining that she had a yeast infection, not her period, she said feelingfully, "I feel like a yo-yo." Leah had been able to ask questions of her doctor who told her she would probably menstruate sometime in the next six months. She asked me when she would get hair under her arms and shared that she already had it "everywhere else." Growing pleasurably excited in anticipation, Leah's hand slipped into the waistband of her pants as she talked again about the TV star she liked. Her reaction to my verbalizing her sexy feelings was to say "Yuck!" but the next hour she brought her diary again and showed me drawings she made in bed at night. In response to a drawing of a woman with breasts and nipples, she said that she hoped her breasts would be big ones.

By this time, Leah had been in analysis for four years. The combination of starting school when she was turning 6 (due to her late fall birthday) and the year in the transitional class meant that she was older than her classmates. Increasingly this contributed to her both feeling, and being regarded as, different. Leah brought this in by saying that she wanted to stop coming to her analysis because it made her feel she was weird. At this juncture, this represented an externalization of her conflict rather than a real push to terminate.

Several other discrepancies in her development contributed to her "weird" feelings. Leah's physical development outdistanced the pace of her intellectual development. Until this point, when Leah was in third grade, her marks from school were A's, B's, and C's and her teachers did not express concern about her performance. Her mother, however, was dissatisfied and critical of her progress. Leah cruelly taunted herself as a "retard," especially when she had more difficulty with math as it became more abstract. This was experienced as another internal discrepancy. Her language skills developed more easily, but comparable effort did not bring improvement in her math abilities. When I commented on how hard she was being on herself, she said straightforwardly that she thought she had a learning disability.

As we focused on this, Leah became increasingly curious both at home and in my office. She snooped through her parents' belongings and old picture albums. She began to explore my building, instead of coming directly to the office as she had always done. Leah steadfastly maintained her idea that her parents had only had sex two times and only to make her and Jacob—not, as I suggested, because it felt good. She told me she was thinking about a girl whose mother got pregnant at the age of 16, but cautioned, "Don't tell my mother, they're just thoughts." Once again, Leah brought material suggestive of her reliance upon knowing and not-knowing.

This defense, frequently erected in response to anxiety aroused by observations of anatomical differences between the sexes, had been evident in her phallic mermaid fantasies and ideas of being a girl with a tail. Now, however, Leah expressed the thought that something had happened to her mother when she was younger. I acknowledged her perception that there was something from her mother's past that had made a difference in the way her mom treated her, something she could not fit together. I added that not knowing some of these things got mixed up with her ability to know things at school and left her feeling confused and stupid. At the end of her hour Leah told her mother what we had been talking about.

A few days later, Leah came to her hour complaining of a stomachache. She had been trying to figure out where babies grow, if not in the mother's stomach. She told me her mother had talked with her about the first pregnancy. The primary effect this had on Leah was to pave the way for reality to gain ascendance over her defensive and wish-fulfilling fantasies. With regard to her learning problems, the subsequent analytic work indicated that both Leah and her mother gradually became better able to relinquish their shared attitude that these represented signs of damage or punishment for sexual misdeeds.

Leah began to talk seriously about finishing her analysis at the end of third grade, one year before she actually ended. When I asked at that time what she felt she still wanted to work on, she wrote down, "My tempure" [sic] and "Hurting myself."

At the beginning of fourth grade, when Leah returned to her analysis after the summer vacation, she grinned broadly and announced, "I've grown a lot." Her unisex outfit was typically adolescent and her face was broken out. With sincerity, she expressed her wish to work toward finishing her analysis, "Not today or tomorrow or next week, but this year." She did not set a definite date then, but put us both on alert that she hoped to finish our work before the start of another school year. In March she proposed that she would come five days a week until June, when school let out, and then she would cut back indefinitely to two days a week. Leah offered her own review of her progress. She was getting along better with Jacob now that "there's more love than hate. We don't fight . . . well, almost." Her temper was better and she and her mother did not fight as much. She realistically noted, however, that some problems remained. She would like to have some girl friends and get better grades. Leah seemed determined to work hard on these problems. She did not fit in well with the other fourth grade girls. She thought they were babyish and they teased her about her clothes. She reflected that she used to act tough, fight, or asked for tasks so she could avoid the playground at recess, but now she wished she could make friends.

Leah brought schoolwork to her hours and was open in showing her efforts and sharing her thoughts. Soon, however, Leah's efforts to work on her troubles turned into complaints that she was being left out, bossed, and treated meanly by the girls at school. In the transference she was provocative and mean to me. I interpreted the passive-into-active defense and the way she turned me into one of the girls with whom she could not get along. Leah turned to drawing and leaving me out during her hours. She critiqued her drawings as evidence of either genius or stupidity. I said that she seemed to feel she had to be perfect or she would be a nothing.

At one of our monthly meetings, her mother let me know that she was not going to involve herself in Leah's homework anymore. I was reminded of when Leah went to first grade and her mother felt abandoned and withdrew resentfully from supporting Leah as she did her first book report. It seemed that Leah's pubertal development represented another loss and threat to her mother. At the same time she wished to allow her daughter ownership of her functions, including learning.

There were a number of times Leah brought math problems to solve in her hours. She had not been able to memorize her math facts. She struggled for days, attempting to figure out a real life problem that involved multiplication. For example, she tried to determine how many miles she rode her bike to school in a week. She knew it was two miles each way, four miles a day, five days a week. After much effort, Leah came up with the number 20, but by then she was lost and unable to say that this was the total number of miles. She blamed her previous teachers for not teaching her anything or caring about her.

Some hours later, Leah wanted to play the card game black jack, which required adding to 21. Every time she had to add a smaller card to one worth 10, she had to count using her fingers. Leah told a joke that reflected how nonsensical math seemed to her: "Two kids get on a bus, four get off, three get on—what color are the bus driver's eyes?" She could not move from the concrete to the abstract, from the physical to the mental. This paralleled her difficulty as a younger child having feelings and fantasies in thought instead of action. At this point, however, I asked about the reality that other kids, with the same teachers, had been able to learn math. Leah was relieved when her mother pressed the school for another evaluation. Further educational testing confirmed that Leah needed tutoring in math.

Soon afterwards, Leah had her first period. She canceled a week of analytic appointments and looked miserable upon her return when she announced, "My period started." Unhappy, she continued to miss many days of school and treatment because of colds. After one three-day absence, Leah busied herself with schoolwork and would not discuss her feelings about being away. She bragged that two-step division was easy for her, but her words quickly revealed this to be her familiar reversal. "Let's see, three goes into five how many times?" she asked aloud. "Let me think." She was strikingly unable to think or recognize the answer. She took out a multiplication chart in order to find out. For the first time she referred to the tutor with whom she had begun to work, implying she was nice, unlike me. According to Leah, her tutor had told her she should not work too hard, again in contrast to me. Leah's loyalty conflict reflected the old split between the good object/ bad object that originated in her early relationship with her mother and which had been repeated in the transference as her analysis got under way.

Leah omnipotently announced that she was going to cut back to three days a week. I pointed out that she treated me like a nothing by leaving me out of the decision making and that she was trying to turn her termination into a fight. Once this was interpreted, she did not need to act out by cutting back. She did, however, decide to stop coming altogether as of the last day of school and she stuck to this plan. With sadness, Leah told about the lonely times at school when she felt left out of things. I said it might be a relief, then, to stay home sick. She became truculent, but was thoughtful when I questioned whether this way of being "on the muscle" actually kept other children from wanting to play with her.

Leah began to think about how it was going to feel when she really did stop coming. She brought her disappointment that her analysis had not done more to change her parents' troubles or her own. Once she began to menstruate, Leah's material reflected a new step in consolidating and accepting her mental representation of her female body. She brought in a basket containing embroidery floss to make friendship bracelets. The careful way she put things in and took them out of this basket could be interpreted as a way to let us know she was wondering about the place inside of her that she could feel but not see. Claiming she was getting her third period, Leah complained of cramps, but was vague about this physical discomfort and could not localize it. She replicated an anatomical drawing from some of the materials she had about menstruation. Although it was accurate, it was obvious that it was still very hard for her to imagine the inside of her body. Leah was surprised when I said that menstrual bleeding comes from a different opening than bowel movement or urine. She did recognize that the pain was lower than her stomach. I asked her whether it was really pain, or whether it was a new, unfamiliar feeling she was having a hard time getting used to. She retreated at this point and said she only wanted to talk about it with her mother.

Leah returned to some math problems she had started earlier. I took this opportunity to interpret how her curiosity could become restricted. I connected her inability to think and know about or accurately feel sensations from her body with her inability to use her mind for learning. Referring to her sewing basket, which at other times had represented her inner genitals, I suggested that part of her does imagine an inside place where one day a baby will be able to grow. This pleased Leah—briefly. However, she began to pull the braid trim from the basket lid and wanted to cut it off. When I asked why she did not glue it, she insisted that it could not be fixed. I recalled her ideas that being a girl means she has had a part cut off and cannot be fixed. Leah retorted, "I'm not a girl, I'm a tomboy!" but grinned when I replied, "A tomboy with her period."

The next day Leah brought her basket again. She enjoyed the work and was patient and encouraging as she taught me how to braid the floss. She said she had formed a club with some girls to make bracelets at recess. Leah suggested I make one to remember her by. I asked if she worried that I would not remember her or that she would not be able to remember me and the work we had done. Leah thought back to some happy memories from our work. She did not have a pin, as she usually did, to hold some of the threads as she worked. When I offered to help, Leah indicated her wish to do it by herself. I asked if she also wanted to work on her troubles by herself now. "Yes, and with my parents." She noted we had only twelve more days as she hummed the Hallelujah Chorus. Her readiness to move ahead independently, using new relationships, was evident as she talked about her tutor and a young teacher she liked.

Leah's mother confirmed that Leah was using her tutor's help well and that she was showing a new interest in doing well in school. She had gotten an A on a project, but chided her mother for getting too involved. Leah asked her to let her work on a story independently so that, if she did well, she could feel she had earned it on her own. By this time her mother could not only honor this request, but also respected and enjoyed it. She agreed with Leah's assessment that family relationships were much improved.

The story Leah was working on was her own version of *The Little Mermaid*. The emphasis was on the mermaid's desire to get away from her father. Now Leah's focus had shifted to a developmentally appropriate push to distance herself from her oedipal objects and her analytic work. She worked on the story with unimpeded pleasure, alone in my presence, during her final hours. She was proud of the result, but clear that it was fantasy. Speaking of mermaids she said, "I know this can't really happen."

Leah was reading a book in school and wanted to tell me how it felt to come to the end. "It's like, when you're reading it, your whole body is filled with thoughts about it and then it's over and you feel, like, blank . . . like, hollow." I wondered with her whether these were the feelings she was having about finishing our work. She expressed the feeling she was leaving me with a cliff hanger. On her last day Leah asked, "How will we say goodbye? Do we just shake hands and say, 'You're nice'?"

When the time came, Leah extended her hand and said, "It was nice working with you." We shook on it.

SUMMARY

Leah's decision to terminate her analysis at the end of five years reflected the developmental pressures from within. Her difficulty with math was neither "cured" nor fully understood analytically, but she seemed able to use the tutorial help that was made available to her. This would not have been possible for her prior to her analytic work. Though she left a "cliff hanger," the criterion of restoring progressive development had been satisfied. Leah's analytic work demonstrated that an early disturbance in her relationship with her mother interfered with Leah achieving adequate drive fusion necessary for integration and the development of the synthetic function. This adversely affected her ability to integrate her harsh superego in early latency. It also resulted in an inadequate supply of neutralized energy at Leah's disposal to put in the service of learning (E. Furman, 1985, 1991).

In Leah's learning problem, this early ego disturbance became elaborated with ego restrictions, inhibitions, fantasies of being damaged, guilt, and an unconscious collusion with her mother to avoid knowledge of sexual secrets. There may have been some neuropsychological basis for her difficulty with quantitative and abstract reasoning, as suggested by the original IQ testing, which might be remediated educationally. Leah's work allows insight into the inner world of a child with a learning disorder and illustrates the complicated interplay of drives, object relations, conflict and endowment.

Chapter 4

Discussion of Leah's Analysis

It is not unusual for the analyst of a child with a neuropsycho-logically based learning disorder to become convinced of that diagnosis rather late in the analysis. This may be due to the analyst's propensity to emphasize psychogenic aspects of his or her patient's pathology. Or the psychologist who is called in to help evaluate the case may refrain from a definitive state-ment of neuropsychological contribution. The tests that are performed may be insufficient to make the diagnosis, or the tester may deemphasize strong preliminary evidence for a neu-ropsychological disorder and not engage in further testing. The analyst, relying on the psychologist's input, may be reluctant to go beyond the tester's conclusions as to whether a neuropsy-chological contribution is present. At times the analyst may also conclude that, on balance, the presence of neurotic inhibitions and conflicts may need to be treated before the patient can benefit from interventions aimed at a learning problem with a neuropsychological component.

Such was the case for Mrs. Barrett's patient, Leah, who was briefly tested three times during the course of her analysis, as part of the routine screening process offered in her school. There was compelling evidence that psychological and environ-mental factors played a palpable and complex role in Leah's psychopathology. In contrast, the neuropsychological contribu-tion was at first given little emphasis. The analyst who recom-mended evaluation for analysis did so because he believed Leah's "symptoms and the learning problems likely repre-sented internalized conflicts which were not amenable to

117

change through guidance alone.'' The test evaluations were circumscribed and did not diagnose specific areas of disability, although they were suggestive of this possibility.

Leah's history, and later her analytic material, provided evidence aplenty for a significant emotional contribution to her learning problems for which analysis was the optimal treatment. Leah could not establish an appropriate learning relationship with her teacher. Nor was her poor performance restricted to her schoolwork. Leah had trouble caring for herself. In general she was excessively dependent on her mother and lacked sufficient autonomy. For example, she could only intermittently tie her shoes and suffered from enuresis. Her mother's need to keep Leah extremely close to her early on, later understood in part as a result of her (i.e., mother's) having lost a previous child through an abortion, provided a basis for an intense preoedipal attachment. So too did the birth of Leah's brother when she was 15 months appear to interfere with the normal course of development of separation-individuation (Mahler, Pine, and Bergman, 1975).

Leah's mother's conflicts about separation were likely to have made it more difficult for her, and then for Leah, to become independent of each other. Not only was a rival brought into the family field, but Leah's mother was also overwhelmed by having to care for two small children. As Mrs. Barrett observed, Leah's mother ''yelled and hit Leah with increased frequency'' and ''her aggression interfered with her assuming the role of the educator of (Leah's) drives and promoter of ego mastery. She was unable to help Leah with her ambivalence toward her and her jealousy toward her little brother.'' Furthermore, she failed to apply appropriate toilet training techniques. Derivatives of conflicts over toileting continued to manifest themselves during the analysis. For example, during the second year of the treatment, Leah ''complained that her mother was nagging her about her homework.'' When Mrs. Barrett, drawing on previous work with Leah, suggested that Leah's ''old memories of fighting about the toilet seemed to get in her way as she tried to remember school things,'' Leah was suddenly able to recall a name she had previously forgotten.

The rapprochement subphase of separation-individuation, which lasts from approximately 15 to 24 months of age, was particularly important for Leah. Her brother was born when she was 15 months and her mother became even more distressed than before as she struggled with rearing her two children in the months that followed. In addition, the rapprochement subphase involves the child's alternately and repeatedly distancing himself from and then clinging to his mother; this must have been an especially threatening experience for Leah's mother.

The impact of disturbances at this age, which Mrs. Barrett wisely did not interpret to her patient, lest the analysis become too intellectualized, is often considerable. Conflicts between desires for close contact with mother and wishes for independence and autonomy, normal in the rapprochement period, may become accentuated when excessive stress occurs at that time. Leah's failure to achieve sufficient autonomy, necessary for learning and caring for herself, was due not merely to her mother's attributes, but also to the specific period in Leah's life during which these difficulties intensified. Eighteen months is also a period of heightened castration anxiety (Roiphe and Galenson, 1981) and awareness of injury to objects such as toys (Kagan, 1981), increased awareness of the self (Kagan, 1981), and the centrality of anal conflicts (Freud, 1905). Kagan (1981) also suggests that early signs of morality appear at this time. Leah's upset during this period of her life seems to have interfered with many of the developmental trends crucial for her learning.

Early in the analysis Mrs. Barrett became convinced that what appeared to be a defensive regression from oedipal conflicts was in fact "an overlay to an ego disturbance dating from the difficulty in her earlier relationship with her mother," a formulation with which we agree. Leah's early experiences with her mother resulted in an oedipal stage strongly influenced by preoedipal determinants and contributed to Leah's penchant for defensive regression. Leah's rage, for instance, occurred in an oedipal context, but also involved a pronounced regression which was at times so intense and untamed that it significantly interfered with her learning. Leah's impulsivity also posed a major interference to her learning.

Another contribution to Leah's learning problems was revealed as the analysis proceeded. Leah's aggressive tendencies came into conflict with her superego. In one session Leah said that she wanted revenge for a mean thing her brother Jacob had done. She then attacked Mrs. Barrett, hitting and biting her. Mrs. Barrett said that she "was sorry that her [Leah's] mean mouth feelings can take over like that, surprising her and then getting the mean mouth yelling at herself." Indeed the harshness of Leah's conscience became more evident as she accused herself of laziness and stupidity.

In our view these psychodynamic and genetic factors combined with solid evidence (in Leah's developmental, family, medical, and academic history, and in the abbreviated diagnostic evaluations and psychoanalytic process material) of neuropsychological contributions to Leah's learning problems. By history, she had respiratory distress at birth. In school (and sometimes in analytic hours) sequential problems in spelling and grasping concepts based on sequence, reversals in writing, and visual processing difficulties were sometimes observed. For example, from the earliest grades Leah could not consistently recognize numbers or letters or grasp prereading concepts. Test findings suggested problems with some aspects of fine motor coordination and revealed weaknesses in immediate memory for visual and auditory stimuli, as well as trouble with mastery of phonic associates and computational math facts.

As Mrs. Barrett noted, she felt reluctant to take an active stance toward Leah's learning and diagnostic evaluation during the course of the analysis; she believed that doing so could have been experienced by Leah as a repetition of mother's chronic intrusiveness into her functioning. In addition, although Mrs. Barrett suspected that neuropsychological factors contributed to Leah's learning problems, she did not seem to be fully convinced of this, even at the conclusion of her case report when she wrote, "There *may have been* some neuropsychological basis for her difficulty with quantitative and abstract reasoning . . . which might be remedied educationally" (emphasis added).

An optimal diagnostic evaluation probably would have permitted clarification of the existence and specific nature of the neuropsychological contribution, supporting the goals of the theoretical perspective Mrs. Barrett outlines in her opening statements. Her sensitive and insightful collaboration with Leah in analyzing the psychodynamic conflicts which compromised her learning—her grasp of the "relative contributions of psychopathology and neuropsychological dysfunction," their interrelationships, and Leah's fantasy elaboration of her learning difficulties—may only have been further enriched.

We will briefly discuss the diagnostic testing evaluations performed from this perspective. The first took place when Leah was a little over 6 years old and at the end of her kindergarten year. This (along with the second evaluation a year later) was part of the routine screening performed at Leah's school and was, therefore, quite limited. It consisted only of an IQ test and an achievement test examining reading, spelling, and math. The initial testing revealed that Leah's intelligence (as measured by the Stanford-Binet) was in the average range, and that "her vocabulary, comprehension of verbal material, and abstract visuospatial reasoning were considerably above expectations for a child her age." However, "oral arithmetic skills and immediate memory for both visual and auditory stimuli" were weak. Similarly, on achievement tests, Leah performed above grade level in general factual information, but below grade level in spelling, mathematics, and reading. These statements notwithstanding, the psychologist appeared to attribute Leah's marked unevenness to anxiety exclusively, perhaps weighing heavily her observation that Leah became upset and gave up when she did not know the right answer. A more comprehensive testing assessment of the reasons for this unevenness was not undertaken. However, Leah was referred for an evaluation for analysis, which was recommended at this time.

On the second set of tests one year later, when the routine screening was readministered because Leah repeated kindergarten, she "still manifested a weakness in immediate memory for visual and auditory stimuli" and her "percentile rankings on the achievement test . . . had fallen." Although the psychologist did not suggest a specific diagnosis, we believe that these evaluations done before the analysis began, and again after one year of treatment, provided strong evidence for a neuropsychological contribution to Leah's learning difficulties (as Mrs. Barrett suggests); more in-depth testing might have clarified matters further.

When Leah was 10 years old, she and her mother were apparently dissatisfied with Leah's academic progress. By then Leah's considerable analytic progress permitted her to be eager to do better in school. Indeed, she was relieved when her mother pressed the school for further testing. The results "confirmed that Leah needed tutoring in math." Mrs. Barrett elected not to receive a copy of the report on this evaluation since she felt that doing so would implicitly be experienced as an intrusion in an area in which Leah was experiencing an active struggle with her own conflicts. Thus we do not know the specific nature of Leah's difficulties with math. What we *do* know is that the tests at this time fortified Mrs. Barrett's previous suspicion that Leah's learning disability contained an important neuropsychologically based element which required more than just analytic intervention. In fact, Leah continued to require academic help after the analysis was terminated.

It was clear that Leah never lost sight of the centrality of her concerns about learning. Her stated motivation for beginning the analysis at the end of kindergarten was "to read"; later it was to do math. At one point in the analysis she reminded Mrs. Barrett of her "I-can't-read feelings." Leah complained that she could not read as some of her classmates could, and wanted to become more proficient. She found writing an effort, partly because she forgot the meanings of words and partly because she had difficulty with the sequence of letters; sometimes she even failed to place letters in the right order when she tried to copy a word. She also reversed individual numbers and letters, for instance "7" and "9" or "p" and "b."

In her case report Mrs. Barrett elegantly delineated the ways in which the sphere of learning became drawn into conflict. Leah unconsciously equated learning with knowing forbidden information, and with independent forays. Her mother misinterpreted Leah's attempts at independence as indications that her daughter no longer needed her, to which she responded by abandoning Leah. Mrs. Barrett also described particular psychodynamic meanings of the types of errors Leah made in her academic work. For example, she read "violence" for "violin," thus expressing warded-off aggressive impulses. Mrs. Barrett also interpreted the conflictual significance of Leah's difficulties in interpreting words, including her tendency to reversal of letters, numbers, and words, as a defense against envy.

In our view the neuropsychological contribution to Leah's learning disability facilitated her making such errors, which could then be analyzed from a psychodynamic perspective as well. In turn her inner conflicts potentiated her slips, malapropisms and other errors reflective of her neuropsychological weaknesses.

More broadly, we believe that the environmental sources of Leah's learning difficulties dovetailed with such neuropsychological determinants of her learning disability. Indeed it is likely that neuropsychological factors not only coexisted with, but in some instances also played a role in the course of, Leah's psychological development. For example, memory problems may have compromised Leah's ability to establish object constancy, and thus contributed to delays in separation-individuation. Furthermore, particular forms of expressing and defending against conflictual wishes (e.g., a proclivity for specific defenses) was potentiated by Leah's neuropsychological picture. Were Mrs. Barrett to have had the benefit of a detailed and comprehensive evaluation of the specific neuropsychologically based cognitive disabilities with which Leah was grappling, she may have been even better able to help Leah integrate these aspects of herself with the conflictual formulations.

We will proceed by sketching some of these possible interrelationships, particularly as they revealed themselves in the analytic process. We will include some of Mrs. Barrett's descriptions of her interventions, as well as several additional perspectives that have occurred to us in view of our conviction about the significance of neuropsychological contributions.

Leah employed a variety of defenses, some of which were facilitated by her neuropsychological vulnerabilities. As noted above, we believe that Leah's possible weaknesses in visual and auditory memory, along with other stresses at that time, would have contributed to difficulty in separating self and object representations, thus compromising separation-individuation (as discussed above). Such developmental experiences would increase her potential for reliance upon projection (attributing one's own characteristics to others) and identification (taking on the traits of others).

Denial was another defense that Leah used prominently. As we will suggest in discussing other cases as well, the neuropsychologically based difficulties with perception associated with some learning disabilities facilitate denial and (as Mrs. Barrett commented) interfere with "ego functions crucial to learning: perception, reality testing and curiosity." There were strong suggestions in Leah's case of problems in visual processing which would have combined with another factor, so astutely noted by Mrs. Barrett, to compromise her patient's learning: "Her identification with her mother's attitude that some things must not be known, such as pregnancy and abortion, had the effect of inhibiting Leah's approach to learning in general."

Some of the above-noted errors in reading and writing probably resulted from several neuropsychological sources (e.g., a failure to know phonic associates, weaknesses in visual discrimination, sequencing, graphomotor coordination, and/or immediate visual and auditory memory), in addition to the psychodynamic conflictual meanings Mrs. Barrett delineated. She found evidence that Leah harbored introjects who burst forth in the form of angry or sexual words. Frequently this took the form of salient wishes and concerns being expressed via errors in reading or language usage. To illustrate, when Leah told the story of *The Princess and the Pea,* in conjunction with drawing a picture of a girl on top of many mattresses, she reversed the letters "b" and "p" and called the story *The Princess and the Bean.* Mrs. Barrett suggested that it was hard for Leah "to know it was a story of a princess and a pea, rather than a bean, because of her own peeing in the bed problem." Soon thereafter when Leah reversed the number "9," she recognized that it looked like a "p" and then said she had wet her bed the night before. Discussing Leah's reversals, Mrs. Barrett noticed that Leah used this type of reversal as a defense. (This is contrasted with another use of the term *reversal*, in which Leah became the active attacker rather than the person attacked.) In a displaced version of this defense, if Leah thought something was pretty, she called it ugly. We believe that this type of defense was promoted by aspects of Leah's neuropsychological predisposition: her graphomotor dyscoordination and visual discrimination difficulties.

Mrs. Barrett also interpreted that Leah's inability to read the word *bad* when practicing for a play (Leah guessed that a passage involved the words *bite, mad,* or *sad* instead) signified that she tried to hide her hatred of her brother whose birth troubled her immensely. On another occasion Leah misread "violence" for "violin"; this could have reflected a failure to know phonic associates (e.g., the sound associated with "e" versus "i") which potentiated the expression of an aggressive wish. In a similar vein, when Mrs. Barrett asked Leah what she called her pacifier, Leah replied, "Some Fucker." This could also have found contribution from the sequencing problems (*some-fuck-er* rather than *th*umb-*s*ucker) suggested by testing, as well as by her teacher's observations (for example, that Leah had difficulty with sequential concepts such as "bigger-smaller," "more-fewer").

Leah's painful awareness of her learning deficiency accentuated her fantasies that she was castrated and her associated penis envy. She continued to feel terrible about her deficient reading and complained that she was "stupid, a zero, a girl." Over time she was greatly distressed to realize that her trouble with mathematics was even greater than her verbal disability. As Leah anticipated the onset of menstruation and then started to have periods, her emerging eagerness to be more mature came into conflict with her fears about bleeding which she experienced as evidence of damage, dirtiness, and inferiority. An easy displacement from concerns about her body to worries about her mind occurred as Leah attacked herself as a retard. Observations that she was not as adept academically as her schoolmates led her to conclude she was mentally deficient and must have facilitated this displacement.

As Leah approached puberty her struggles with oedipal wishes grew. She became anxious about her sexual urges, which made her feel "hot" and "sizzling" as she thought about boys and her father. Her guilt over these feelings surfaced as she became provocative, inviting punishment. She discussed her theory that masturbation caused her learning problems, and experienced her forthcoming period as a punishment. Leah retreated to homosexual feelings and wanted to end the analysis. Her initial retreat from the frightening aspects of her discoveries was followed by a serious determination to terminate, and an actual termination a year later.

At the same time, Leah's entry into menarche during the termination phase propelled her analysis. She took steps toward "accepting rather than denying her mental representation of her female body." This was seen in her reworking of the story of *The Little Mermaid,* which she had introduced earlier in the analysis. This tale expressed conflicts about sexuality with which Leah grappled. At first the outcome was sad. The mermaid, with whom Leah identified, lost the prince she loved to a real human princess. As the analysis progressed the mermaid represented the castrated girl, as well as a defense against being defective; she was the girl with a penis Leah wished to be. At the end of the treatment Leah worked on her own version of the story. She emphasized the mermaid's desire to get away from her father. As Mrs. Barrett states, "Leah had shifted to a developmentally appropriate push to distance herself from her oedipal objects and her analytic work." She also demonstrated a remarkable capacity to sublimate as she wrote a creative version of *The Little Mermaid.*

This coincided with Leah's development of an active stance toward learning. Once the unconscious fantasies had been analyzed, she could have a more reality-based recognition of her strengths and weaknesses. The analysis was essential to her ability to make use of the educational and tutorial interventions offered to her, just as the tutoring was essential to Leah's being able to master the academic material. It is unlikely that analysis alone, extraordinarily valuable as it was, would have been sufficient to treat the neuropsychologically based aspects of Leah's learning disability.

Some analysts feel concern that the presence of another treating professional who facilitates the patient's competence will contribute to a split transference. Indeed there is evidence that this occurred to some degree in Leah's case. However, the coexistence of the tutor and analyst did not seem to pose a major problem. Leah brought her schoolwork into the analysis, just as she engaged in similar work with her tutor. It seems likely that Leah used her tutor as a substitute for the analyst she was losing during the termination period. In our opinion, Leah's achievement outweighed any possible analytic loss. Leah was becoming an independent person. Her constructive discussions of her difficulties with math, both in the analysis and with her tutor, demonstrated that at the end of the analysis she could develop a fruitful academic working alliance with an adult. This constituted quite a remarkable progressive departure from her earlier failure to establish an appropriate learning relationship with her teacher prior to her analysis.

Chapter 5

Julia's Analysis

Jill M. Miller, Ph.D.

INTRODUCTION

This chapter describes the courageous journey of a young girl through three-and-a-half years of her analysis. When she began at $5^1/2$ years of age Julia had already been subjected to multiple surgeries as a result of a stroke and shunt implant in the first months of her life. During the first year of the analysis she developed epilepsy. The focus will be on Julia's mind and the way it worked which was dependent on the intertwining of neurological and psychological factors. My technical approach, as well as the overarching themes of defense management, conflicts over aggression, and the nature of Julia's changing internal representations of self and objects will be detailed.

Whilst analysis was the intervention which served to organize Julia's experiences, both past and ongoing, and to help her structure and make sense of her world, it was not the only intervention. The contribution of medical professionals, EEG neurofeedback, special education, optometric vision therapy,

Acknowledgments. The author is indebted to Dr. Carla Elliott-Neely for her many helpful discussions and to Dr. Ted Gaensbauer for his comments on an earlier version of this paper.

and occupational therapy also played a significant role. In addition, the family's (especially her mother's) work with Julia and with me were vital to the positive outcome.

Julie was a little girl who felt lost. She struggled to find ways to master her internal world, her brain, and the world around her in order to find her place in it and to grow up. This is her story.

CONSULTATION

Presenting Problems

Julia's parents first consulted me three days after her most recent surgery. They described how their 5½-year-old daughter was in a state of panic, at times hysterical and inconsolable. She could not be left alone and was having nightmares.

Developmental and Medical History

Painfully, Julia's parents described her long history of medical complications. Julia, the family's second child, was born after a full-term pregnancy. Labor and delivery were uncomplicated. Julia had a birth weight of 6 pounds, 3 ounces and her Apgar scores were within the normal range. She was born a healthy baby and her parents were delighted. Initially, she did well.

Twenty days after her birth, Julia developed greenish watery diarrhea, had projectile vomiting twice, and a urinary tract infection. When she awoke one morning irritable with decreased appetite, increased fever, and generalized stiffness in her extremities and neck, she was hospitalized. Doctors suspected spinal meningitis. Once admitted, she was found to be alert and attentive, with normal leg and arm movements. An ultrasound study indicated blood in the ventricles, and a CAT scan demonstrated a bilateral intraventricular hemorrhage. Julia remained in the hospital for eight days, her mother staying

with her most of the time. Whilst the cause of Julia's hemorrhage was not ascertained with certainty, according to her medical records she probably had a choroid plexus hemorrhage or
possibly bleeding from a venous angioma.

Julia was released and seemed to do well. At 12 weeks, due
to the development of hydrocephalus, a ventriculoperitoneal
shunt was implanted.[1] This surgical procedure was performed
under general inhalation anesthesia and involved injections
(i.e., intravenous). Julia's parents were told that cerebral palsy
and retardation were strong possibilities, and that Julia might
never walk. However, the predictions of medical professionals
did not deter these grief-stricken parents. They talked to other
professionals, researched the field, and took Julia to a speciality
clinic for brain injured children to teach her to crawl. To everyone's surprise, she made remarkable progress, with the help of
her mother and physical therapy from 16 weeks to 21 months
of age. At 18 months Julia began to walk, and her once limp
body aligned itself. By 2 years of age she was thought to have
completely recovered.

Julia grew into a happy and bubbly toddler. She displayed
no noticeable difficulties, was developmentally on target, and
began preschool at 2 years. At 2 years, 9 months she required
her first shunt revision, but continued to do well. Albeit jealous,
she was also pleased when her brother was born when she was
3 years, 10 months.

Six months later Julia (4 years, 4 months) had her second
shunt failure, the first in a series of five in fourteen months.
Because the induction room at the hospital was not available,
Julia was taken from her parents before she was anesthetized.
It was then that she first became anxious, having sleep and
separation difficulties. These responses subsided, but did not
disappear.

The first indication that Julia's shunt was failing was a
headache which eventually brought her to tears. She required
immediate surgery. Except for once, Julia was anesthetized in

---

[1]This is a shunt which drained fluid from the ventricles to the peritoneum. Its purpose
was to repair the disruption of the free flow of cerebral spinal fluid, which was producing hydrocephalus and an increase in cerebral spinal fluid pressure.

her mother's arms, and she always woke up there. Admissions were short (two days) and her parents stayed with her. The surgeries and hospitalizations went smoothly, void of complications. Once home, Julia could be more aggressive and tearful, responses with which her parents appropriately and patiently helped her.

Julia's developmental progress remained within normal bounds. She did well in preschool, and there were no noticeable signs of cognitive changes or impairments. At 4 years, 8 months she obtained a General Cognitive Index on the McCarthy Scales of Children's Abilities of 113, in the Bright Normal range (her subscale scores were: verbal 60, perceptual performance 46, quantitative 70, memory 59).

Julia's third shunt failure occurred at 4 years, 9 months, followed by a fourth failure two months later. She began to exhibit difficulty finding her way around and locating things when, at 5 years, 3 months, the family moved to a new house. The next month her shunt failed for the fifth time. When, a month later, she started kindergarten, Julia was quickly overwhelmed. She got lost going from room to room at school, was easily confused about where things were, and had trouble remembering. At the same time, she could do puzzles, knew her letters, and had an uncanny ability to recall in detail stories which were read to her. The following month (5 years, 6 months) her shunt failed again. It was then that her parents contacted me knowing she needed help.

Evaluation

I saw Julia in three evaluation sessions. As I walked into my waiting room that first day I found a tiny little girl, with frail features, dark hair, and dark, frightened eyes, who looked far younger than her chronological years. She huddled against her father, holding his hand tightly. As he introduced us, Julia smiled and nodded, drawing closer to him.

We sat at the table in my playroom, Julia on her father's lap, hiding in his coat and chewing on its strings, or sucking on his fingers. At times she tried to unbutton her father's shirt, as if getting closer to his skin would make her safer. With reassurances about not being the kind of doctor she was used to, and addressing her anxieties about meeting a stranger, Julia slowly began to talk. Anxiously and bitterly she complained about her 7-year-old sister hitting her, calling her crazy, and hating her. I said I could see how much she disliked her sister for these things. Julia nodded, and her rebukes continued. When I commented that maybe she was a bit worried that she was, indeed, crazy, Julia gave a quick affirmation of "uh huh," and began to draw, slowly moving off her father's lap.

Her drawings were like those of a younger child. Legs were directly attached to heads with eyes, a nose, and smiling mouth; bodies, arms, and hands were conspicuously missing until one figure was made into a mother, arms added to hold the baby. Julia accompanied her drawing with constant, anxious chatter.

It became clear Julia was a girl with a great deal on her mind. There was more about her sister hating her, admonishments which were equaled by retorts of her 20-month-old brother. Julia's anger at her siblings extended to her mother. She didn't want to leave kindergarten, which was being considered, adding crossly, "My mother made me!" Her sense of unfairness and feeling rejected further extended to the world at large, as she talked about friends. A girl who had been her best friend didn't want to be anymore, so now she had no friends. "I'm my own friend now," was Julia's sad solution. As the childish figures in her drawings became more like scribbles, anxious words like "pea brain," "upside down," and "backwards" were uttered. I verbalized her feeling that she was upside down and that her brain was on backwards. Nodding, Julia told me a confused story of how she had been very sick as a baby, but now was better; she repeatedly added, "I didn't know where I was." She gave a wide-eyed nod to my comment that maybe she felt that way now, and we could talk about how confused and mixed up she got, often forgetting things.

This was my first contact with this young girl whom I came to respect for her fortitude, perseverance, and determination, characteristics also found in her caring and psychologically minded parents. Over the next two sessions Julia proceeded to let me into her inner world.

Julia's concern that she couldn't remember things was quickly evident in the second session. However, when she talked about a finger puppet she had like mine, she described it in detail. She wanted me to understand that she could re- member what it looked like, she just didn't know what to call it. Slowly Julia moved from her mother to the floor with me, in closer and closer proximity, as she relaxed and became more animated, eventually allowing her mother to leave. Julia intro- duced a game of "let's pretend," repeating this reminder so as to keep her feet firmly planted in what was real and what wasn't. This helped her contain her anxiety to a degree. A girl went to the zoo to pick out an animal. All the animals craved to be the chosen one, crying "Pick me! Pick me!" In the end the girl picked them all so as not to hurt anyone's feelings. Julia's fears of attacking and being attacked soon followed, as the girl maliciously teased the animals, saying she would never come back again. The animals who bit the girl were sent back to the zoo. The story ended tragically as the girl was eaten.

In our third session Julia began to approach the traumas she had experienced, as she attempted to put order to her chaos and help me understand. The baby doll fell out of bed, then crawled out of the house into traffic. The mother repeat- edly rescued her from this dangerous situation, but in the end was unable to, and the baby was run over by a car. As the baby was rushed to the hospital, Julia reminded us we were pretending. The baby overheard the doctors say she would have to have an operation. Then she was snatched from her mother's arms and taken away. Quickly Julia had the family at home all secure, and changed the play. Again the girl was at the zoo to pick an animal, sending the ones back who bit, but this time she remained safe as Julia sat close to me touching my fingers. She complained that her thumbs itched, then her back, scratching and lifting her dress to reveal her stomach. "I have something to show you that you have never seen before," she told me, pointing to her scar. When I asked she explained that this was from an operation a long time ago. She continued by noting with pleasure that they didn't have to operate on her

last time. I said that she was a girl who had had lots of operations. "No!" she said, quickly followed by yes and complaints
of a rash. She agreed when I verbalized that she had many
concerns about her body that she wanted to talk about, and
many mixed up feelings she wanted to sort out.

Recommendation for Analysis

The assessment revealed how confused and disoriented Julia
was internally. She felt lost, couldn't make sense of things, was
frightened she was crazy and damaged, as well as being terrified
of abandonment. Like a deer frozen in the headlights of an
oncoming car, she had called a halt to thinking and feeling,
and tried to remove herself mentally. She felt at the mercy of
her own aggressive impulses which found expression in her
fears of attacking and being attacked. At the same time, Julia
exhibited enormous strengths. Despite the early traumata of
her surgeries, her development had proceeded relatively
smoothly from 18 months to 4 years due to the good parenting
she had received. Julia's attachments were strong and secure,
seen in her ability to trust me and her wish for my help.

With the necessity of five emergency surgeries in 14
months her parents, who had provided her with a secure holding environment, were no longer able to protect her and keep
her safe. In addition, they too were anxious as Julia's future
was uncertain. Julia's adaptation of making the best out of
things was now failing her and had a brittle and false quality
used to mask her affect; it could no longer be used in the
service of mastery. Furthermore, Julia's more recent traumas
recapitulated the early ones which had previously been mastered, causing them to become an issue retrospectively. Her
development, which was now lagging, was in jeopardy.

One issue to consider was what impact Julia's original hemorrhage, hydrocephalus, and shunt failures had on her brain.
How much of her getting lost and forgetting was due to her
massive internal psychological disorganization, or to what
might be the result of neurological damage with subsequent

learning disabilities? This was an open question. Thus, neuro-psychological testing was indicated. Educationally this was not immediately necessary since it was decided that Julia would be placed back in preschool. Kindergarten had become too much for her to handle. Other children were beginning to make fun of Julia and to victimize her. The return to preschool also gave us time to help Julia settle within herself, to see how much integration would occur, and to evaluate further. If neurologi-cal damage was evident, this would not only add complications and considerations as to the way in which the work was ap-proached. It could also be used by Julia in the construction of fantasies and internal representations, and influence her developmental progression.

My initial aim was to contain Julia's anxiety and affects, thus relieving some of the strain she and her family were under. I was aware that multiple evaluations and testing by medical professionals would be required in the near future. These could retraumatize Julia and serve as organizers for pathological solu-tions. Additional aims were also clear. One was to disinhibit Julia's thinking and emotional life, thus helping her give up her frozen position and utilize her mind and feelings in the service of her development and mastery. Other aims were to assess and address the impact of Julia's illness on her develop-mental progression, representational world, and ego develop-ment. Furthermore, we had to ascertain what Julia's unconscious fantasies were about her illness in order to allevi-ate any distortions they were causing.

In order to meet the initial and subsequent aims, I believed that analysis, which deals with all areas of the personality (A. Freud, 1965; Sandler, Kennedy, and Tyson, 1980; Moran, 1984) was the treatment of choice. In this model the technical ap-proach focuses both on interpretation and work in the transfer-ence, and the correction of developmental imbalances which, for Julia, were induced by neurological assaults on her brain (A. Freud, 1974; Edgcumbe, 1993; Fonagy, Moran, Edgcumbe, Kennedy, and Target, 1993; J. Miller, 1996). It was my assess-ment that Julia could understand and make use of these types of interventions. Julia's parents concurred and she began seeing me four times a week. In addition, I had frequent sessions with one or both of Julia's parents. Initially I met with her mother weekly, eventually reducing these parent meetings to an as-needed basis.

COURSE OF THE ANALYSIS

It is difficult to convey what it was like to enter the mind of this young child and to be in it with her. Putting sessions to paper orders the material in a way which does not capture the experience we both had. Sequential themes through a series of sessions were eventually evident, but within any one session she would flip from one thing to another, all of which seemed unconnected. I was able to follow her lead, when suddenly I felt as lost and confused as she did. I fought to stay with her, reengaging my mind to pull out of the chaos and confusion. I redirected my thoughts to try and catch up, and if possible, to sort out what had prompted the switch, confusion, or lost feeling.

I attempted to offer Julia my mind and to do the thinking for both of us as we worked to disinhibit this crucial mental process in a way which felt safe to her. In parallel, we identified what scared her so. Slowly and cautiously she took what I offered, as she began to wonder, to ask questions of herself and me, and to have ideas. She was eager for my help and had not yet lost hope, which proved to be one of her greatest strengths. She wanted me to understand, to make sense of her inner world and what had happened to her, and she exhibited a strong push toward mastery.

With an excited nervous quality, Julia came into her sessions on her own. Whilst she felt safe enough with me, leaving her mother made her anxious; she reassured herself about where her mother would be. Julia denied she had any feelings whatsoever, and diverted to lovely games. Any anxiety provoking material resulted in difficulties in her getting words out and remembering what she was doing. My interventions focused on the identification of her constant anxiety, her fear of talking or thinking about anything in case doing so might make it worse. I also described the way in which she forgot when she felt so nervous and scared.

As the treatment alliance strengthened, Julia began to allow herself to feel and to think. "I have five feelings to tell you. Remember the day I had none?" she announced. Cautiously she allowed some awareness of the meaning she had given to her experiences, both past and ongoing, to enter her conscious mind. This served to move the analysis forward, and also prevented retraumatization as a result of the multiple evaluations and tests she was undergoing.[2]

Julia brought me a picture of a boat looking distinctly like a person in a box. When I interpreted the defensive nature of her nice play, she said, "I have two feelings to tell you. When I have an operation and they call my name I get scared. I hope I never have to have another operation again. When they put me to sleep . . . ," but she could not go on. "I can't get my words out right." I suggested we draw as a way to help her. She drew herself in a hospital bed and asked me to write the words, "Doctors, will you promise not to do it to me again? Sometimes I'm afraid I'm going to die." We could then identify how afraid she was to go to sleep for fear she would not wake up again. She talked further about her operations, the smells of the room, and going to sleep in her mother's arms. She added, "Once when I was a baby the doctor snatched me away from mommy, mommy told me so," revealing her terror of a repetition. She stacked blocks, seeing how many she could carry, but they all fell. Then she asked if I could hold them all. When I verbalized her wish to know if I could hold all of her scary feelings, she said, "Oh, oh! Something is going to come out of my mouth. I get scared they'll operate and not even tell me." We identified her desire to know what was going on, and have no surprises, and her fear of an MRI was not what mommy said, but instead an operation.

The process of identifying and containing her affects, and

---

[2]In the first year of her analysis Julia had two consultations in other states, an MRI, two CAT scans, two EEGs, neuropsychological and occupational therapy evaluations, a number of blood tests, and neurological examinations.

offering her my mind within a safe and consistent environment, helped Julia feel more secure. As I linked her anxiety to her forgetting and feeling lost, it was possible to interpret the ways in which her defenses against thoughts and affects were not working. The alternative of thinking, feeling, and talking, Julia found, led to understanding and a decrease in anxiety.

Julia's conflict over knowing and not knowing then surfaced. Following a consultation, I interpreted how part of her wanted to hear and understand what was said to her, but part of her did not because it made her scared. Julia admitted she ran away when her mother talked to her, and I clarified that she ran away in her mind. Slowly and cautiously Julia opened the door to the experience of thoughts and feelings, and to self observation. Now she wanted to come out of hiding, as her wish to know strengthened.

Fears of object loss were pronounced, an anxiety which was multidetermined. Julia had ample evidence that when her objects disappeared, frightening medical interventions occurred which dictated an experience of danger in the absence of her objects. The fact that she could get lost in her physical surroundings, and feel lost internally, compounded her anxiety and fears of losing her objects. In addition, Julia's best efforts to cope with her overwhelming anxiety further exacerbated her fears of losing those she most needed. As her primary defensive maneuvers were reversals, wishes to attack or separate from the object were quickly followed by fears of being attacked or abandoned. Furthermore, by removing herself mentally she could avoid both thinking and feelings, which provided some sense of safety; however, this also resulted in the loss of her internal object representations.

By the third week of analysis the primary theme in Julia's play was of parents who were lost, leaving baby all alone. Transitions were the hardest. Julia would sit down defiantly, refusing to move, complaining that her mother was crazy. Her anxiety soared toward the end of her sessions. "This is hard," she would say. "You tell me when time is up and I'll run and jump in mommy's lap," as she tried to physically retain her objects. With interpretations of her feeling that I was sending her away and didn't want to be with her anymore, like the animals who were sent back to the zoo, endings became easier. Interpretations of her fears of where she would be taken helped with transitions.

As Julia began to relinquish her frozen position and disinhibit her mind, her anger with her mother surfaced in the material. I interpreted her fear that, because she wanted to get rid of her mother at times, she would indeed feel she lost her. We could examine in a clearer way how Julia ran away in her mind, using her metaphor: the baby who ran away to the mountains. Now firmly engaged in the analytic process, Julia also often played the perplexed mother who tried to gently talk to baby and to help baby talk, and was left wondering what was wrong with her child who kept running away to the mountains.

Our first extended break four months into the analysis brought Julia's fears of object loss to the forefront. "This is the saddest day of my life," she said, expressing her longing and fear I would not return. When I did, Julia was pleased to see me and complained of "owies" (physical injuries) and falling down. In her play baby asked me to take her to the mountains. Julia, also the mother, told me to watch baby carefully so she did not fall. When, following her directions, I did not pay attention and baby fell (luckily into her mother's arms), I interpreted how it felt as if I had dropped her and did not protect her. "That's why baby goes to the mountains by herself," was Julia's response, explaining how going away in her mind felt safer than the reality of her life. Over the next few days Julia also demonstrated how baby ran away out of anger, leaving me as I had left her.

Julia's reaction to my being away demonstrated a shift. Not only were her affects felt and experienced, but she was able to identify them. She had not lost me in her mind, but rather had missed me and felt I had not protected her. She let me know how angry she was. Whereas previously Julia played games where the mother was lost forever, leaving the baby all alone, now there was a change. It was not that the mother was lost, it was that we were not looking in the right place. Search and search we did; mother was in the one place we forgot to look.

More secure in her ability to retain her internal object representations, Julia brought her fear she had lost herself, given all that had happened to her. This fear was first represented in a worry that she had lost her brain, which was why she could not use it. To Julia, forgetting came to mean that her brain fell out and she lost it. Julia had a number of theories about what caused her brain to get lost. One was that when the doctors operated, her brain fell out. When she would forget what we were doing, she would say, "Oops, my brain fell out"; then she picked it up and stitched it back in. Another theory was that it was too scary and painful to feel and to think. When we talked about her difficulties sleeping, Julia said her brain fell out; then she lost track of what we were talking about, and tried to go on to something else. When I verbalized how nervous she had gotten talking about sleeping, she spoke of bad dreams where spiders and lizards were in her bed trying to get her. An additional, but related, theory was that her angry feelings were the cause. When Julia talked about "stinky doctors" whom she wanted to kill, she lost her brain. In all of this we could discuss how it was not her brain that was missing or broken, but all of her feelings and worries that made her forget and run to the mountains for safety.

Julia's mind was now engaged in the process. We had analyzed her defenses and the consequences of this management enough to help her move forward. She could retain her internal object representations and was no longer as lost in the external world. She had faced the first level of her fear that she had lost herself. This was concretely expressed in the form of losing her brain, the part of her body which had been assaulted by hemorrhages, shunt failures, and medical interventions, and represented the mind she felt she no longer had. Whilst still prone to inhibiting her thinking and feelings, thus losing her representations of self and others when anxiety or intense affects were experienced, Julia had gained some control over her internal and external worlds. She could now allow herself to utter the previously unthinkable question, what is wrong with me?

In response to beginning to express this question, Julia's aggression and ambivalence entered the transference. She had the baby taunt me, singing, "Na, na, na, na, na, put your head in dodo." She then defended against these aggressive attacks both by regression and progression. The baby became a new-born and Julia was her loving mother. The beaver bit me and kissed me simultaneously, and then was blown away by a wild wind, unable to get home. Julia quietly confirmed my interpretation of beaver's fears of what he would do to me, and of what I would do to him in return. She initiated games of catch, wildly throwing the ball at me whilst making fun of me and then giving me a big hug. Julia also played games of my pursuing her as she tried to keep her angry feelings in hiding. As Sissy she looked very upset and sad, leaving baby and me to go to her room. Playing both the pursuer and the pursued, baby ran after Sissy asking, "Okay, what's wrong? You're not going to run from your old pal are you?" But Sissy did, locking us out.

To tolerate her aggression and to allow herself to express it, underpinned as it was by terror, Julia overwhelmed this affective state with excitement. Now baby no longer ran away to the mountains. Instead, she defiantly jumped into a swimming pool with gales of excited laughter.

Five months into the analysis Julia's parents and I decided the time was right to pursue a neuropsychological evaluation. Although precarious at times, Julia was more settled within herself. She had made numerous gains, but the question of neurological damage remained, and plans for the coming school year needed to be made. Unlike previous evaluations and tests Julia had undergone, this time she was able to retain her mother's explanation and relate it to me. At the same time, her underlying fears and traumas were revived in full force. Once again her play involved sick newborn babies who were rushed to the hospital, ran away, and jumped into their mothers' arms because they were so scared. Julia admitted that whenever she got into the car to go to a doctor she was afraid they would operate. We differentiated surgery from the evaluation, and talked about its purpose.

Julia completely fell apart at home during the three-week period that it took to complete the evaluation. She could no longer sleep, collapsing at night in tears, and needing reassurance that her mother would be there when she woke up. At school she was lost and disoriented. With me Julia's fears of loss and damage, that her brain was broken, and that she was an incapable girl were once gain dominant themes. We talked about these to some extent, but in order to manage her overwhelming anxiety Julia was primarily absorbed in wish-fulfillment games. Occasionally she could talk about the testing. She explained that when the evaluator asked her to do something and she did not hear, she told the lady she did not know how to do it. We concluded this meant she was too afraid to take in the information.

The results of Julia's neuropsychological evaluation were not optimistic.[3] On the WPPSI-R Julia attained a Verbal IQ of 87 (in the Low Average range) and a Performance IQ of 78 (in the Borderline range), giving her a Full Scale IQ of 81 (in the Low Average range). Whilst many of her verbal subtests were performed at a level average for her age, she demonstrated weakness on tests requiring spatial reasoning ability. As Julia was still in preschool, and thus her academic skills could only be measured in a rudimentary way, test scores were in the average range for preacademic skills. Nevertheless, it was predicted she would have difficulty both acquiring reading skills (as she was unable to do tests of phoneme awareness) and with math (because of her spatial reasoning difficulties). Julia's strongest performance was on tests of receptive language. She also did quite well on several tests of short-term verbal memory. Most concerning was the evaluator's conclusion that Julia demonstrated significant impairment on tests of both long-term verbal and nonverbal memory.

Based on my clinical observations, I had a number of questions about these test results. First of all, from the way Julia worked within the analysis I felt her IQ scores underestimated her intellect. Second, I was confused about how one could be so certain at this time about Julia's memory functioning. It was clear that trauma was, in part, responsible for knocking out some of her memory, and that her thinking was being compromised internally. In the analysis her recall and thinking abilities seemed to come and go dependent on her internal state. In

---

[3]The test battery included: selected tests of the Expanded Halstead Reitan Neuropsychological Battery for Young Children, the Wechsler Preschool and Primary Scale of Intelligence-Revised and selected portions (cognitive and academic subtests) of the Kaufman Assessment Battery for Children.

addition, observations of her functioning at home were also suggestive of fluctuations in her memory. Because Julia's behavior at home had been so difficult, her mother and I had worked on ways to handle this, such as engaging Julia's verbal capacities. When Julia could describe in words what she had done, she was less prone to bypass her thinking and to forget, and thus better able to own her actions. This approach of expecting her to think and to remember was working, and Julia's behavior had settled considerably. Furthermore, Julia's ability to recall in detail stories which had been read to her and movies she had seen was excellent. Julia also seemed to be aware that her verbal capacities were her strength. She commented, "I'll tell you the whole story (of what happened to me), and then I will remember." Third, during the three weeks of the neuropsychological testing Julia was in a pronounced state of internal chaos, disorientation, and terror, since the evaluation retraumatized her.

It was my view that the tester had exaggerated Julia's verbal memory difficulties.[4] A further complicating feature was the fact that two months following this evaluation Julia had a grand mal seizure and epilepsy was diagnosed. It is possible that prior to this diagnosis, she was experiencing absente seizures which went undetected. If so, this would have influenced the test results.

Even though I carefully prepared the parents for what they would hear at the interpretative interview, and gave them my thoughts on the matter, they were devastated. Julia's mother, herself retraumatized, felt it was like hearing that Julia might never walk, and that her future prospects in terms of learning and career were extremely poor. As we sorted through their and Julia's reaction to the experience of the evaluation, her parents implemented the recommendations they could. Julia was enrolled in a special school for children with learning disabilities to begin in the autumn, and intensive help from an occupational therapist was arranged for the summer. Once the

---

[4]Arden Rothstein's review of the data detailed in the test reports also suggested this conclusion. In a letter to me, she stated, "The data suggested that Julia did have significant problems in memory for visual (and especially visuospatial) stimuli, but that her auditory memory was intact and even an area of strength."

evaluation was completed, Julia calmed down considerably and quickly returned to the level of functioning she had previously attained.

Almost six years to the day of her first hospitalization, Julia was subjected to yet further trauma. She had a grand mal seizure. An EEG confirmed the presence of epilepsy, and Depakote, an antiseizure medication, was prescribed. Whilst Julia did not have another grand mal seizure, she did suffer from frequent absente seizures. When I first saw Julia following this seizure she was overwhelmed and withdrawn. Her fear of dying was reactivated, but now it clearly incorporated her conflicts over aggression.

Julia and I worked to get herself in order, to calm down. She counted dominoes and built structures, demonstrating a number of activities which looked distinctly like tasks from the neuropsychological evaluation two months earlier. I told her I knew how frightened she was, so much so she could hardly talk, sleep, or think, and that I knew what she was frightened of. "Operations?" she asked. Yes, I continued, but even more than that you are afraid of dying. Julia looked at me for the first time and said, "I tell mommy that all the time and she says I won't and to get that idea right out of my head." I agreed with her mother, that she wouldn't die, but, I continued, "You are still scared of dying because sometimes you wish others would be dead. Then you are afraid it will all come back at you." Julia's relief was enormous. She took out the baby and played eating meals, bedtime, and being together.

Julia continued to try and approach her rage. In her play, baby wanted to run away to the mountains, but now I was to hold onto her tightly so she couldn't. The alternative was the swimming pool, called "diving heaven." Julia also desperately tried to rid herself of these feelings as baby was locked in the cupboard, thrown across the room, or abandoned in the pool to drown as I rushed to rescue her. It was tough going; much of Julia's material was scattered, her memory was not functioning as well as it had been, and she was lost at times.

Julia's parents consulted a specialty clinic for epilepsy and were told that Julia was having absente seizures every three to five minutes. These doctors concluded that the seizures could be controlled with medication until Julia outgrew them. They thought her spaciness was due to stress and emotional difficulties. Her parents were relieved and optimistic. Two months later Julia's mother and I again discussed her state. Whilst it was clear that intense affect disorganized her, we wondered how controlled Julia's seizures actually were.

I supported her parents' arranging for a consultation with another neurologist. He concluded that Julia was having hundreds of absente seizures a day, each lasting a split second and manifested by a sudden and brief glassy-eyed stare. He increased her Depakote. A year after the diagnosis of epilepsy Julia's absente seizures were still evident. As her Depakote was further increased, her seizures were initially controlled, but they eventually broke through again. There had been no evidence of seizures for several weeks, until the following session. It was then possible to observe what seemed like an interrelationship of the affective state of anger and seizure activity.

Julia's mother and I talked in the waiting room after a session; this was an occasional occurrence. Julia waited for a while, then took off down the hall. When we heard the muffled cries of a child, her mother raced off to find her.

The next day, to my surprise, Julia retained the experience, and could tell me what had happened. She was going to the car because "you and mommy were talking forever." She agreed she did not like this one bit. Then she described how she got into the elevator, pounded on the door to get out, sat down, and almost cried, revealing her fear of being trapped. "I yelled for mommy and then she came, but she was mad at me." As we explored this, Julia agreed that she was the one who was angry. Every time we approached her rage, Julia attempted to divert to something else more pleasurable. Each time I brought her back. In this context, her absente seizures began, becoming frequent and rapid. She would either stop for a minute, interrupted by a seizure, and then go on or, at other times, would lose what we were talking about and we would have to begin again. Julia was in constant motion and had trouble speaking. She agreed with a wide-eyed panic that talking about the angry part was the hardest of all.

I took her hands and held them, stressing how very important this all was. I talked about how she became very mad, then scared by her feelings; then she couldn't think, and was afraid to be away from mommy. This, I added, was what we had to work on. She took out the farm animals and played in a disjointed way, with frequent seizures. The babies could not find their mother. She was in the thicket dying. The story changed as the babies, who were lost, called for mommy. With urgency, Julia tried to draw a picture for her mother, but returned to the animals. I said the babies were very mad at mommy. Then they worried that something awful would happen to her because of how they felt. When I told Julia our time was almost up for that day, she quickly finished her picture and said that mommy had gone away on a trip. She recalled, when I reminded her, that mommy was at home. I interpreted that when she was not with mommy, especially when she was so angry with her, she lost mommy in her mind and felt she was gone. "Yes," said Julia, "gone forever."

Julia slowly tried to understand her feelings of aggression and torture. Now, not only doctors, medical interventions, and seizures motivated these affects. She experienced them any time she had hurt or angry feelings, or thought others were being mean to her. A sadomasochistic organization surfaced as she yelled at me, "Just do it, do the operation," lifting up her shirt; she laid across my lap excitedly, wanting me to spank her.

We now faced an unavoidable interruption. As Julia's seizures were still not controlled consistently with medication, her parents opted to try a somewhat unconventional approach: EEG neurofeedback (neurotherapy). This treatment method is based on the concept of normalizing an EEG by either enhancing certain brain waves or inhibiting others. The theory is that certain types of abnormal brain functioning can be corrected by learning to condition the brain's electrical activity. This is accomplished through visual or auditory feedback received from a computerized EEG machine which shows electrical activity as it occurs (for more detailed information see Lubar and Shouse, 1976; Sterman and Macdonald, 1978; Hoffman, Stockdale, Hicks, and Schwaninger, 1995). For Julia this meant wires being connected from her head to a computer where she could observe her brain's electrical activity. She was told to concentrate on keeping a light on or to play a computer game. Completing the task meant she was inhibiting theta, which was the aim. She was then rewarded with a prize.

Over the summer Julia, now 7 years old, went to another state every other week for treatments. My aim was to try and help her contain her rage enough so she could participate, which she wanted to do, feeling the treatment could help her. At the same time, enactments of unconscious fantasies emerged at home. She cut her hair with garden shears. Having found her father's razor, she thought she would shave but her mother caught her just in time. With both new rules at home about playing with sharp objects (which were placed out of her reach), and my interpretations that Julia was trying to cut herself as others had done to her, these fantasies and actions went underground. Julia cooperated with the neurotherapy which proved to be quite successful.

The weeks I did see Julia we talked about the process of the neurotherapy and she told me about the fun things she also did. Clearly exhausted, analysis provided a holding and secure environment where she relaxed and we played games of caring for baby. She had frequent seizures.

It is difficult to describe what it was like for Julia when she had a seizure, or my experience of being with her. Her eyes glassed over, occasionally her eyelids fluttered, and she was blank for a second or two. When there was a succession of seizures, Julia was rapidly in and out of awareness, which she struggled to regain. At times she felt able to hold onto her thoughts, but at others she was lost and asked me to remind her of what we were doing. Seizures left her with holes in her experience so that she missed out, could not sequence, and was profoundly lost.

Beginning with the first time I observed a seizure, I tried to talk to Julia about what was happening to her. In response, she ignored me and my words, continuing with what we were doing as if nothing had happened. Now it had become possible to talk about seizures, a process aided by the neurotherapy. By watching a computerized EEG Julia established both a visual representation of her brain and the idea that she could control it. Feeling not so helpless, and therefore somewhat less frightened, she could tolerate words being attached to her experience. "Seizure" started to take on meaning. I began to describe my sense of the experience of a seizure to Julia. Initially she was resistant, but slowly she, too, began to wonder what was happening to her.

Following a seizure, the children in Julia's play were suddenly lost. She agreed when I said that this was rather confusing, as the children had previously known where they were. "What happened?" she wondered. On another day, following a seizure, she had the two of us and the dolls spin round in a circle in order to find the one who was lost. Then she seizured again. "Now who got lost?" I asked. "I did," she exclaimed, "but I'm not lost. I know where I am." Yes, I said, you aren't lost, you just had a seizure. This work enabled Julia to identify for herself when she had a seizure, to utilize some cognitive understanding of what happened to her, and to retain her representations of herself, thus countering her feelings of anxiety, helplessness, and loss of control. Julia was pleased when her mother was impressed with her new ability.

The neurotherapy ended after the summer as Julia entered her third year of analysis.[5] Upon returning from her last session, she fell into my arms and clung to me. Julia wanted to surprise me by setting up the toys on her own. Then she called me in to look, seemingly pleased with herself. I entered to a mess of piles and things scattered everywhere with which she demonstrated her sense of internal disorganization. Julia and I spent some time creating order as I talked about how upside down she felt inside, following which she reorganized. Her seizures then stopped.

No evidence of seizures has been observed since then, and over time Julia's medication has been reduced. When she was forgetful or confused, it was clearly related to a specific internal

---

[5]When Julia began her fourth year of analysis she resumed neurotherapy locally. Her seizures were not visibly evident and Julia was on the lowest therapeutic dose of Depakote possible. Julia's parents hoped that the medication could be discontinued and that the neurotherapy would help with her learning disabilities. To accommodate Julia's twice weekly neurotherapy appointments, her analytic sessions were reduced to three times a week.

psychological state rather than seizures. Julia and I began to make this distinction.

Prior to a family trip to familiar surroundings Julia was lost. She continually forgot where she was going and asked me many times. I identified her lost, confused feeling, and told her it was not due to seizures because she was not having seizures. It was, I said, because she was worried about something; that worry kept her from thinking and remembering. Baby began asking Sissy what she was worried about, and I interpreted her fear that she was going off to see another doctor. This trip, I told her, was a vacation. When my words suddenly found their way through her fog, she asked in disbelief, ''You mean I'm not going to the doctor?'' Her mind now freed, Julia described all of the fun things she would do. She told me the number of days she would be away, and said she would miss me, but then added, ''Maybe I'll have such fun I won't even think about you!''

The idea of seizures became something Julia used on occasion in the service of defense. When, for example, I would interpret her lost and confused state as a way to keep a thought, worry, or feeling out of her mind, she angrily retorted; ''That's not why I forget. I forget because of seizures.''

As a result of medical interventions and seizures, Julia's self representation was no longer that of a capable girl. Instead, she felt incompetent, helpless, humiliated, as if she had no control over her mind, body, or emotional life. She defended against these intolerable states with fantasies of omnipotence. In her play she insisted she be the best and most admired, and that I be the one who was excluded, incapable, helpless, or had hurt feelings. Without her sense of omnipotence, she was left vulnerable to her anxieties and a self representation of an incapable child with problems, which prompted her to fall apart as the baby in despair.

Early in the second year of Julia's analysis, when she was still experiencing seizures, it became clear that she had no way to resolve her omnipotence. Analyzing her terror of helplessness was not enough. Julia needed concrete things to hold onto, skills and compensations of which she could be proud. I worked with her parents on ways to aid her with this. They helped Julia find realistic things she was good at and supported them. I also directed my interventions toward this aim.

The resulting depletion of omnipotence resurrected Julia's fears of self and object loss. However, her ability to find adaptations which alleviated her sense of loss or rendered her feelings about missing others tolerable was now evident. Her fears, as well as seizures, contributed to Julia's sense of losing herself and her surroundings. Added to this was the fact that she continued to inhibit her mind when anxious. My interventions were once again aimed at helping her engage her mind, which would in turn diminish her need for omnipotent solutions.

Julia now sometimes felt she had some real accomplishments to hold onto and be proud of. Whereas previously she, as Sissy, put on performances which were silly, obnoxious, and wild, now baby and I could honestly clap and admire her for her lovely songs. But in another game in which a house was on fire, Julia demonstrated the dangers she still felt. As Sissy she was able to get out of the fire safely, but when baby got out Julia looked at me puzzled and said, "She's not our baby." Our baby was still trapped in the burning house. Julia's need to dominate and control once again became a feature in the transference. I was locked out by Sissy, the babies locked me in the basement. Julia also locked me out by ignoring my words, as she tried to lock her feelings away and hold onto her omnipotence.

To relinquish her omnipotence meant taking responsibility for herself and growing up. As yet, the risks involved were too great since they touched on the issue of blame and Julia's deeper question, who is to blame for what happened to me? In turn, this question activated both her rage and fear about the possible answers.

Early in the third year of her analysis there was a change. Through the neurotherapy Julia had learned that she could make things happen by using her mind, concentrating, and paying attention. This seemed to strengthen her feelings of omnipotence. Her helplessness was diminished and her feeling of control over her mind was intensified. Thus her conflict over her omnipotent solutions was more readily accessible to be analyzed. At the same time, due to her question of blame, Julia's murderous rage, accompanied as it was by excitement, was enormous. Now I began to interpret more directly the consequences of her behavior and help her confront her fears.

Julia threw the baby and banged her on the table. She started to besiege me, squeezing my neck and laughing. I said, "I wasn't fooled. These hugs were not loving hugs, but attempts to choke me. When you act this way, pushing others around and trying to hurt them, they don't like it. Other children then don't want to play with you, and you feel hurt because you don't have friends which you so much want." Julia tried to get away, hid her face, and attempted to retreat to nice fantasies, revealing her shame and the defenses against it. I acknowledged how much she hated hearing this because then she felt so bad about how she acted. When I mentioned her mother, Julia interrupted, "Mommy likes it!" "No," I said, "you want to think she does so you won't feel bad, but she doesn't." "It's show time," Julia insisted, and sang a song. I interpreted that when she felt bad about herself it was an awful feeling and she believed she could not do anything. Then she needed to show me and herself the things she could do well.

As Julia presented further material on being lost and confused, I took up her feeling that she had lost herself with all that had happened to her. She made up a nonsensical song about booboos, falling on heads, smacking babies, death, and broken bones. "When you feel lost," I told her, "it feels like a booboo and you wonder what is wrong with you, is your brain broken, are you dying or dead, is someone else dead?" "Oh, be quiet," she insisted, but then asked, "What's wrong? I don't know what to do." We could then define the problem, the big question in her muddle. What was wrong with her, with her brain, with the mind that she felt like she was losing, and why did she get lost when she hadn't gotten lost previously. "Why?" she asked, "Why, why, why?" "Yes," I added, "why you, why has this happened to you? Why have you had all these operations, tests, and seizures?"

The impact of neurological difficulties on Julia's emotional life now came more to the forefront. We began to sort out what was her "brain" and what was her confusion, in an effort to help her separate out the aspect of confusion which served as a defense against intolerable affect. In addition, before Julia could approach her feelings about herself and her own sense of blame, she needed to further strengthen her sense of self.

Julia and I continued to identify areas of competence as her repertoire increased. We also began to clarify what was understandable confusion and what was part of her memory and brain problem. There were many times she attributed her confusion to her "silly, broken brain," when the reality was anyone would have gotten confused. For example, when we went to get a glass of water, she naturally went to the water fountain when I intended to go to the water cooler. When she reprimanded herself, I explained I could see how she would think we were going to the fountain. She was not confused. We were going to the cooler because the water was colder there. The next day she wanted to do this again and found her own way.

Julia's loss of her previous sense of self with the bombardment of shunt revisions and seizures had made her uncomfortable and insecure in her body. The material began to focus on how to do physical things safely, an area further exacerbated by an unconscious fantasy which was to appear in a clearer way later. We worked to help her talk herself through things, how to use her brain to think, to plan ahead, and to listen to her own feelings. For example, Julia could jump off the table safely when she planned it first in her mind and felt calm enough inside. "Wait, wait," she excitedly told herself, "my feet aren't listening yet." Then she calmed herself down and jumped successfully.

Julia was thrilled with her accomplishments. Using her mind, having ideas, making plans, and thinking things through became something she was proud of. This could be used in the service of increasing her self-esteem, rather than something to be avoided out of anxiety and terror. She began to retain events in her mind and to remember things from the past, for example, what had happened when she fell and lost her front teeth over a year ago. She told her mother with pride, "You'll have

to stop calling me Miss Forgetful, and call me Miss Remembering." She often sang new songs or told me what she was learning in school, and what she could and could not remember,
which was appropriately thought of in the context of just learning and needing to practice.

The ability to contain feelings and tolerate overwhelming
affects became a focus. Julia put baby to bed, playing both the
role of the caring mother and the baby. Baby cried and Julia
tried to comfort her. She asked baby what was wrong, but she
only cried more. When I said we could help baby use her words
because then she felt better, baby told us how sad she was
because her friend moved away. Julia tried to console baby by
telling her it would be all right because she would make new
friends, but baby said, "That doesn't help. My friend moved
and now I don't know anyone." Julia looked at me wide-eyed
saying, "This is a mix-up. I don't know what to do." I agreed,
saying she wanted to help baby by taking the sad feelings away,
but she could not. It would help baby to know that we understood how sad she felt and would be here with her. Eventually
the feeling would not be as big and strong as it was right now.

Throughout the analysis the theme of falling and getting
hurt had appeared in subtle and sporadic ways. As Julia began
to ask questions about what happened to her and why, another
theme surfaced; who is responsible? The contribution of her
aggression made these questions extremely dangerous because
of its relationship with annihilation and loss.

Now, in the third year of analysis, Julia's mind was clearer
and her seizures were consistently controlled. With no further
medical difficulties, traumas, or upheavals occurring, Julia had
the resources, opportunity, and time to do the parallel work
of facing her rage in a new way and using her intellect in the
service of sorting out her questions. The meanings of falling,
jumping, and being dropped then entered her play, as Julia's
unconscious fantasy of the cause of her brain injury surfaced
within the context of blame.

Julia began to ask, "Why did I get sick?" which we both
agreed was a very good question. A beaver puppet came into
her play as one who could help us sort this out. But beaver was
locked in a cage and the question became, would we let him

out? Julia spent sessions hiding from a dangerous monster. Each attempt to move forward was met with resistance, and we were all to be afraid.

The monster Julia feared and hid from encapsulated her questions and theories, and the rage which they motivated. This compounded her feeling lost internally and her fear of losing her objects. With these kinds of interpretations, Julia quit hiding, and her sadism entered once more in full force. Like previous phases in the analysis, what she needed was to be the baby whom I would keep safe; she also wished me to know and to feel both what she felt, and what she thought others felt when they hurt her. Now there were differences as well. Julia was conflicted about her aggression and, in displacement, the idea of blame was tolerable. There was also evidence of attempts to contain her affects rather than being overwhelmed or inhibiting them.

Julia worked to keep herself contained. Together we identified how she stuffed her mouth with food so no words and feelings could come out. When she stopped eating, her aggression entered as babies were thrown; there was wild and excited swimming, and attempts to fight with me. She asked, "How do you be a big girl and a baby?" as the part of her that wanted to grow up strengthened. In parallel she brought a series of questions: "What will happen when I get home?" and "What should we play next?" I elicited her thoughts, helping her think these through. When the questions persisted, I linked them to her other questions, the ones which were not so easy to answer and terrified her.

Beaver got very wild, which was followed by an interesting condensation where he was both dropped by someone and fell by himself. Julia and I talked with beaver about what happened. As Julia spoke for the beaver, he described how he got wild, jumped, and I didn't catch him. I took up how angry beaver was with me, and I must be to blame for his injuries. As beaver lashed out at me, Julia tried to gently explain to him that no one was to blame, but beaver only cried more. "I don't think beaver believes you," I said, adding, "he thinks someone must be to blame." When beaver smothered me with sadistic kisses, Julia threw him, and then he fell on his own. I rescued beaver and made him cry. "Little beaver, what's wrong?" Julia asked with concern, looking at me. I now spoke for beaver, sobbing, "It's me, I did it, I got wild and fell and hurt myself. I'm to blame." Julia reassured him over and over that no one was to blame; at the same time she asked me to make him cry and say that he did not believe us.

With this interpretation in displacement of Julia's theory of jumping and falling, she became more invested in putting forth effort at school. She arrived with a badge from her teacher which said "Super Job," and told her mother and me with pride, "I worked really hard in school today." Julia, now 8 years old, made other developmental steps as well. Having had difficulty with peer relationships, which were inevitably linked to her questions of blame, she struggled to confront the reality of how she acted; she felt insulted by and concerned about her behavior. Julia wanted to grow up and to have friends. She also began sleeping consistently in her own bed. As we had analyzed the multiple meanings of her sleep difficulties, she began to try to give up her transitional object. Her Depakote was reduced.

Julia began planning out what we would do, in an attempt to keep everything nice. At the same time she told me how she ran up the stairs of my building, adding sadly, "It was very hard. This is what my life is like." In sessions she played *Alice in Wonderland* who sat daydreaming; she had so many things on her mind that she could not listen or think. She angrily confronted people who would not answer her questions. Punishments were frequent, and tricking and torturing me continued. Not only was Julia afraid I could not tolerate her rage and attacks on me, but her conflicts over her aggression had grown stronger and now met head on with the structuralization of her superego and her investment in being a good girl. Being angry meant being mean and going against values she had incorporated, which contributed to her forming better relationships. Julia, who wanted to be a nice, kind, and good girl, experienced being angry as a narcissistic injury. What had begun as a wish to please her objects, had grown into a pleasure in their pride in her, and now, pride in herself. In addition, her rage continued to usher in fears of loss and annihilation, of both herself and her objects.

Julia marched into a session looking very upset. In an impressive way she told me what happened, all the while pacing and looking scared. "The reason we were late," she began, "is because, by accident, I lost control of myself." Accepting responsibility for what she had done, Julia explained how she had gone into the neighbor's house without telling anyone, thus breaking the family's biggest rule. Her mother became furious when she finally found her. Worried about the consequences of her actions, Julia added; "Mommy will tell everyone what I did." I verbalized her humiliation and fear that I and others would not be proud of her. In her play an orphan boy got mad and sobbed so hard that no one could console him; he screamed, "I want my mommy." His mother suddenly appeared and they were joyously reunited. I interpreted how the boy, like Julia, got so mad that he felt he had killed off his mother. Then he was scared because he was all alone. But, I added, neither his mommy nor Julia's were dead, and Julia was not dead either. As we ended she thanked me in sign language.

Julia began asking where we left off the day before, she wanted to continue, but then came up with the idea that we write ourselves a note. We talked about how much she hated being told she forgot something, because it reminded her of what it used to be like to have so much trouble remembering.

Julia turned to the story of Heidi as a metaphor for the analysis. But now there was a change. Feeling more secure in her sense of self and less helpless, Julia had relinquished her sense of omnipotence and was better able to take responsibility and control. Thus she rarely felt herself to be a victim at the hand of others; she was no longer fearful that anger meant death, her own or someone else's. Playing both the victim and the aggressor, Julia was Heidi and the nanny. The nanny took Heidi away when I, the grandfather, was out chopping wood. Before she allowed herself to be carted off, Heidi wrote a note telling me where she would be. I ran off in search of her, pounded on the door of Clara's house, but no one would let me in. The nanny tricked Heidi, saying she would take her home, but took her to the Gypsies instead. Heidi formulated a plan which she then carried out. She bit the Gypsy and then the nanny, following which she ran into my arms. We raced back to the mountains, locking the cabin door, safe at last. Happy, we went for a sleigh ride, singing *Rudolph the Red Nosed Reindeer*. However, Julia could not get the last stanza right. Rather than the other reindeers cheering Rudolph, they still laughed at him and called him names. Julia giggled at her mistake and tried again, but she still could not get the song out properly. I said, "Poor Rudolph feels that no matter what he does, he will never have friends, that he will always be hated and miserable." The play then took a drastic change. Fairies suddenly appeared and sprinkled fairy dust on Julia who floated away. The kids and I tried desperately to get her back, using all kinds of methods as Julia gave us ideas. There was enormous urgency as Julia shouted, "Try this." The kids and I screamed, "Oh no, now what? We're losing her again. Come back Julia!" Suddenly Julia was captured in a bubble. We tried popping it with a pin and then a pencil, all to no avail. When I let Julia know we had very little time, she started yelling at the fairies, "Stop it! Leave me alone! You stupid fairies. Why are you doing this to me?" "Yes, why?" we wondered, as we ended. Julia and I agreed this was a very important game. "Write a note," she insisted.

This was a profound and deeply moving moment in the analysis. It seemed that Julia tried to convey her internal experience of what it was like to float away in her mind, represented as fairy dust and entrapment in a bubble, a process activated by both her misery and terror. It was the inner experience of running away to the mountains, the earlier representation of her defense of inhibiting her mind. Not only psychological factors contributed to Julia floating away, but also neurological ones. The experience of seizures may also have been what Julia was trying to express. No longer feeling as helpless in the face of either of these processes, Julia could express her anger and take charge of herself. Now she could begin to confront what had scared her the most: that she was to blame.

Over the next few days Julia began dropping things. When I pointed this out, baby jumped off the table into my arms. In the middle of the night she sneaked out of bed, jumped off the table on her own, and was badly hurt. I rushed the sobbing baby to the hospital, where her injuries were minimized, and

Julia wandered off. I said I seemed to be the only one who could feel worried. As sadistic, excited play ensued, I identified the terror Julia felt when she thought of baby being responsible for her injuries.

The following day there were many things the children were frightened of. Although Julia's play was jumbled, she was no longer scared of getting lost or losing her self. Baby wanted to go to a friend's house to play. She walked down the street mumbling to herself that she did not know the way. She got lost and then tried to recall the way mommy drove her. Whereas usually baby was completely lost and scared, this time she knew exactly where she had made a wrong turn, and could tell me where she was when she phoned. Baby was very pleased with herself.

As the analysis progressed, and these changes occurred, Julia seldom played the role of a little girl or a baby. She became an older girl with the promise of a future. But before she could move ahead, she had one final task to complete. For this, she once again turned to the beaver.

Julia was beaver and his mother was the rabbit. I was beaver's friend, the grasshopper. Beaver climbed on grasshopper's back and they played "bucking bronco." The play got wild, beaver fell, was knocked out briefly, and awakened. For the first time, clearly and calmly, Julia explained that beaver got too wild and out of control, fell, and hurt himself. Suddenly, beaver and grasshopper were in a strange place. "Where are we?" asked beaver. "It kind of looks familiar, but where is it?" Together we contemplated, wondered, and beaver said, "I woke up and don't know where we are." We quickly determined that wherever it was, it was dangerous, and the hyenas were after us. We ran, terrified, trying to get to the mountains and screaming for mommy to help us, with the hyenas on our tails. A frantic mommy appeared, but she could not save us both. She got grasshopper out and then returned, gallantly saving her child. But beaver had been hurt, scratched on the head by the hyenas, and he was bleeding. We were all terrified, but incredibly relieved.

This session marked a profound shift. Julia had faced her inner terror that she was responsible for her brain injury. She allowed full voice to her fantasy of causing herself to fall which resulted in the nightmare of her life, the subsequent dangers, disorientation, and feeling lost. When I next saw her she opened the cupboard (which looked the same as it always did), and commented, "It's so neat! I've never seen it like this." She took out the phones and told me, "I bet I can spell phones, f-o-n-s." I told her she was almost right. That was how it sounded. I asked if she had learned about those funny words that sound like "f," but are spelled "ph." "Not yet," she said, "but don't worry, I will." I said I was not worried, and she was not either, because now learning was not so hard.

FOLLOW-UP

Julia, who is still in treatment, is now on the lowest therapeutic dose of Depakote possible. The neurologist's impression of a waking EEG was that it was only moderately abnormal. It contained irregular brief spike wave discharges anteriorly and off to the right side posteriorly, with occasional runs of theta activity more prominent on the right side. The background in the EEG was otherwise normal and no actual electrical or clinical seizures occurred.

Educationally Julia is doing well. According to her teacher she now works independently without difficulty, can find her way around the school on her own, plays with the other children, and is well liked. Sequencing remains a problem, but only on some days and nothing like it used to be. If any of Julia's capacities is unstable, it is her ability to stay focused. An evaluation of Julia's basic skills, as measured by the Illinois Test of Psycholinguistic Abilities, indicated that her visual abilities are generally stronger than her auditory capacities, except in memory where she is stronger in the auditory sphere; weaknesses are evident primarily in visuomotor levels.[6] Academically, Julia is $1^1/_2$ to 2 years behind in her basic skills, but is

---

[6]Adequate scaled scores range between 32 and 38. Areas of strength include visual reception (39), visual association (33), grammatic closure (36), sound blending (46), and auditory memory (35). Areas of weakness include auditory reception (19), visual memory (19), visual closure which is a timed process (23), and auditory association (28).

quickly catching up. To quote her school report: "Julia is a smart little girl. She is no longer 'Little girl lost but little girl found!' She is now beginning to apply her energy to developing social and academic skills rather than fighting fears others never have to experience. She has made very positive strides in all areas this year."

Chapter 6

Discussion of Julia's Analysis

Dr. Miller's report of the analysis of Julia, a patient who presented clearly documented evidence of frank cerebral damage and associated cerebral discharge phenomena producing seizures, demonstrates *in relief* certain problems typical of patients with milder neuropsychologically determined learning disabilities. From this perspective, we emphasize several aspects of the case.

One is the importance of working to understand how *specific* cognitive disturbances affect the patient's experience of the functioning of his or her mind. Dr. Miller provides a beautiful explication of her attempt to grasp "what it was like to live in Julia's mind." A second is the crucial value of appreciating that findings of damage (or dysfunction) are necessarily woven into the patient's fantasies, thus shaping development in fundamental ways. This is something Dr. Miller well appreciated from the outset of the analysis with Julia. Related to this is the very interesting question of how and when it is valuable (and indeed even possible) to make differentiations between symptoms attributable to cerebral pathology, as contrasted with those of purely psychogenic origin. The analysis of Julia also demonstrates the importance of exploring with the patient the specific cognitive findings as they emerge.

Third, Dr. Miller's case highlights several common fantasies experienced by learning disabled patients, most particularly their unconscious fantasies about who "caused " the damage. Fourth, the issue of concomitant interventions (i.e., those in addition to analysis) can be fruitfully examined in the context of this case. Do these necessarily dilute, or in some other way conflict with, the analytic work?[1] In our view, while they are of course crucial and necessary regardless of their impact on the analysis, they *can* become a valuable focus of analytic understanding and thus forward analytic goals.

We will discuss these four aspects of Julia's analysis in sequence.

"ENTERING THE MIND OF THE CHILD"

The organic difficulties with which Julia had to cope were of several types. From the beginning of her life, when she was only 20 days old, Julia suffered from hemorrhage into her cerebral ventricles. While that alone might have caused brain damage, a further complication ensued. Scarring and/or interference with arachnoid villa (a part of the cerebral ventricles) functioning disrupted the free flow of cerebral spinal fluid, producing hydrocephalus with an accompanying increase in cerebral spinal fluid pressure. Fortunately the neurosurgeon constructed a shunt which drained fluid from the ventricles to the peritoneum, thus preventing further damage to the brain. Julia was subjected to six shunt failures which occurred between the ages of 2 and about 5; five took place within only a fourteen-month period, prior to consultation with Dr. Miller. These required

---

[1]Some readers may question whether the treatment was truly psychoanalysis. More than with other patients described in this book, Dr. Miller had to reassure and teach her patient and help her patient's parents in realistic ways. Furthermore, some may raise a question as to whether Julia's difficulties prevented sufficient insight, which is an essential aspect of psychoanalysis. In addition, other modalities (e.g., medication, neurofeedback) supplemented the psychotherapeutic intervention.

We believe that from a practical point of view, such doubts are semantic and irrelevant. However one labels Julia's treatment, it consisted largely of interpretation of defenses, drive derivatives, inner conflict, and unconscious fantasies in the context of her present and past life situations. Insight enabled Julia to cope with extraordinarily difficult circumstances and to benefit from other therapeutic modalities. Her symptoms diminished and her adaptive behavior was enhanced. It is true that the full range of preoedipal and oedipal conflicts was not dealt with; there was a greater focus on conflicts over aggressive impulses than libidinal ones. But since the treatment was still ongoing (although diminished to three times a week), we can expect more extensive interpretive work and insight.

surgical procedures which involved terrible head pain, general anesthesia (in one instance, while held down), and experiencing the loss of her parents as she became unconscious. Following this, Julia had a grand mal seizure followed by multiple (as many as a hundred a day) absentes (petit mal seizures) that plagued her for over a year following diagnosis until they were brought under control with medication. She now experienced organically based periods of feeling lost, of failing to perceive herself and her environment, and repeatedly losing her memory of and access to representations of those upon whom she desperately needed to rely, most centrally her parents. This contributed to further feelings of abandonment, terror, fury, and confusion.

Dr. Miller exquisitely portrays what it was like to "enter Julia's mind and be in it with her." She reported her efforts, as Julia's analyst, to cope with her own experience of sessions as lacking in sequential organizations or themes. Julia seemed to flip from one thing to another, all in a seemingly unconnected way, which elicited a sense of chaos, confusion, helplessness, and anxiety in the analyst. In many respects Julia's thinking was more like that of a prelatency child in whom primary process thinking (which is disorganized, illogical, meandering, with relatively rapid shifts of one thought or representation to another) predominates over secondary process.[2] Julia often had the experience of not knowing where she was or where others were. She was not always able to differentiate between what was real and what was not.

Julia's first consultation session is illustrative. As she started to talk, she said that her older sister hated her, calling her crazy and hitting her. She soon became angry at her sister and brother who also attacked her. Her anger switched from being directed toward her siblings and herself and turned toward her mother who, she said, made her stay in kindergarten. Switching again, Julia targeted a schoolmate who did not want to be her

---

[2]Dr. Miller commented that in writing up this case, it was not always possible for her to convey the degree of confusion and disorganization which actually characterized the early hours with Julia. That is, in the very act of writing, of putting the experience into words, she could not help but impose some degree of organization on what was in reality far more chaotic.

best friend anymore. Finally, as she scribbled, she anxiously said words like "peabrain," "upside down," and "backwards." When Dr. Miller said that Julia must feel "upside down" and as though her brain were on backwards, Julia told a confused story about being sick as a baby and not knowing where she was.

Dr. Miller came to realize that in many ways her own experience in the hours mirrored Julia's fundamental experience of her life. Initially the best she could do was to empathize with her patient and then help her begin to identify and verbalize the anguish, confusion, rage and terror with which she had so long lived. For example, when Julia recalled that she had been sick as a baby and did not know where she was, Dr. Miller responded, "Maybe she felt that way now, and we can talk about how confused and mixed up she got, often forgetting things." As Dr. Miller was better able to get her bearings, over time, she could increasingly help Julia make sense of her world and her own experience of it. She could gradually locate what set off the confusion and sense of loss. Similarly, when Julia's seizure activity began, Dr. Miller attempted to talk to her about what was happening to her. This included analyzing the interweaving of the biological in the development of Julia's fantasies.

INTERRELATIONSHIPS BETWEEN THE BIOLOGICAL AND PSYCHOLOGICAL

From the outset of the analysis, Dr. Miller was aware of Julia's "massive internal disorientation," which included her tendency to walk in the wrong direction, her difficulty finding things, her confusion in general and about spatial orientation in particular, and her terror of being crazy and damaged. The likelihood that these were related to neurological damage, which could also contribute to subsequent learning disabilities, was clear to Dr. Miller as well. She wrote, "this would not only add complications and considerations as to the ways in which the work was approached, but also be used by Julia in the construction of fantasies and internal representations and influence her developmental progression."

Dr. Miller believed that neuropsychological testing (when Julia could withstand this procedure) would be necessary to help make these determinations. She probably appreciated that if such an evaluation were not performed, there would be less clarity on the part of both analyst and patient. The potential for under- or overgeneralizing the damage (its scope and degree) would be increased, and the possibility of comprehensively appreciating the interrelationships between the biological and psychological would be reduced. In addition, testing was necessary to help define educational plans and approaches.

Julia had several diagnostic psychological evaluations prior to and relatively early in the analysis which indicated that specific problems in visuospatial reasoning and visual memory existed. Before the consultation with Dr. Miller, at the age of $4^1/_2$ (in a screening for application to kindergarten for the following school year), Julia displayed a meaningful disparity between her higher verbal and quantitative functioning, as compared to her perceptual and perceptual-motor functioning. At that time Julia scored somewhat above average overall.

After several months of analysis, when Julia was nearly 6 years old, she presented a considerably worse picture on a more extensive neuropsychological evaluation. By that time Julia, who had entered kindergarten the previous fall, had to return to preschool because she suffered panic reactions. Probably contributory was the clear loss of function evident on the new tests that were administered; this was possibly the result of several additional shunt failures and the surgery required to repair them. Not only did the testing procedure revive Julia's earlier terror about the many surgical procedures to which she had been subjected (as Dr. Miller poignantly describes), but it probably also evoked a catastrophic reaction in Julia as she was confronted with being unable to do what she had previously been capable of doing. She scored overall only at the lower end of the "Low Average" range (albeit on a different intelligence test), with a pronounced degree of variability on the individual subtests of which this test is comprised. Julia functioned at an average or just above average level on most verbal tests (including one of immediate auditory sequential memory, repeating sentences), with the exception of two which involved reasoning

(Arithmetic and Comprehension). These lowered scores could also have reflected the interference of anxiety, which was reportedly severe.[3] In contrast, Julia had a striking degree of difficulty on tests which measured visual memory, and visuospatial (including visual sequential) memory.

We agree with Dr. Miller that the reported diagnostic impression that she suffered from memory problems (as a whole) seems, therefore, partially incorrect. It was *visual* memory that was at issue, while *auditory* memory seemed to be intact; indeed Julia attained her very highest score on a test which measured this function. This corroborated Dr. Miller's clinical impression of the intactness of Julia's auditory memory, and was further borne out by teacher observations (e.g., that Julia's spelling improved when she was first allowed to spell words orally and then to write them down).

Keeping in mind these specific findings, we can discuss Julia's compromise formations from several perspectives: (1) the psychological derivatives (in the form of unconscious fantasies) of biological contributions of her experience of herself and others; (2) the ways in which specific aspects of her cognitive dysfunction, or the general experience of being "defective," can be employed for defensive purposes; and (3) features of the patient which are seemingly uninformed by having biological (organic or neuropsychological) difficulties. We can be on shaky ground when we make interpretations of purely psychogenic causation about features of the patient which find some contribution from biological difficulties, the first two of these three perspectives.

There were at least several psychological derivatives of Julia's severe visual memory and visuospatial reasoning problems reported in this account, which were perhaps not fully identified as such. These included Julia's fears of object loss and of getting lost, which were associated, for her, with frightening things happening. Julia's self-experience of being a "pea-brain," "backwards," and "upside down," which Dr. Miller

---

[3]Dr. Miller wrote in a letter to us that "I cannot emphasize enough how anxious she was. At home, school, and with me she was a basket case for the three weeks it [the evaluation] took, as bad as she was when she first came to me. She was sure her brain was broken, and acted as if it was, and was all over the place."

helped her verbalize, probably related to her *general* sense of having severe cognitive difficulties. However, it may also have been an expression of her *specific* deficits in grasping and retaining visuospatial matters. It is noteworthy in this regard that Julia was first reported to have psychological difficulties in the context of moving to a new house at the age of 5 years, 11 months, two months after which she started a new school in September in which she got lost. Julia was unable to learn the location of things both at home and at school. One month later (in October) she was brought to Dr. Miller in a panic. As the neuropsychologist (who evaluated Julia) commented, "having difficulty remembering locations and how to get from one place to another can be extremely anxiety-provoking for a young child in a new setting." We can add to this the likelihood that Julia's profound specific cognitive disabilities (in visual memory and visuospatial reasoning) greatly increased these normal concerns and potentiated her intense sense of loss, helplessness, and the like.

Difficulties in the development of libidinal object constancy, which involves the psychological retention of representations (including visual images) of significant others, is necessarily compromised by major visual memory impairments. Of course, fears of object loss also found contribution from Julia's anger at her mother, including her wishes for her to disappear. Such fantasies then, in turn, terrified her and prompted fears of being attacked or abandoned. It was as if, in fantasy, the punishment fit the crime. Julia's cognitive disability and the fantasies which surrounded it also became interwoven with terrifying memories of surgery. Julia remembered how she lost her mother before she was able to go to sleep in her mother's arms; she associated this with the doctor's snatching her away from mommy for an emergency procedure, an event she had also heard about. In addition, the experience of surgery on her head and her brain was elaborated into a theory about the etiology of her memory impairments; Julia explained that she forgot things because her brain had fallen out.

Dr. Miller also worked interpretively to help Julia appreciate the relationship she observed between Julia's rage and her seizure activity. The more prominent was her rage, the more frequent was the recurrence of seizure activity. Another important line of interpretation was Dr. Miller's effort to help Julia to appreciate the use she made of her biologically based disorders for defensive purposes. This was seen in the context of the neurofeedback which helped Julia control her seizures. Initially Dr. Miller meaningfully assisted Julia in observing the nature of her seizures. She told Julia that, "[F]ollowing a seizure children are [i.e., feel] suddenly lost," and Julia took a step forward. She could distinguish between a seizure and a confused or forgetful state due to internal turmoil involving conflict. Then, in the absence of seizure activity, Dr. Miller focused with Julia on emotionally determined states which they were able to compare to past seizure experiences.

However, even once Julia's seizures became controlled, at times she tried to attribute her nonseizure lapses to seizures. This was a defense against recognizing emotional conflicts. Julia sometimes used the seizure experience of being suddenly lost (in a fog) to prevent the appearance in consciousness of one or another worry or feeling. In order to help Julia identify and work with these defenses, Dr. Miller undertook to help her distinguish between feelings caused by the malfunctioning of her injured and disordered brain and the strange sensations that arose from psychic conflict or remembrances of disturbing experiences. Dr. Miller helped Julia reflect on her sense of being out of control and its relationship to her denial of responsibility for aggressive feelings and wishes; that is, Julia produced mock seizures to deny her aggression. Another example was Julia's sense of confusion prior to a trip. As Dr. Miller wrote, "Prior to a family trip, Julia was lost. She continually forgot where she was going. I identified her lost, confused feeling, and told her it wasn't due to seizures because she wasn't having seizures. She was worried about something, and that worry kept her from thinking and remembering." Indeed Dr. Miller and her patient ultimately ascertained that Julia imagined the trip was to a doctor; when she realized it was not, her confusion lifted and she looked forward to a happy vacation.

Via interpretation of these unconscious fantasies and other aspects of her compromise formations, particularly her central defenses, the analysis facilitated many facets of Julia's functioning which were associated with areas of organic damage. Her capacity to maintain her internal object representations, and to use them to soothe herself, was greatly ameliorated. This was despite her major impairments in visual memory and spatial organization. Julia had far more flexibility in her repertoire of defenses. She no longer had such a heavy reliance upon reversal (being the hurter, the abandoner) with the fears of being attacked or abandoned as a result of this. Her tolerance of knowing, without the experience of overwhelming affects, was also enhanced.

Dr. Miller also emphasized the importance of actual experiences of competence in facilitating Julia's progress. For some time Julia mobilized fantasies of omnipotence to counteract her sense of herself as a powerless and incapable person who could not control her seizures or other traumatic and disturbing events. While interpretation diminished this maladaptive defense, realistic achievement was needed to supplement interpretation. For example, the success of neurofeedback afforded Julia the feeling she could actually control seizures by willing this; concentration and sustaining her attention paid off.

Thus in some instances it was extremely useful to make distinctions between "brain" and psychological phenomena. However, there are other times that making such distinctions can leave one on shaky ground. Moreover, doing so may unnecessarily limit the scope of analytic inquiry, and somewhat oversimplify what are truly more complex phenomena. There were several subtle suggestions of this possibility in Dr. Miller's report. For example, Dr. Miller describes helping her patient begin to sort out "what was her brain and what was her confusion, helping her separate out the aspect of confusion which served as a defense against intolerable affect. . . . We also began to clarify what was understandable confusion and what was part of her memory and brain problem."

It was also extremely valuable to help Julia explore how organic phenomena, such as the experience of seizures, affected her sense of self. In this regard, Dr. Miller commented that there were many times Julia attributed her confusion to her "silly, broken brain," when the reality was anyone would have gotten confused. In another context, Dr. Miller states, "In all this we could discuss how it wasn't her brain that was missing or broken, but all of her feelings and worries that made her forget and run to the mountains" and "It was too scary and painful to think and feel."

When taken to an extreme, there may be a problem with this. In some respects Julia's brain *was* "broken." Similarly, Julia described to Dr. Miller that when the testing evaluator asked her to do something, she "did not hear" and therefore "told the lady she did not know how to do it." Dr. Miller interpreted, "this meant she [Julia] was too afraid to take in the information." It is important to keep in mind that this could *also* mean that Julia really could *not* do it and instead wished to attribute her failure to not having heard. Another example was the exchange which took place between Julia and Dr. Miller about the water cooler. Julia may have been conveying her experience of organically based spatial disorientation; in this sense it may not have been entirely natural that she went to the wrong place for water. At some juncture in the analysis, Julia's memory problems were viewed as her attempts to not think, which ultimately caused eruptions, confusion, forgetting, and nightmares. There were gains reported in Julia's memory functioning as her defenses against thinking and remembering and the interference of her anxiety were explored. Nevertheless it is important to keep in view that Julia *did* have specific kinds of persistent memory problems which were severe and organically based.

Thus we believe it would not be accurate to conceptualize these as examples of conflict of a *purely* psychogenic nature. Probably Dr. Miller would agree with us but may have been emphasizing one facet of these complex phenomena. This is often all that we can do, pragmatically speaking, at any moment in time in an analysis and in a case report. However, it is crucial that, in our conceptualizations of such patients, we bear in mind the persistent effects of their specific types of cognitive dysfunction as they become interlaced with the patient's wishes, defenses, superego injunctions, and the like.

COMMON FANTASIES ABOUT ORGANIC AND
NEUROPSYCHOLOGICAL DYSFUNCTION

In the third year of analysis Julia directly tackled the question of blame. Why had this happened to her? Why did she have "all these operations, tests, and seizures?" Variations on these questions are typical of patients with neuropsychologically based learning disabilities, whether at a conscious or unconscious level. They evidence ideas about having brought their disabilities upon themselves as punishments for forbidden libidinal or aggressive wishes. At the same time, they harbor fantasies that loved ones "caused" the damage. Common is the associated rage they experience toward loved ones for "unfair" punishment, for not protecting the patient or indeed for not preventing the danger posed by others.

While Julia's questions had been foreshadowed earlier in the analysis, it is probable that the degree of panic, rage, and despair associated with these questions was too overwhelming to permit her, with Dr. Miller's assistance, to pursue them more systematically at that time. After a period of growing self-confidence, which seemed to strengthen her, she could delve further and ask who was responsible. This question evoked rage and fears of annihilation and loss. Dr. Miller also suggests that the absence of further medical procedures or other types of upheavals permitted Julia to more effectively use her resources to grapple with her fantasies about this in a new way.

Julia's efforts are exemplified in clinical process material such as the following. With the help of a beaver puppet that Julia brought into her play, they tried to sort things out. First beaver, locked in a cage, was associated with a monster that contained the questions, theories, and rage that Julia feared and wanted to keep hidden. Then beaver became very wild, an expression of the rage, sadism, and fear Julia tried to contain. Embedded in this material is Julia's fantasy (expressed elsewhere more clearly) that she got wild and jumped and fell because of her angry feelings. A related fantasy was that her brain fell out and was missing when the doctors operated. Beaver was angry at Dr. Miller who, beaver thought, was to blame for the injuries she had permitted by failing to catch him when he fell. This is most likely a displaced expression of a fantasy that mother caused the injury by omission or commission. After a while beaver blamed himself. Because he was wild, he fell and hurt himself.

It may be difficult for the reader to follow Julia's meandering thoughts. Eventually it became clear that the beaver represented Julia, who blamed others and then herself for her failure to control her impulses, particularly her rage and sadism. Blaming others defended against self-reproaches, but was also an expression of her genuine fury, probably at the doctors and her parents, which was displaced onto Dr. Miller. In the transference, Julia feared Dr. Miller would not tolerate her rage and attacks on her. She played this out as she enacted *Alice in Wonderland* during which Julia, as Alice, daydreamed so that she could not listen to people. This included fantasies of tricking and torturing, and anxious expectations that she and others would be annihilated.

There are strong hints that Julia was struggling with other wishes as well. She may have blamed herself because of her sexual feelings, still hidden and unanalyzed but coming closer to consciousness. Most likely her excitement, her falling, her changes of consciousness, her piercing of a bubble she was in, and her looking into the neat cupboard where there are phones are derivatives of sexual feelings. Dr. Miller pointed out that Julia's superego was becoming more structuralized. It seems likely that sexual as well as aggressive wishes came into conflict with her conscience.

In none of the other cases reported in this book did severe shock trauma (E. Kris, 1956) play such an important part as a codeterminant of the effects of the patient's problems in learning. We define shock trauma as severe sudden overstimulation of the organism beyond the organism's capability of dealing with it by means of its usual defenses. Shock trauma is different from stress trauma in which the stimulation is less intense and usually more prolonged.

Julia was severely psychologically traumatized in several different ways: (1) by each of the operations and the associated anesthesia; (2) by the actual separation from her parents during the surgery (children may suffer from the internal buildup of tension when drives cannot be satisfied after they lose their parents; the anxiety following loss can also be overstimulating); (3) through the loss of object representations (experienced as object loss) due to unconsciousness at the time of surgery and during seizures (combined with severe visual memory problems); and (4) by the overwhelming overstimulation during Julia's seizures.

Shock trauma causes immediate confusion and diminution or distortion of cognition including perception. Hence it accentuates the other types of cognitive difficulties which are experienced by patients who are learning disabled. Further, the intense anxiety generated by the traumata can interfere with cognition. Defenses following trauma include regression (involving ego regression with cognitive decline), denial (which interferes with perception), and active repetition of the traumatic experience, often in disguised form, in an attempt to master it. Frequently such attempts at mastery fail, and the patient experiences the repetition itself as terrifying and traumatic.

Julia had all of the above experiences. She became confused and disoriented at the time of the traumata and during repetitions, including situations like psychological testing, which reminded her of the surgery. She at first remained relatively calm during other repetitions, as when she cut her hair or tried to use a razor. However, she simultaneously created a confusing and frightening situation as she alarmed her parents.

QUESTIONS OF THE IMPACT OF CONCOMITANT INTERVENTIONS

In Julia's case other modalities (medication, EEG neurofeedback, neurological examination, diagnostic testing, special education) necessarily supplemented the psychoanalytic intervention. Some analysts might question the possibility of creating an analytic situation under these circumstances. Most notably, they may be concerned about the potential for splitting or in some other way diluting the transference and for significant interruptions in the treatment. Their doubts about working with such a patient might be compounded by reservations about being able to engage a child whose "equipment" is compromised in an analytic treatment. We believe that this case illustrates, *in bold relief,* the ways in which Dr. Miller and her patient made use of these necessary experiences for the analytic aims of furthering Julia's insight. Two interventions will serve as examples.

Psychological testing as a diagnostic tool was necessary to evaluate the degree of cognitive disturbance with which Julia was coping and to aid in selecting an appropriate educational environment for her. It was initially delayed because Dr. Miller and Julia's parents judged that the testing process would upset Julia too much because of its resonances with her repeated surgeries. When it *was* undertaken, this provided an opportunity to differentiate a psychological evaluation from the surgery Julia feared, and to help her see that she responded to other events as if they were invasive medical procedures. In anticipation, Julia not only feared the testing procedure, but also "fell apart" and felt lost and disoriented. She feared that it would reveal that her brain was broken and that she was incapable. Reality testing and interpretation of Julia's tendency to connect relatively benign procedures with dangerous ones contributed to the diminution of her anxiety over time.

The treatment for the absentes included medication (Depakote) prescribed by physicians who had to examine Julia, and EEG neurofeedback. This was an unconventional approach which required that Julia and her mother go to another city for a period of time, thus interrupting the analysis. Dr. Miller's work was cut out for her and Julia, brave warrior that she was, engaged in it valiantly. Dr. Miller saw her immediate task as trying to help Julia control her rage so that she could participate in the neurofeedback. To accomplish this Julia used the analytic situation as a comforting, reassuring environment.

But the neurofeedback treatment was also a focus of continuing interpretation and insight which promoted the analysis in the long run, as well as helped Julia confront her immediate anxiety. It was at this point that Julia tried to cut her hair with garden shears, thus symbolically repeating her surgical experiences actively (she was the surgeon) in an ill-conceived attempt at mastery, which her analyst interpreted. It is also noteworthy that, as Dr. Miller reported, it was not until the introduction of EEG neurofeedback (a procedure which Julia viewed with hopefulness, since it involved the idea that she could exercise some control over her body), that she and her patient could truly talk about the seizures. This was despite the fact that Dr. Miller had tried to explore with Julia what was happening to her from the onset of the seizure activity within the analytic hours. The neurofeedback also helped Julia recognize the presence of seizures and to differentiate confusion, failure to perceive, and memory loss due to absentes from similar symptoms due to emotional conflict.

Whatever lies ahead in the therapy, Julia is doing remarkably well. The multifaceted approach to treatment is succeeding. Julia's parents' devotion to their child, their willingness to undertake many interventions, including analysis, is paying off. Her seizures are under control and she does well in school. She is much less fearful, and able to sleep in her own bed and to recognize that reality imposes difficult tasks. To quote Dr. Miller: "According to her teacher she now works independently without difficulty, can find her way around the school on her own, plays with the other children, and is well liked." This is true despite the fact that Julia still has serious persistent cognitive deficiencies, as would be expected in a child who has sustained significant cerebral damage.

Chapter 7

Andy's Analysis

Morris L. Peltz, M.D.

INTRODUCTION

When parents consult child therapists because their son or daughter has learning problems, we rely on as complete a diagnostic evaluation as is possible given the limitations of our current knowledge. My approach to the clinical investigation of learning problems includes several interviews with both parents and often as many as six to ten unstructured sessions with the child. I augment this clinical appraisal with psychological and educational testing. Concluding this preliminary exploration, I may still only have a largely descriptive portrait, but I have nonetheless a picture of what treatment I will recommend to the parents. Most often, the plan includes some combination of psychotherapy and tutoring or (when there is a specific learning disability) remediation.

In Andy's case, the scope of the evaluation and range of interventions fell short of this ideal. My work with Andy ended well over ten years ago. Testing for and evaluating learning disabilities have become much more refined and sophisticated in the ensuing decade. It is conceivable that had Andy been examined by modern tools, discrete problems in reading or other academic skills would have been detected. From the very first, I strongly advocated tutoring in reading. However, Andy's parents never implemented this recommendation because, they said, he adamantly refused this help.

Thus Andy, a boy with serious reading and other types of learning problems, was treated only with psychoanalysis. I was not happy with this prescription, but it was the only one open to Andy and me. Incomplete as a therapeutic psychoanalysis without the tutoring in reading that I recommended, the treatment did conclude successfully. I could not have foreseen this result, and am unable to entirely explain it. Nor is it clear whether the treatment outcome would have been significantly different, had a discrete reading problem been diagnosed and treated educationally.

CONSULTATION PROCESS

Presenting Problems

Andy's parents were very despairing about their $8^1/2$-year-old son when they first consulted me. They felt completely alienated from him and were bewildered by his silly and often out-of-control behavior. Further, they feared he was exerting an increasingly destructive influence within the family. In addition to these behavioral symptoms, Andy was having serious learning problems in school. In the third grade, he was barely able to read and was struggling to keep at grade level in all other requisite skills. His intellectual parents felt especially wounded by this aspect of Andy's difficulties.

Andy's mother elaborated. She dreaded his coming home from school. He would be deliberately provocative with both his sisters and parents. He would so tease Janet, fourteen months older than he, that she would angrily denounce him as being crazy. This would enrage Andy, driving him to further escalate his tormenting behavior. He had no friends at school and played only with younger children. He had a very aloof relationship with his mother. When he turned to his father for help with his homework, as he often did, these encounters ended badly for both. Typically Andy soon became very excited and silly as he attempted to crawl into his father's lap. Imitating the family dog, he would try to lick his father's face as he drooled saliva. Sadly, his most constant friend in the family was the dog. Often, however, he would roll on the floor with her, rub her vulva, and become increasingly excited, much to the family's dismay. Only with his younger sister, Peggy, could he occasionally be sweet without regressing or teasing. Andy resented both parents, especially his mother. He often accused her of being unfair and unnecessarily punishing. Andy was also quite fearful. He was terrified of being arrested by the police, dreaded going to his pediatrician because of his fears of shots, and was worried about catching germs from his mother and sisters.

Andy's teachers described his trouble working in the classroom. Occasionally, he was disruptive but this was not regarded as the major problem. Rather his teachers emphasized that instead of concentrating, he spent his time daydreaming. He refused remedial tutoring at home, hated being read to, and stubbornly resisted most of his parents' attempts to help him with his schoolwork.

Developmental and Family History

Andy's story of developmental problems and impaired family relations had a long, painful history. Andy was born under circumstances that were quite different from his older sister's birth. At the time, his family was living in a foreign country under somewhat primitive conditions. The labor was long (more than twelve hours), painful, and frightening. Weighing in at 6 pounds, Andy was small and jaundiced (APGAR scores were not available). He was born with a neonatal staphylococcal infection of his eyes and toenails which delayed the ritual circumcision.

However, Andy soon became a good-natured baby who rapidly gained weight. His early motor development was within normal limits. He turned over at 5 to 6 weeks, sat without support at 8 months, and walked at $13^1/_2$ months. Although speech was delayed (as will soon be discussed) mother fondly remembered what a happy and cheerful infant he was during his first year.

Andy's mother became pregnant for the third time one month after Andy's first birthday. The birth of his sister Peggy seemed to mark the onset of Andy's developmental problems. Mother initially explained that because Andy was so content and self-sufficient she believed he could do well on his own, she thus felt free to take care of the new baby. Mother also began toilet training Andy shortly after Peggy's birth. Andy easily achieved bladder control, but became very symptomatic in trying to master bowel control. He was frequently constipated, retaining stool for two or three days before having a painful movement. This state of affairs persisted for more than a year when (only fortuitously) Andy's mother helped him resolve the symptoms. One day, with an abdomen distended with feces, Andy anxiously asked his mother, "I'm not going to have a baby, am I?" "No," answered his mother, "Boys and children do not have babies."

As pleased as she was with her reply and its ameliorative effect, Andy's mother sadly described that by this time she felt she had lost all emotional contact with him. He had become distant and self-absorbed. This was his mother's view of the beginning of their impaired relationship. The troubles with his older sister Janet followed very soon.

In addition to these beginning strained object relations, his mother described his other developmental problems. He had been very slow to acquire language; the quality of his speech was problematic as well. Andy was $2\frac{1}{2}$ before he even tried to speak and 3 before he could be understood. Speech therapy before he was 5 helped him, but there were still residuals of infantile speech three years later.

When Andy was in the first grade, his parents first learned of the behavioral and learning problems he was having. In contrast to his older sister who performed very well and had many friends, Andy was shy, often silly, and giggly. Hoping Andy would mature, secretly fearing he was organically damaged, his parents delayed taking action for two more years.

Initial Interviews with the Analyst

When I first met Andy he was a sturdy, well-built boy whose good looks were marred by his vacuous grin and his drooling saliva. His clothes were dirty and shabby, giving him the waiflike appearance of a poorly cared for child. He claimed to have no idea about any problem he might have, insisting rather that what he needed were toys and money from me. As he left the first consultation hour, Andy fingered a dent in the side of a toy rubber cow. He reflected with little emotion, "Skinny cow. No milk."

Andy's behavior during the two-month diagnostic study confirmed the dismal portrait painted by his parents. Often Andy acted as if he hadn't a care in the world. He would begin hours lying on the floor slowly eating a candy bar. Never satisfied when he had finished, he asked if I had anything else he might eat, and acted truly aggrieved that I did not. He was uninterested in toys and only mildly curious about the objects on my desk. He sometimes asked for drawing paper, but growing bored with the task, he would begin to scribble. What truly interested him was the amount of letterhead stationery he could cajole from me. Easily becoming restless, he would bounce on my couch, jump from the cabinets, and dart out of the office to check on his mother's whereabouts. Beneath this apparently aimless behavior, I sensed a sad and frightened child.

Psychological Testing

Because of the complex clinical picture of overlapping developmental and psychological symptoms, I concluded my study by obtaining psychological testing. I will cite from the test results:

In the office he was initially quite tense, wore the same fixed smile, said very little, and periodically wrapped his legs around the legs of the table at which he was seated, as we talked briefly about why he came to see me. As testing proceeded he became progressively more restless, flipping the extension-wings of the typewriter table at which he sat, up and down in rapid and noisy successions, played "bass fiddle" on the vertical window blinds, reached across four feet of desk to grab a stopwatch, squirmed under the desk to retrieve a broken pencil point, knocking furniture noisily as he went, and in general gave a picture of an extremely anxious and hyperactive child for whom verbal constraints seemed relatively ineffective. However, parts of his test performance revealed a rather different picture, one of a boy who despite his hyperactivity can, under certain circumstances, tolerate delay and persist in a goal-directed task orientation until closure is achieved.

The psychologist concluded:

The test picture is one of anxiety and considerable depression in a boy of potentially Bright Normal to Superior intelligence. His anxiety and low self-esteem interfere with his cognitive functioning at times, inducing regression to infantile speech and a feigned helplessness and ignorance. His attention to his surroundings, his social judgment, and his capacity for new learning are impaired by anxiety and dynamically his anxiety and depression appear rooted in his intense ambivalent feelings about his parents.

While the total picture is one of considerable ideational and emotional impoverishment, and aggressive discharge of anxiety and unconscious hostility, this boy's intellectual potential, his still intact capacity for persistent goal-direction in problem solving, and his wish and capacity for object relations make him a relatively promising candidate for intensive analytic therapy.

Recommendations

After completing this diagnostic evaluation, my working diagnosis was one of a mixed neurosis (anxiety and depression) in a developmentally compromised boy. Attention Deficit/Hyperactivity Disorder was not available as a diagnosis at the time I worked with Andy. Although Andy could be hyperactive both at home and in my office, at school he was often subdued and withdrawn. I decided the intermittent hyperactivity was driven by a defensive regression in the face of potentially overwhelming affects.

I never considered using medication with Andy. There was insufficient evidence of an Attention Deficit/Hyperactivity Disorder. While he did have significant anxiety and depression, anxiolytic and antidepressive medications were only beginning to be used by child psychiatrists at the time I was treating him.

Buoyed both by the psychological test report and by the fact that Andy could be a sweet and engaging child, albeit for brief moments, I recommended as the treatment of choice an analysis at a frequency of four times a week. I explained to Andy's parents that I would also need to meet with them on a monthly basis for some time, and subsequently on a bimonthly schedule. After some consideration, Andy's parents agreed and the work continued over the next five years when it successfully concluded.

COURSE OF THE ANALYSIS

During the opening phase of the analysis, my interventions were aimed at two goals: establishing a working relationship with Andy and interpreting conflict whenever possible. Neither proved an easy task.

Andy's begging behavior that had emerged during the consultation persisted for months. He endlessly pestered me for money. "Please, won't you say yes. I'll do anything you want if you give me that dollar bill." In many variations, I interpreted his belief that I could make him feel better with gifts which he imagined would fill him and take away his anger and fear. He became furious with my refusals. He threatened and sometimes attempted to destroy objects in my office. When I asked him to put his angry feelings into words instead of trying to break things, he would fill his mouth with wads of tissue which both gagged him and enacted the fantasy that I was filling his mouth and satisfying his intense longings.

During this early work, I decided my principal task was to help Andy accept the limits, frustrations, and possibilities of the analytic situation. I did not give Andy the food and money he attempted to extort from me. I did not let him dig through my pockets nor wreck my office and its contents. I set firm but flexible limits which I had to physically enforce from time to time. Of course, Andy treated me as if I were the cruelest, most stingy man he had ever met. At the same time, less consciously experienced, I believe Andy was reassured that I would not punish or reject him because of his emotionally driven behavior.

Because of his psychopathology and developmental delays, Andy was unable to engage in any symbolic play or games which could have permitted him to express his feelings in a more socially conventional fashion. Moreover, he could not engage in any phase appropriate latency activity, so urgent and compelling was his conviction that only redress and restitution could make him better. Andy could not comfort himself, could not be comforted by his mother, and could not be comforted by me. His self-esteem had been damaged as a result of his bad relations with his family, his school failures, and his inability to obtain mastery over his drives. He could not stop his constant teasing of his sister, his slobbering over his father, and his masturbatory play with his dog. Andy believed his only hope for comfort and repair was restitution with gifts.

For months I simply persisted in my hope that Andy would form an attachment to me which could include the experience of being correctly understood and calmed by me. What I am describing is what Freud (1912) called the simple positive transference. It is characterized by the patient's largely unconflicted affectionate feelings for the analyst. In children like Andy, who are so angry, depressed, and anxious, I expect the simple positive transference to exert a consoling effect. I have called this aspect of the positive transference the "soothing transference" which becomes an important tool in clearing the path for interpretive work (Peltz, 1992).

During the first eight months of the therapy, Andy learned how to comfort himself, and to feel comforted by me, and an affectionate bond developed between us. This is how this sequence of events took place. After several months Andy found a game which comforted him: hide and seek. There was no place in my office which concealed his large frame, but that made no difference. He hid himself, I found him, and he was content. He did not easily tolerate my interpretation that in hiding himself he hoped to hide his bad and frightening feelings. He appeared indifferent to my idea that his pleasure in being found must be like the way a lost child feels when he is found by his mother. (Of course, early on, I tried to interpret to Andy whenever I thought it could conceivably help.)

The game and my interpretations evidently enabled Andy to resort less to the defensive regressions which fueled his begging and poorly controlled behavior. Andy began to play cards. Sometimes he would play with me, but more often he played by himself. His favorite game was solitaire in which he engaged with quiet concentration. Deeply engrossed in his game, he did not respond to my observations or questions. But he was calmed! He had found a way to soothe himself, and peace reigned in the office. His newly developed capacity to soothe himself, coupled with his increasing comfort in being with me, permitted me greater opportunity for interpretive work.

Second Year of the Analysis

Becoming bored with card games, he switched to making paper airplanes. He sailed these planes through the office hoping they would fly out the open window, both in spite of and because of my request that he confine their flight paths within the office. Over several months, as this play continued intermittently, I was able to observe to Andy that his airplane factory was busiest when his father was about to fly to a distant city on a business trip. I further ventured that he must get frightened when his father had to go away.

When his father left for a two-and-a-half-month trip during the second year of analysis, Andy doubled his aircraft production and disclosed the particulars of his fears. He was worried about mental patients who kill presidents. "Do you see mental patients?" he anxiously asked. He next dictated a story to me about a messy boy who left home because his father became mad at him. The boy spent the night in a church terrified as he watched cats eat rats. Soon Andy asked me to draw a picture of a serial killer, then retracted the request and made the drawing himself. He said of his picture, "He's drunk so he's crazy in the head." He captioned a second drawing of a balloon-headed monster with a serrated head and huge teeth, "Time Bomb." "That's a picture of me," he reflected.

During this period of the analysis things with Andy's parents were not always smooth. Andy's father was, in general, more benignly inclined toward the continuing work than was his mother. She, on the other hand, although more psychologically minded, was more frequently doubtful about the value of the work and critical of what seemed to be its early failures. She was often hostile and rejecting when I tried to reassure her. Yet Andy's mother not only had to bear the brunt of Andy's hostility, she had the complete burden of getting an often reluctant child to his treatment hours.

Furthermore, early during the second year, Andy's mother bitterly complained that Andy had become more overtly defiant and argumentative. She was losing patience with his one-sided view of justice. He demanded that all treats which came into the house be scrupulously divided between children and parents. At the same time, he staunchly refused to share when he came into some windfall. I tried to reassure his mother that as Andy came to know more about his warded off hostility, it would be inevitable that family members would be his first targets. I explained that as Andy felt less deprived and aggrieved, he could become more generous. His mother was not mollified.

As the analysis continued, Andy stopped begging for money and instead began begging for answers to his questions. Andy had long ago implied that being "dumb" was an inexcusable sin. He reaffirmed this opinion many times, as he made his paper airplanes. Crushing an airplane which didn't fly properly, he said, "Stupid airplane, it doesn't even know how to fly!" I told Andy, "You want answers to your questions because then you hope you won't feel dumb. But my giving you answers will never really make you feel better about your worries and sad feelings. The problem is you believe you cannot think for yourself." Thus we began to see how Andy's problems had succeeded in encroaching upon his cognitive and intellectual skills.

Andy next played out his demands for answers which replaced his whiney verbal requests. He began darting out of the office, insisting he had to go to the bathroom. Instead he would hide outside the door spying on me through a crack in the door. During one of the many hours in which he played this game, he excitedly reported watching a couple get married on TV. He was indignant that "Here Comes the Bride" was not played.

I talked with Andy about his wish to peek at me. I told him I knew he wanted answers to his questions. But peeking might also be connected with something that had really happened but confused him. I conjectured, "I can imagine you were peeking into a room, and you weren't sure what you were seeing. (His mother had told me that for a long time Andy was convinced he needed glasses and occasionally wore lensless spectacles around the house.) You rubbed your eyes. Maybe they burned. Perhaps you saw something going into or coming out of a person's mouth. You were frightened and wondered how much you had seen and how much you were imagining."

Andy confirmed part of this construction in the following way. He argued, "No, that didn't happen. But I did see once, I can't remember where it was, this guy who put a sword into his mouth. Except the sword kind of rolled up on itself like this tissue does, though it really wasn't going inside of him." He added, parenthetically, "But I didn't tell you my eyes burned when I read too much—I told you they hurt." Sometime later he additionally confirmed my construction. He remembered when he was about 4, he wanted to look into a darkened horse trailer. His father picked him up so he could look over the tailgate. Out of the darkness a dog leapt at him, biting him near his eye.[1]

In contrast to this sequence, the occasions when Andy actively participated in the analytic work were few. He was pleased

---

[1]Although derivatives of primal scene excitement and anxiety recurred throughout the analysis I did not further or more explicitly reconstruct the primal scene.

enough simply to come to his hours and be with me. I remained vigilant for the opportunity of interpreting whenever I could. When he was not insisting that we play quietly without talking, Andy busied himself folding origami birds intended as gifts for his mother. Yet the transference wishes asserted themselves and the begging frequently recurred. When his anger and frustration with me got the upper hand, Andy would wage a war of stony silence. I told him he was not giving me anything because he felt I was not giving him anything. He must experience me as he does his teachers at school and his mother at home. I wouldn't give him things because I was stingy and because I preferred girls to boys.

Andy immediately knew what I was talking about. Many times before he had insisted that I close my eyes so he could scamper into my lap to hug me and speak in a girlish falsetto voice. His longed-for but dreaded wish to be a girl was dramatized more explicitly in play when his dog became pregnant. Andy lay on the couch, encircling with his arms the space above his abdomen. The fantasy was enacted in the transference as Andy came to hours with his pockets stuffed with sundry items. He insisted I guess what was inside of his pockets, just as he was constantly guessing at how many pups his dog would have. This was expressed in the ghost stories he recounted to me. His favorite was *The Monkey's Paw* in which the first of three wishes granted to a mother results in the amputation of her son's hand, and the third leads to his death.

Third Year of the Analysis

As the fourth grade drew to a close, Andy was a remarkably changed boy. He no longer arrived for his appointments in dirty clothes and unkempt hair. He no longer regressively clung to his family but played out-of-doors with boys his own age. Occasionally he could even play with his older sister. He was reading at grade level as measured by standardized state tests and, remarkably, had made the honor roll at school. At this time Andy's former refusal to be read to began to wane.

Grudgingly, he began to allow his father to read to him. Interestingly, for a very long time the only book he would listen to was Jack London's *Call of the Wild.*

It never became clear how Andy learned to read. His interest in reading appeared to be announced by his willingness to listen to his father read to him. He occasionally took the risk and read to his father. Once this happened, and as the analysis progressed, he achieved grade level reading (and writing) during the third year of the analysis. I am convinced that the resolution of Andy's anxiety about looking and thinking allowed him to acquire the reading skills he needed. But I have wondered what else contributed to this development. I know that Andy was helped at school. I have also wondered if Andy developed his own techniques to facilitate the task of learning to read. Only retrospectively at the conclusion of the analysis did I venture this conclusion. I became persuaded that the therapeutic action of the analysis succeeded in greatly diminishing the anxiety and depression that fueled Andy's regressed and driven behavior. Less crippled by psychological turmoil, Andy was enabled to address his wish that he could read and the reality demand that he must by whatever means became available to him.

Fourth Year of the Analysis

Andy continued to explore his fear that he was dangerous and a potential crazed killer who would be punished. Ultimately he was able to reconcile for himself that volatile anger was compatible with a sound mind. A typical sequence follows.

Reporting the latest news of a serial murderer, and seemingly unrelated, he asked, "Did you ever cut yourself so that the blood came gushing out?" I answered, "Sure," and showed him a small thumb scar. He confided, "I got a fish hook caught in my head once." He parted his hair so that I could see the scar. Soon he regressed and became silly and wild. He threw a can against the wall which nicked the paint. He looked at me apprehensively, expecting me to admonish him. I talked with him about this sequence: first fear of crazed killers, then silliness and its consequences, and then the expectation that he would be punished.

During the prior couple of years, Andy had been frightened and angry at a neighbor, a cross old woman who frequently scolded Andy and his friends. Now, two years older, he reported that he and his friends were simply playing catch in front of her house when she yelled at them and threatened to call the police. Andy could not understand why she wanted to take such drastic action. Andy commented, "She's mental, she's stupid, she's crazy, and she's always yelling at us." I reminded him that when he first came to my office he thought he was mental and stupid because he had to see a "feeling doctor." Andy smiled and knowingly replied, "I know I'm not mental, but she really is." A couple of days later Andy related some news as if it were a cautionary tale. The mother of his best friend had to go to a mental hospital for a week because she had such a bad temper!

Still later we were able to more explicitly examine Andy's volatile temper. Andy described a camp experience from the prior summer. Andy and his cabin mates brought firecrackers to camp with them. Secretly, when alone, they placed a firecracker in a glass bottle, topped by a tennis ball. In awe, Andy exclaimed, "The ball went so high I lost sight of it." The camp director found Andy's firecrackers and confiscated three packs, which he promised to return when Andy left camp. Fiercely, Andy exclaimed, "And he didn't. He broke his promise!" I told Andy I knew he felt as if he were an exploding firecracker when promises to him were broken.

At this time, Andy developed a new way of torturing family members, which raised questions in their minds about whether he *was* "mental." He endlessly repeated an apparently meaningless random phrase, which the entire family found crazy. "Is he schizophrenic?" his mother angrily demanded. She was somewhat pacified when, with complete confidence, I told her I knew he was not. I reminded her that he was beginning to read at near grade level which spoke to the integrity of his mind.

Although Andy had become reassured that he did not have a damaged mind, he continued to believe that the forbidden act of looking would be punished by injury to his eyes. This fear impacted upon and intensified his immense castration anxiety. As we analyzed these issues, Andy remembered additional traumatic scenes. The revival of these memories not only helped Andy to master the trauma, but explained, in part, his counterphobic defensive stance.

Andy, who spent much of his recreational time at the ocean, had become very interested in its lore. After returning from Disneyland, he described his submarine ride in detail. He mused about the creatures of the deep. He recalled once seeing a shark through the porthole of a sailboat. "No," he asserted, "I wouldn't be scared of one even if I saw it when I was swimming." But he cautioned, "Even if there is one drop of blood, then the shark gets you and there will be a whole bunch of sharks coming right away. And that's for true."

We pursued this issue over many months. Once, as we played cards, Andy twice encircled his wrist with a rubberband. He said, "You know if you stop the blood from going into your hand, it will be like your hand is dead and you won't be able to move it anymore." He added, "That's what happens when half of the people die. Their hearts stop pumping blood and they can't move anymore."

I reminded Andy that only recently he had spoken the word *death* in such a quiet whisper that I was almost unable to hear him. "Death must frighten you," I said. In a mock and condescending tone Andy retorted, "You say such stupid things sometimes." Sprawling on the floor, he added, "Do you know what the Indians used to do? They used to cut open their chest and put a stone inside and sew it up again, just to show how brave they were." I told Andy I thought he had often done similar things. He did frightening things bravely to show his courage. Andy again retorted, "You say such stupid and dumb things."

Some weeks later, after telling me about catching some sharks, he played the following game. He interlaced his fingers, keeping one cupped out of sight within his folded hands. I was to guess which finger was missing, which I could not do. I then asked Andy about his fear of accidents, including loss of fingers or arms, reminding him of several of his shark stories. Andy responded with a never-before-reported memory which he dated to age 6: "I saw this accident where a man's head rolled off. I really didn't see that; someone told me about it. What I saw was this horrible wreck and the guy's hand sticking out of the window. Blood was covering the back seat. It was really gross. We were traveling in Europe then."

Andy's next association was remarkable: "That was the time we went in this cave and inside there were these things like icicles hanging from the ceiling and coming up from the floor of that dark cave." I responded, "Some boys and men believe a woman's vagina is like that: a dark cave with teeth inside." Andy replied, "That's interesting," and drew a picture of sharks' teeth.

Several months later, after seeing a video of *King Lear,* he reported, "Especially after they pick the guy's eyes out. Ugh! Sick! Everyone in that picture gets stabbed and dies." He then asked, "Have you ever seen anyone without an eye?" He recalled, "Once at a service station I saw a man without an eye. Just skin. It didn't look too bad." (I did not believe he was convinced.) Andy excitedly associated to watching firecrackers explode. I told him, "I believe you are afraid that if you see something very exciting you will get punished and lose an eye."

Andy's anxiety about injury to his eyes, although muted, persisted. Typically, Andy announced his fear by using Kleenex to shield his eyes. Most frequently, his worry surfaced as we explored his curiosity in general and his sexual curiosity in particular. Yet alongside the exploration of this anxiety, Andy at age 11, was making rapid intellectual and social strides. He felt increasingly competent in school, maintained his reading skills, and very impressively, for me, became able to clearly summarize and narrate the stories of the television shows he watched.

There is no question in my mind that real traumata impacted Andy's use of his eyes, his target organ so to speak. These traumata were also incorporated into his primal scene fantasies. Andy's memory of the dog who leapt at him out of the dark also proved to be a screen memory for a strain trauma which had taken place at roughly the same time. During the second year of analysis, Andy's father, evidently in association to my asking about primal scene exposure, had told me a significant piece of history.

When Andy was about 6 his great uncle and his adult daughter paid the family an extended visit. The great uncle had been blinded by failed surgeries for detached retinas. The daughter who accompanied him had one glass eye. No derivative of this material emerged until very late in the analysis when Andy spoke of seeing a man with a yawning eye socket covered by skin. By that time I had completely forgotten that piece of history and so could not exploit an opportunity to integrate an historical trauma with a contemporary experience.[2]

Evidently not all aspects of trauma need to be revived in an analysis. Andy and I apparently did enough work to vitiate the effects of the eye traumata. Andy could begin using his eyes aggressively, as in reading, without fear of blindness. He felt as if he were now allowed to use his eyes.

This permission was extended to Andy's thinking. It allowed him to become convinced that his mind was intact and that he was not a crazed serial killer. In turn, his capacity to tolerate anxiety was increased so that we could investigate his emotional conflicts. Working together interpretively, we explored the layers of compromise formations embedded in his symptoms and his character traits.

Andy's cupped hand trick with the disappearing finger prefigured his disclosure of his masturbation and his anxiety over phallic competence. In the prior several months, Andy had

---

[2]To clarify the chronology, I will list Andy's infantile visual trauma and their temporal relation to the onset of Andy's learning problems. Andy's teachers reported Andy's classroom difficulties when Andy was 6 and in the first grade. The reading problem was grossly apparent by the end of second grade, and the parents first consulted with me as Andy began third grade. Andy remembered that he was 4 when he peeked into the darkened horse trailer. (I did not confirm this age with the parents.) Further, Andy, again unconfirmed by me, believed he was 6 when he witnessed the bloody automobile accident. The parents place Andy's age at 6 when the blind great uncle and glass-eyed aunt paid their visit.

There was never any doubt in my mind of the interrelatedness between primal scene fantasy and anxiety and visual trauma. I believe Andy and I were able to sufficiently analyze both elements, fantasy and trauma, thereby enabling Andy to make better adaptive compromise formations.

been preoccupied with the consequences of bad habits, like smoking and drinking. Finding a right moment, I asked if he were worried that he had some habits that he believed might damage his health. He scoffed, "What bad habits are you talking about?" This was followed by a seemingly innocent question. "Do you want me to take my shoes off?" Andy immediately pulled off his boots, smelled them, and exclaimed, "Phew!" He then began rubbing his feet. I told him, "I believe you are telling me about your habits. You rub yourself and then get very frightened that something bad will happen to you."

Following this, he brought in one of his recent gifts, a fountain pen. He insisted that he compare his pen to mine. During this inspection, he reflected, "My father has a fountain pen too, except that the point of his pen is different." As he concluded his comparison, he decided his pen was fatter and made a darker line than mine. I wondered aloud that even though this was the case, he still might have doubts about whose pen was the best: my pen, his father's or his. Andy stoutly denied he had any question. His pen was the bigger and better. Yet he also offered to trade pens. Later, in the same hour, he disclosed that after a lot of tugging he allowed his father to pull out a wiggly molar tooth. A week passed and Andy reported his first dream of the analysis, now in its fourth year. In the dream he was brushing his teeth when the alarm awakened him. He associated that he knew his dad liked him to brush his teeth.

Andy's increasingly tamed sadomasochistic love for his father was a constant presence. When he was in a good mood, he gently teased his father as he found the opportunity. For example, when his father drove him to his appointment, Andy would attempt to leave the hour, unnoticed by his father. His father would have to find him outside the building, and joined in the game in good spirits. I observed to Andy that in these games, "Your dad has to wait for *you* and find *you*, much as you have to wait for him during his many trips."

When we began to face the fourth year summer break, Andy was confronted with a double loss: his father left for a month's trip and there was the prospect of my month's vacation. He wondered both about what I would be doing and where his father would be traveling. He reported that his mother cried as his dad boarded the airplane, which startled him. Then he found tears running from his eyes. Defensively, Andy claimed the sun must have shined in his eyes. I reflected that I thought he was sad because both his dad and I were going to be away at the same time.

Andy's feelings about me were not pure and unalloyed. Although he liked me, he remained convinced I was a stingy, rich man who only cared about him because of the money his parents paid me. He expressed his idea that rich men also had worries. They lived in fear of robbers who would kidnap and/ or steal all their money. Somewhat fearfully Andy confided, in spite of such fears, he hoped he would become a rich man.

His recurrent transference love surfaced, from time to time, usually accompanied by displays of castration anxiety. On Valentine's Day, he brought me a card which read, "Don't keep me up in the air. Be my valentine." He then began to play with some toy soldiers, engaging them in war games. I reflected that although soldiers are trained to fight, they might also love each other. Maybe they even gave valentines to their best friends. Almost immediately Andy asked, "Do you know where the main artery of the heart is?" Correcting me when I pointed to my chest, he held out his wrist. "If you cut this, you could die!"

Andy's hostility toward me surfaced in anxious forebodings. He made daily trips to my calendar that led him to reflect on the year 2000. "Who will be alive?" he wondered. "Will my father, my grandfather, or you still be alive?" His mood promptly flattened as he assured himself that he certainly would be alive into the next century.

Andy's sisters were also never far from his thoughts. Again as he was leafing through my desk calendar, he spotted my reminder, "Sue's birthday." He angrily asked, "Who is Sue?" When I did not answer, he grabbed a pair of scissors and began cutting his sneakers. I told him my calendar note reminded him of the girls who came to my office. He must feel very angry and jealous of them. In response he wrote the words *love* and *peace* on separate pieces of paper and stuffed them under my eyeglasses. I acknowledged, "I know you love me and want peace in the office. Yet when you become jealous and angry, you forget about your loving and peaceful feelings."

Very soon, Andy became able to experience and speak of his jealousy without regressing. We had begun to play poker through many of his hours. I finally insisted we reserve at least some time at the end of the hour to talk. When for the first time I enforced this rule, Andy angrily turned his back to me and cried. These were the first acknowledged tears he had ever shed in my office. I told him I knew it saddened him when we couldn't play cards all the time. He turned around, faced me, and said, "You probably play poker all the time with the girls, and then you don't feel like playing with me." He insisted I promise to play poker for all the time he wanted.

As the analysis progressed, Andy's relations with his parents vastly improved. I cannot emphasize enough Andy's mother's pleasure when she could begin to feel that her son was not damaged. In the prior year, she reported that Andy's overt sexual play with the dog had virtually stopped. She glowed when she reported Andy's progress in reading, further confirming to her that Andy was a healthy boy.

As Andy became more affectionate and less sullen with his mother, she was able to respond reciprocally. In the comfort of their newfound relationship, the mother confessed to me a secret she had consciously withheld. She acknowledged her responsibility for the emotional distance between herself and Andy when he was a toddler. Andy had become identified in her mind with her older brother who had died when she was 3 years old. The mother had grown up increasingly embittered that she had never been able to compete for her parents' love because of their preoccupation with the dead, idealized brother.

Even given Andy's improved relationships at home, his tendency to defensive regression recurred when his father traveled away from home for more than a week. Then Andy would target his mother with angry tirades and belligerent behavior. For example, he berated her when she failed to take him shopping with her if he wanted to go. Scenes like this would end with Andy's rageful complaints that he simply hated both his mother and father. He would become unbearable to his mother (less so to his sisters) until his father returned. I could only sympathize with Andy's mother during these terrible times.

In my opinion, the heart of the work during the second half of the analysis, which heightened during the termination phase, was Andy's struggles with his feelings about his mother: his deep hostility, his fear, and ultimately his sense of her betrayal. This nexus of affects and fantasies, which comprised the core of Andy's depression, was consciously experienced and explored most often in relation to his school principal and the crabby neighbor. Andy was convinced both women hated boys. In this context, he reported that his friend's cat ate two kittens of her recent litter. He remembered that a friend's rabbit ate all her bunnies. He lay on the couch and imagined again that he was pregnant. Pretending that he was karate chopping his abdomen, he exclaimed, "You hit her in the liver, you hit her in the gut, and then you hit her in the kidneys." I responded, "I think you believe that is what should happen to a mother who eats her babies. And I know you want to be very strong and good at karate to protect yourself from women like your principal and your neighbor who hate boys."

A week later Andy wondered aloud what an abortion was, having watched a television hospital show which dramatized this procedure. He was clearly puzzled. When I asked him about it, he answered, "It's when a baby gets born before it's born." He immediately associated to some recent bad news. Three children of family friends would be spending the weekend at his house because their mother had just died of cancer.

Having become more tolerant of his anxiety when learning about frightening events, Andy pursued the abortion issue over the next several weeks. He was able to think clearly as he mastered the information. After a nocturnal nose bleed, he came to his appointment anxious and excited. "Hey, do you want me to tell you something gross?" "Sure" I answered. "Well, last night my nose bled all over the sheets. It was a mess. In the morning when I blew my nose, big bloody globs came out."

I told Andy I guessed his worry about nose bleeds must be connected to his curiosity about abortions which we had been talking about lately. After some haggling, Andy told me what he learned. "It must be very bloody, a big bloody mess. The doctor cuts the woman open and then pulls it out and then sews her up." Under his breath, he muttered, "Cuts her with a dull knife and takes out the bloody mess." I felt triumphant that Andy had allowed himself to know so much in spite of his anxiety. I believed Andy shared this feeling.

The Termination

In retrospect, the termination occupied the last year and a half of the analysis. Toward the end of the fifth grade, Andy declared he would not be returning when he was in the sixth grade. He mounted a vigorous campaign on behalf of his conviction. "I'm not going to come here in sixth grade! You promised me!" I acknowledged we had talked about it, but told Andy I was afraid we didn't have time to finish our work before the sixth grade. "What work?" he scornfully replied. He remained angry and sullen for days.

Andy did return in the sixth grade, but the analytic year proved to be grim for both of us. I only began to understand its meaning as we lived through it together. Immediately upon returning from the summer break, Andy angrily demanded to know why he was still coming to see me. He insisted I had promised he would not have to come during the sixth grade.

Although I had made no such promise, I also understood that this was Andy's psychic reality. He believed I had, and he felt betrayed by me. During many of the hours of that year, Andy sat in the swivel chair at my desk, his back to me, silently fiddling with the objects on my desk. In the analytic hours he seemed overall downcast and withdrawn. Often he complained of stomachaches and would leave the office for the bathroom. I felt locked out, discouraged, and sad for Andy. I was perplexed about how to reengage him. Little of what I said seemed to make a significant impact. I felt as if we were on opposite sides of a great divide. From time to time, the only words he uttered were, "I wasn't supposed to come here in the sixth grade." I repeatedly made the same interpretation, varying it as I could. "I understand you are furious with me because you believe I made a promise and broke it. I've disappointed you and you feel you cannot trust me." This scenario dominated the stage throughout the year. (There were brief interludes when Andy relaxed his intransigent stance and we briefly reconnected. During these breaks we resumed analysis of those conflicts that drove his anxiety.)

By midyear, there was some change. Andy seemed less angry, and more depressed. No longer sitting with his back to me, he often engaged in some mindless activity, or briefly described activities with his friends or family. From time to time, Andy would even read aloud to me from the newspaper or share a school assignment. During the sixth and seventh grades, his life outside the analysis continued to improve as did his self-esteem. He developed close friendships with peers. With them he fished, played individual and group sports, and began noticing the girls in his classes.

Pari passu with these developmental advances, Andy and I revisited and further analyzed conflicts and anxieties previously known. We also investigated issues that had previously been warded off: masturbatory anxieties, his transference love and hatred, and finally his war against the analysis and its meaning to him. This was the prelude to the termination phase proper.

Slowly, the meaning of the transference–countertransference engagement became clearer to me, if not to Andy. I understood the accusation of a broken promise to include much more than returning during the sixth grade. Evidently, I had become for Andy his mother as he experienced her when he was a toddler. She had broken an implicit promise to be there for him when he needed her. She had not been there. She had withdrawn from him.

I began reconstructing, in small segments, this piece of Andy's childhood experience. Armored by his maturity and our prior analytic work, Andy could better tolerate intense depressive affects without resorting to defensive regression. I told Andy I knew he believed I could never treat him fairly because he was convinced I preferred girls over boys. I became for Andy the hostile mother who, for no apparent reason other than my preference for girls and hatred for boys, broke my promises to him. Andy's claims for justice and redress were no better satisfied by me than they had been by his mother. Andy became filled with loathing and despair for himself, for me, and less consciously for his mother.

Thus the central trauma of Andy's infancy and toddlerhood, and his fantasied elaboration of it, was lived out during that painful year. It is not enough, in my opinion, to explain Andy's reactions simply on the basis of turning passive into active. Rather, I believe the more complete explanation is in the inevitability of the revival of this early maternal experience. It was the only way open to Andy and me if we were to analyze the depressive core of his neurosis. And this he accomplished with my help: analyst as transference object, analyst as the interpreter of unconscious mental life, and analyst as new object. Parenthetically, I do not believe my reconstructions of his mother's withdrawal from him to have been the mutative agent. Rather, it was our lived-out experience.

In spite of his great anger and sense of betrayal, Andy agreed to return the following fall as he entered seventh grade, so that we had time to say good-bye. This last phase of our work was concluded in four months. As we began, he disclosed his anxiety about going to high school the following year. Although he had stopped playing with toys several years before, he staged his apprehension with small plastic animals and toy soldiers. With their bayonets, the soldiers began poking the animals' anuses. I commented to Andy, "I guess you have heard high school guys horse around and sometimes goose each other." He had heard that. Deflecting, he demurred, "I'm not afraid of those high school kids."

After we agreed on a termination date, Andy responded by regressing. He teased and begged for my spare change. I reminded him of the very first time he came to my office. He had left the hour, holding up the skinny cow, and said, "Skinny cow. No milk!" I added I thought he was feeling like that now: empty and in need of refilling. He did not remember this experience, but was intrigued with my recalling of that first hour. I added I also thought he had forgotten the many times he had been left wanting by his mother. A couple of weeks later, after seeing *The Scarlet Pimpernel,* he spoke of the old hags who glee-fully watched men being beheaded by the guillotine. Andy re-newed his preoccupation with my calendar, always an indicator of his jealousy of the other children who came to my office. I told him he must be worried and sad that when he left, some other child would take his place.

As the end grew near, Andy became concerned about aging men and their illnesses. He reported a couple of events. An art teacher whom everyone hated had to leave school be-cause of a heart attack. And the very rich father of a family he knew also had a heart attack. That man was hospitalized for a month because of complications. I reflected to Andy that he probably was worried about me because he would no longer be seeing me. Andy responded that he thought he might want to be a doctor or a veterinarian when he grew up.

During the last couple of hours, we made mazes for each other, an activity we had abandoned years before. My final interpretations to Andy concerned his sadness and mine. Yet together we finally had found our way out of the maze of his troubles and of the tangles of our attachment to each other.

At the end of the analysis, Andy was mildly depressed but triumphant. He had made a best friend and, with him, experi-enced the joy and pain of intimacy. He became more interested in girls. In his analytic hours he could think clearly and coher-ently. He no longer needed prodding from his parents to com-plete his homework but promptly tackled it as soon as he arrived home. He was not afraid to compete academically and often made the honor roll. He even believed he would go to college. He could tolerate anxious and depressive affects with-out regressing. He could laugh at his failures instead of acting the clown. He largely stopped begging me for gifts, saving his money instead for the things he wanted. More confident of his mind and body, he was ready to take on the challenge of adolescence.

As Andy concluded the analysis, his maturity was a source of great pride and joy for his mother, his father, and for me. When his father traveled Andy was no longer terrified of step-ping into his shoes. His mother began to depend on him in many different ways and he fulfilled her expectations. What

mother enjoyed most was the increasing intimacy between the
two of them. He was able to talk with her about his feelings.
She had recaptured the son she lost when he was 3.

CONCLUDING THOUGHTS ON ANDY'S LEARNING PROBLEMS

Even at the conclusion of the analysis, I was unable to implicate
a specific etiologic factor underlying Andy's learning problems.
On the one hand the initial psychological testing did not disclose any underlying organic basis. Rather it suggested a causal
relation between Andy's severe neurotic problems and his
learning problems. On the other hand, one could make a case
for organicity pointing to the long and painful labor, Andy's
low birth weight, and his delayed acquisition of language and
the immaturity of his speech. Yet analysts and disabilities specialists often evaluate and treat children with learning disabilities in whom there is no history of perinatal trauma or low
Apgar scores. Nonetheless, these children develop symptoms
very similar to Andy's. Motor development proceeds normally
but is delayed. A delay in acquiring language may later be followed by reading and other types of learning problems. When
these children enter kindergarten, or shortly thereafter, their
teachers report the hyperactivity and difficulty in concentrating that leads to a diagnosis of Attention Deficit/Hyperactiv-
ity Disorder.

Even among this group of children, refined psychological
and educational testing frequently does not disclose any underlying neuropsychological problem. We are inevitably led to an
assumption of a neuropsychological underpinning as the etiology of the disorder. But we do not as yet have the knowledge
which allows us to know where and what has gone awry. I think
it would be fair to state that whatever the neuropsychological
underpinnings of Andy's learning problems, emotional factors
made a significant contribution.

With or without neuropsychological underpinnings, Andy's experience was that his mind was damaged. This view was

strongly reinforced by his mother's perception (and to a lesser degree by his older sister) that Andy was a damaged child: retarded at best, schizophrenic at worst. Andy, as he began the analysis, held the same view. He believed he was both stupid and/or had the potential for becoming a crazed serial killer. Andy's anxiety about the intactness of his mind was always very much in the background of our analytic work, and was subjected from time to time to analytic scrutiny. By the fourth year he told me he knew he was not "mental," but that his neighbor was. He had by this time developed the retrospective understanding that he, like a firecracker, could explode because of the bright burning fury and excitement within him. Andy's anxiety about the integrity of his mind was heightened by the anxiety stream which was manifested in his sensitivity to separation and fears of injury to his body.

The analysis successfully enabled Andy to restore a sense of calm as his previously intense anxiety and depression receded. As this happened, Andy became confident of his mind and body.

Chapter 8

Discussion of Andy's Analysis

Dr. Peltz's report of the analysis of Andy provides an experiment in nature. It poses the question of whether a psychoanalysis alone, without remedial instruction or other related interventions, can successfully treat a patient with a learning disability, and other possible manifestations of neuropsychological dysfunction. The resounding answer is that at least in some cases analysis alone can be extremely useful. Dr. Peltz agrees, as he indicated: "Incomplete as a therapeutic psychoanalysis without the tutoring in reading that I recommended, the treatment did conclude successfully. I could not have foreseen this result, and am unable to entirely explain it. Nor is it clear whether the treatment outcome would have been significantly different, had a discrete reading problem been diagnosed. . .''

A careful study of this analysis raises as many interesting questions as it answers. Andy's parents consulted with Dr. Peltz approximately fifteen years ago, at a time when a diagnosis of "organic" problems was typically viewed as a contraindication to analysis. (See also the discussion of Dr. Waldron's case in chapter 6.) Working in this climate Dr. Peltz concluded, upon completion of an extended consultation including a diagnostic testing evaluation, that Andy's hyperactivity and poor concentration were due to his rage and anxiety, and that his regressed behavior was defensive in nature.

Dr. Peltz believed that there was insufficient clinical evidence of a neuropsychological substrate, what would have been called "Minimal Brain Dysfunction" at the time, and therefore did not prescribe Ritalin or some other related medication. He felt that tutoring was advisable, which he recommended to Andy's parents, who did not implement this suggestion. They explained this on the basis of their son's refusal; we can speculate, however, that in light of their earlier fear that he was "damaged" and their delay in having him evaluated, Dr. Peltz's recommendation may have evoked in them feelings of intense anxiety and depressive affect.

The psychologist who tested Andy as part of Dr. Peltz's consultation reached the same diagnostic conclusion; indeed Dr. Peltz's clinical impressions were in part informed by the testing evaluation. In his view Andy's self-esteem problems and intense anxiety compromised what he believed to be Andy's greater potential: in the "Bright Normal" (above average) or "Superior" range. The examiner felt that Andy's earned IQ levels in the Average range were not a measure of his full potential. Andy's behavioral problems were also conceptualized as one manifestation of his anxiety and "considerable depression."

As Dr. Peltz has indicated, the evaluation performed was insufficient to carefully diagnose the reasons for Andy's academic difficulties. In reporting his findings, the psychologist emphasized Andy's clinical presentation of pronounced hyperactivity and anxiety. He was noted to be "squirmy" and "restless," "flip[ping] extension-wings of the typewriter table," playing with vertical window blinds and "knock[ing] into furniture." Andy clung to his mother, had a "fixed smile," expected failure, and "feigned dumbness rather than risk failure." However, hyperactivity was not incorporated into the diagnostic impression, for example, in the form of a diagnosis equivalent to what we now call Attention Deficit/Hyperactivity Disorder (a diagnosis which did not exist at that time).

It is true (as Dr. Peltz wrote) that the typical diagnostician at that time (15 years ago) did not have access to the full range of diagnostic tests and concepts available to us today. However, the evaluation performed with Andy was unnecessarily limited, even for that time. The battery administered to Andy consisted only of the standard IQ test for his age and an array of projective tests. Achievement tests of reading, math, and writing were not included. (Unfortunately, today, too, it is all too often the case that diagnostic evaluation of a patient's learning disability does not include a full examination of academic functioning.) Nor did it encompass more specialized tests of the individual building blocks for these complex tasks, which would permit a detailed assessment of the specific nature of Andy's learning problems from a neuropsychological perspective. Furthermore, the psychologist did not use the data he *did* have to maximum advantage. An analysis of the patterns of individual subtest scores of which the Wechsler IQ test is comprised, and/or a neuropsychological perspective on Andy's methods of accomplishing specific tasks, and the implications of these for an understanding of his academic problems, was not reported.[1]

Indeed Andy's problems in reading and other academic subjects were not even mentioned in the conclusions and recommendations which grew out of this evaluation. Attention was paid only to Andy's psychodynamic constellation and the adequacy of his psychological structure to permit him to make use of intensive analytic therapy. Andy's difficulties were attributed to his anxiety and depression, and thus the sole recommendation was for intensive treatment. This must have been a relief to Andy's parents who were so panicked by their secret belief that he was "organically damaged" that they had delayed having him evaluated for two years; Andy's behavioral and learning problems had initially been brought to their attention by his first grade teacher.

At the same time, Dr. Peltz's diagnosis of "mixed neurosis (anxiety and depression) in a developmentally compromised boy" implies that he considered Andy's neurosis to have developed within a constitutional framework. In this sense Dr. Peltz implies a dual cause of Andy's condition.

In our view Andy's history was highly suggestive of maturational difficulties, which were likely to have laid the groundwork for the (we believe, at least in part neuropsychologically

---

[1]An effort was made to contact the psychologist who did the original diagnostic work, in order to obtain subtest scores and any other data pertinent to our understanding of Andy's reading and other academic problems. However, given the large interval of time that had elapsed, the raw data had not been preserved.

based) learning difficulties which became evident in Andy's early school years. Dr. Peltz suggests that Andy's twelve-hour long labor and 6-pound birthweight might point to "organicity," although neither provides unequivocal evidence of such an etiology. More suggestive of a constitutional substrate for Andy's difficulties were delays in his development. He was $2^{1}/_{2}$ years old before he tried to speak, and 3 years old before his language could be understood. As early as first grade, Andy's teachers reported behavioral and learning problems. These were not evaluated, but rather avoided, by Andy's parents who feared he was organically damaged. By third grade Andy was virtually a nonreader and was functioning barely at grade level in other academic skills as well. Andy was also sometimes disruptive in the classroom, had difficulty concentrating, and was prone to daydream.

Although strictly speaking the information presented does not meet the current diagnostic requirements for ADHD, we believe that more detailed data from Andy's history meet the criteria for an Attention Deficit/Hyperactivity Disorder, Predominantly Inattentive Type as delineated in DSM-IV (see chapter 1). Dr. Peltz did not believe the diagnosis should be made by recipe without taking the entire history and psychiatric examination into account; with this general point of view, we concur. Dr. Peltz has indicated that, in the absence of consistent hyperactivity in the classroom (Andy was often subdued and withdrawn rather than hyperactive), he viewed the "intermittent hyperactivity" as defensive in nature. Thus he felt he could rule out what would have been called "Minimal Brain Dysfunction" at the time he saw Andy; clinically evident hyperactivity *was* considered crucial to make this diagnosis. Today, we are no longer faced with making such forced choices. That is, we do not have to automatically dismiss the neuropsychological basis of attentional problems when hyperactivity is clinically absent or only intermittently observable; we have the possibility of diagnosing an Attention Deficit/Hyperactivity Disorder with *or* without hyperactivity.

At the beginning of the analysis Andy behaved like a deprived animal who stuffed things into his mouth and could not tolerate deprivation or frustration for long (these, incidentally, are among the criteria for an Attention Deficit/Hyperactivity Disorder). Indeed Andy *had been* deprived. When his sister was born his mother, viewing him as self-sufficient, ignored and neglected him. Later she considered her son to be biologically impaired and must have communicated this to him in some manner.

The initial phase of the analysis involved Andy's "form-[ing] an attachment to his analyst which . . . include[d] the experience of being correctly understood and calmed" by him. Also central were Dr. Peltz's interpretations of Andy's wish to hide his bad and frightening feelings, his pleasure in being found in hide-and-seek games (as a child feels when he is found by his mother), and his fears of losing his father. Andy began to recognize his own anger, referring to himself as a "serial killer." He was also more angry at home; his mother in turn became angry at him for his selfishness and greed.

And greedy Andy was. In the analysis, he replaced his initial demands for food and money with begging for answers to questions. Andy felt defective mentally, as well as deprived of love and comfort. As his analyst said, "You want answers to your questions because then you won't feel dumb. . . . The problem is you believe you cannot think for yourself."

At this point we may wonder whether Andy was recognizing the existence of a (at least in part) neuropsychologically based problem in learning and controlling his impulses, which could have been addressed. Dr. Peltz (possibly intentionally avoiding a humiliating and devastating emphasis on an innate defect) put it another way. Emphasizing the conflictual aspect, he stated, "Andy's problems had succeeded in encroaching upon his cognitive and intellectual skills." This statement, while undoubtedly true, does not take into account (even if possibly wisely) a neuropsychological aspect of the equation.

We favor the view that neuropsychological factors played an important, but by no means exclusive, role in Andy's learning problems in particular and his psychopathology in general. It is also significant, as Dr. Peltz observed, that Andy reacted to his mother's view of him as defective. Further, Andy's mother's withdrawal from him after his sister's birth must have accentuated his feeling incomplete and therefore deficient. In contrast,

Dr. Peltz almost exclusively emphasized the psychogenesis of Andy's cognitive difficulties.

As the second year of the analysis came to a close, another determinant of Andy's cognitive difficulty came to the fore: the role of sudden and frightening traumata. Dr. Peltz responded to Andy's playing games in which he peeked at Dr. Peltz with a partial reconstruction of a primal scene experience he believed Andy to have had: "You were peeking into a room, and you weren't sure what you were seeing. . . . You rubbed your eyes. Maybe they burned. Perhaps you saw something going into or coming out of a person's mouth. You were frightened . . . " Although Andy at first rejected the reconstruction, he then recalled seeing a sword swallower and even connected Dr. Peltz's suggestion with his own reading difficulties; his eyes hurt when he read. Further, Andy recalled a frightening experience in which a dog leaped out of a dark truck and bit him near his eye.

This spectacular reconstruction and memory contrasted with the more manifestly humdrum nature of the analytic hours. Although much of Andy's activity appeared to lack drama, his playing and talking revealed an inner oedipal turmoil in which love for mother was experienced as dangerous and could lead to amputation, loss of one's eye, and even death. Along with this dynamic Dr. Peltz could interpret Andy's desire to be a girl as a defense against the imagined perils of being manly, but also as a result of Andy's awareness of his parents' preference for his sister. Andy's anxiety diminished as he mastered the shock trauma involving his eyes, and as he dealt with past primal scene experiences (involving vision and therefore his eyes) and their oedipal implications.

As this analytic work proceeded, Andy changed in a number of ways. He became much neater and friendlier. He learned to read (he was reportedly on grade level in reading and writing by the end of fourth grade), allowed his father to read to him, and occasionally took the risk of reading to father.

During the second half of the analysis, especially during the termination phase, the heart of the work had to do with Andy's struggles with his feelings about his mother: his deep hostility toward her, his fear of her, and ultimately his sense of her "betrayal." At the end of the treatment Andy was triumphant. Commenting on Andy's scholastic achievement, Dr. Peltz writes: "He no longer needed prodding by parents to complete his homework but promptly tackled it as soon as he arrived home. He was not afraid to compete academically and often made the honor roll."

Thus, Andy's learning problems were a central focus of the first years of the analysis, but they receded in importance during the second half. As Andy was less troubled by his school difficulties, he naturally had less need to talk about them. Nevertheless his analyst clearly maintained an awareness of the marked improvement in his patient's performance.

Although we can be sure that the analysis was having a distinctly positive effect, Dr. Peltz was not sure whether, and how, other factors contributed to Andy's improved academic achievement. Along with Dr. Peltz, we may ask what made for the amelioration? It would be of great interest to know more about the specific factors which enabled Andy to read. A number of considerations require discussion.

One is the interpretive analytic work per se; for example, the facilitation of Andy's use of organs associated with the fantasied dangers of the forbidden activity of looking. As Andy developed more effective ways of managing his anxiety and depressive affect, making drive and ego regression less necessary and potent, he was able to use his previously failed cognitive capacities. There certainly was a more adaptive balance and more flexible use of a wider variety of defenses. He was more organized, more able to see, and more able to recognize his urges. Correspondingly, he was likely to have been less afraid of the experience of active and passive intake necessary for reading and assimilation of other kinds of knowledge.

Also, as an outgrowth of the analytic work, Andy was better able to use his teachers' and his parents' help now that he felt more comfortable with them, less humiliated by receiving help, and more able to tolerate oedipal closeness without excessive fear of punishment through bodily injury. His relationship with his parents improved to their great pleasure. Although the clinical data do not permit us to know with certainty, we speculate that because of his improved interpersonal relations with his parents and teachers, Andy was better able to learn from them and engage with and apply himself to schoolwork, thus enhancing his scholastic achievement. Dr. Peltz had the impression that this was so. In addition, Andy may have (as Dr. Peltz suggests) "developed his own techniques to facilitate the task of learning to read."

In contrast to his effective and vigorous analytic exploration of the above-mentioned compromise formations, we note Dr. Peltz's caution in viewing, and then in talking about, the sources of Andy's learning problems. Although he thought that an "organic" component may have played an etiological role (based on a difficult and prolonged birth and a delay in development), Dr. Peltz never mentioned anything related to this perspective to his patient. In part, he was probably extremely cautious about this because the psychological test evaluation did not support such a point of view. Furthermore, Dr. Peltz would have been likely to downplay this possible source, even if he were certain that a birth injury was, in part, responsible for Andy's learning problems in particular, and aspects of his psychopathology in general. We imagine that he would have been concerned that telling Andy about this could have been misconstrued concretely to imply there was something wrong with his brain; this would have been experienced as a terrible narcissistic blow to Andy's already shaky self-esteem, and a repetition of his parents' view of him as deficient. Furthermore, hearing anything that could be interpreted as a statement of damage might have discouraged the patient, leading him to believe he could not change.

However, Dr. Peltz did *not* ignore Andy's recognition that he was defective in some sense; he worked with this interpretively in a number of ways. Andy himself thought there was something basic (if not biologically) wrong with him. He especially noted his temper and difficulty with control. In this context Dr. Peltz discussed Andy's worries about being unable to check himself. In addition, he emphasized the fact that Andy's parents thought him deficient, as well as their preference for his sister, as determinants of his feelings of deficiency. Dr. Peltz explored with Andy how their attitude had facilitated his use of feeling (and even wishing to be) defective, feminine, and castrated as a defense against the more dangerous masculine strivings of his Oedipus complex. Thus Andy's imagined or real limitations may well have served as fantasied punishments for forbidden wishes, as well as defenses against them.

One question sparked by a reading of this case is, Are we justified in not informing a patient of actual brain damage or neuropsychological dysfunction, in the service of protecting the patient against the humiliation of knowing about an actual "defect"? We wish to make it clear that Dr. Peltz did not feel convinced of a neuropsychological contribution, either in the form of an Attention Deficit/Hyperactivity Disorder (a diagnosis not available at the time) or a specific learning disability. Therefore, while his report enables us to discuss this question, it does not truly exemplify the process of making this clinical decision. In our experience, when the specific features of the neuropsychological dysfunction have been diagnosed, the injurious potential of making an otherwise more global statement of "defect" is reduced. While a confrontation with the fact of disability may be painful, a frank discussion of its nature and extent may also convey a tone of hopefulness, in that the problem is identifiable and, therefore, at least to some degree treatable. Often the disability is of lesser scope or degree than the patient has heretofore imagined. In fact, in our view not discussing with a patient his deficiency may be experienced as a confirmation of his humiliating sense of defect and may foster a maladaptive use of denial.

In studying the cases in this volume (as well as others not included in this book), one observes that analysts of patients with neuropsychologically based learning disorders tend to be cautious and often avoid a direct confrontation with the existence of this dysfunction. Psychological determinants tend to be emphasized. Ignoring neuropsychological factors may be difficult when the patient is taking medication for his disturbance, but even this sometimes occurs. Such sharing of denial by patient and analyst lends itself to an incomplete analysis. Even worse, it may repeat what the patient has experienced with his parents.

In working with such patients, the analyst must decide on how to strike a balance between stating the truth about a neuropsychologically based disorder and traumatizing the patient.

We believe that it is entirely possible to tactfully convey what is wrong and thus help the child to master the more or less serious consequences of such a disorder. In this regard, see Dr. Miller's report (chapter 4) of the case of Julia, a child who had suffered from a ventricular hemorrhage and consequent hydrocephalus, seizures, and learning disabilities. With gratifying results, a major focus of her analysis consisted of confronting and understanding her areas of disability, and the ways in which she both needed to defend against them and to employ them for defensive purposes.

Inevitably a person with a learning disorder, whether it is biologically based or results from psychic conflict, will suffer from the secondary effects of having such a disturbance. Optimally, the analyst and his patient will discuss how the patient's problems in learning, perceiving, and modulating impulses contribute to feelings of inferiority, sadness, and anxiety.

Chapter 9

Frank's Analysis

Sherwood Waldron, Jr., M.D.

PRESENTING PROBLEMS

Frank was $6^3/4$ years old when he was brought for consultation. He had become increasingly anxious in the previous few months, fearing skeletons and goblins at night, and having many nightmares. He also tended to be demanding, unhappy, and angry. When feeling anxious Frank often climbed into bed with his twenty-one-month-older brother, Chris.

Frank's unhappiness seemed linked to Chris' recent improvement. Frank's parents, Mr. and Mrs. Jay, reported that after two years of analysis, which had ended three months earlier, Chris had overcome much of his previous massive disturbance in functioning. Most central had been Chris' failure to handle the normal demands of school, which was associated with developmental lags and graphomotor disturbances. Previously Mr. and Mrs. Jay's feelings toward their two sons had been polarized. Mrs. Jay had felt angry and disappointed with her first child and preferred Frank. Mr. Jay tended to feel closer to Chris and annoyed at Frank's disrespectfulness toward him. Now, as Chris' functioning improved, Frank was losing (to some degree) his special status as mother's favorite.

Mr. and Mrs. Jay reported that two events preceded the onset of Frank's nightmares, although they were not sure if either one had contributed to their son's fearfulness: a teacher in his school fell down the stairs and was out of school recovering, and Frank's father went on a three-week business trip.

DEVELOPMENTAL AND FAMILY HISTORY

Frank's developmental history was unremarkable, with two exceptions. Frank still tended to suck his thumb, which he had done since being weaned from a bottle at one year of age. For many weeks after he started nursery school, Frank was unwilling to separate from his mother.

In giving a history, Mr. and Mrs. Jay described serious difficulties in their own lives, as well as in the lives of their parents. Mrs. Jay had a traumatic early childhood. Her parents had fled their native country when she was first born. When her father died shortly thereafter, Mrs. Jay's older sister was able to remain with their mother, because her being of school age permitted their mother to work during school hours; but Mrs. Jay who was younger had to be placed in foster care.

Frank's mother had always felt a sense of envy and of having been left out in comparison with her sister. She attributed her habitually permitting Frank's older brother to come into her bed to her own early experiences. Mrs. Jay showed a considerable naiveté and seeming lack of awareness of the effect of such experiences. Similarly she never found it important to regulate her children's TV exposure. Because of the many traumata of her early life, Mrs. Jay feared any change. She had been very tearful with her older son's analyst, leading to a referral for treatment about a year before Frank's initial consultation.

Mr. Jay had also suffered childhood traumata. His father, a successful professional who often did not have enough time for his children, died during Mr. Jay's adolescence. Mr. Jay had always had difficulty in school and did not like to read. He wondered whether *he* had had dyslexia. He showed even more difficulty in performing successfully following the death of his father. Despite his inability to complete his education, Mr. Jay functioned adequately at work. His mother, a dominant and proud figure, brought him into the family business. Despite his success, Mr. Jay regarded himself as having "relative ability" and difficulty in self-assertion. He was also markedly over-weight. In fact, *he* sought psychiatric referral from me during the consultation regarding Frank.

CONSULTATION

When I first saw Frank, he was a very polite boy who needed to be neat and clean. A timid and sad boy, he complained that his mother was away a great deal and did not pay enough attention to him when she *was* there. Furthermore, he felt that his father almost never played with him because he was too busy. Soon Frank described his fear that robbers would enter his house in the evening when his mother was away and kill him. He said he had nightmares about skeletons and worried about people dying, especially his parents and his friends. When during the session we played checkers and I won a few games, he grew agitated.

The immature and regressive elements in Frank's initial presentation, and my impression that he had a limited capacity to grasp or respond productively to my comments (there was even a certain obtuseness about him), made me feel hesitant to take him on for analysis. Despite my doubts, my supervisor (I was then a candidate in child analytic training) felt that the disturbances in Frank's communication patterns might well yield to analysis. Although Frank had had an initial evaluation at 4 years, 8 months by a group specializing in learning difficulties, we recommended further psychological testing. We hoped that a second evaluation would further assess Frank's potential and resources, and assist in deciding whether to recommend analysis.

First and Second Psychological Testing Evaluations

Frank's initial psychological testing evaluation, at 4 years, 8 months, took place prior to consultation with me. His mother explained that she took Frank for testing as a precaution, since some of his behavior patterns were like those of his brother. I only learned later, while reading the test report, that Mrs. Jay initiated this evaluation after the private school of her first choice had rejected Frank; he was considered too immature for their beginning grade. Mrs. Jay sought the help of the group of learning specialists who had been working with Frank's brother, in conjunction with the brother's recent analytic treatment.

The first evaluation showed that Frank was reasonably well-coordinated except for some trouble with throwing and catching a ball and with pencil control. Because of fine motor difficulties, his drawings gave an impression of primitivity, with few details. His Bender designs were also poorly executed; there were problems with organization of his work on a page.

Frank's language functioning was variable. He appeared to have adequate language comprehension, auditory discrimination, and sound blending. He had some difficulties in expressive language skills. While Frank was not markedly dysnomic on a formal test of naming, he occasionally misnamed animals when telling stories. He also sometimes had trouble formulating what he wanted to say and produced verbal constructions that were often immature in form. Frank attained a marginal score on a syntax screening test. His functioning on pattern and word matching activities left a great deal to be desired, as did his imitations of tapped sound patterns. While sentence memory was not very good, Frank's memory for verbal patterns was strong.

The projective material was not very informative, despite Frank's evident wish to please the examiner. This was not viewed as a manifestation of expressive language problems, but rather of his anxiety. The examiner had the impression Frank was "terribly nice," and that he probably suppressed and projected his aggression extensively, which contributed to his bad dreams and fearfulness. For example, in interpreting CAT pictures, Frank was troubled that the bears were in the child's bed; in another context, he was upset about a fire sequence. In completing a fable, he said that the child was most scared because "he didn't know he could make fire." A tendency to flight of ideas with a loosening of secondary process was noted, along with magical thinking. To illustrate, in one of Frank's productions an elephant changed into a magic lamb: "He could make some fire and he could make himself into a swimming pool and a fireman and change 'em back to a lamb."

The consultant then suggested to Frank's mother that he be seen again six months later for further evaluation. However, this did not occur, perhaps because Mrs. Jay felt she had her hands full with the analysis and tutoring of Frank's brother. In addition, Frank's mother had an investment in seeing Frank as the healthy one. She was extremely distressed about the difficulties of her first child.

When I recommended psychological testing, Frank's mother indicated her wish to consult a psychologist who did not have a particular bias toward learning difficulties. She chose the same person who had tested Frank's brother three years before, and whose work I also respected. This second testing, which took place when Frank was 6 years, 9 months, consisted of the WISC, Rorschach, CAT, figure drawings, and the Bender-Gestalt. Frank was described as behaving in a somewhat infantile way, with considerable apprehension and a wish to please the examiner. This was regarded in part as a defense; Frank appeared to prefer being seen as the baby, quickly retreating from competition, which was unconsciously associated with castration anxiety. The psychologist believed his immaturity to be related to certain weaknesses in language function, and other cognitive aspects of his test performance.

On the WISC Frank attained a Verbal IQ of only 106 (in the Average range) and a Performance IQ of 127 (in the Superior range), giving him a Full Scale IQ of 117 (in the High Average range). Frank's command of general information and number skills was mediocre. The examiner felt he was selective about what he wanted to know and not to know. In the preliminary interview, he did not know his birthday, and gave an impression of passive negativism rooted in conflicts over sexual and aggressive wishes. A high score in the Picture Arrangement subtest suggested a good understanding of social relationships that was at odds with Frank's surface immaturity. The content of his responses to verbal subtest items of the WISC often involved catastrophes. A tendency toward passivity and helplessness rather than self-reliance was evident. For instance, when asked "What is the thing to do if you lose one of your friend's balls?" Frank suggested calling for the police to help, or that mother would buy another ball. In response to a question about ways in which a brick or stone house is better than one made of wood, Frank emphasized strength and warmth: "A wooden house has leaks—in the snow time it could blow out your fire and you have no matches."

Projective material was suggestive of Frank's sexual identity confusion. His figure drawings included an ill-defined male figure and a devouring female figure with phallic extensions. There were errors in the use of personal pronouns. Frank also showed a tendency to exclude his father and put him at a distance from the family constellation. When asked what his three wishes were, he developed a flood of ideas, as he repeatedly fashioned each group of three wishes to include a final one for three more wishes. Considerable sadomasochistic preoccupation emerged as well, in an array of frightening and exciting fantasies. These were, in part, related to considerable overstimulation at home.

The examiner did not mention the existence of specific learning difficulties. Rather she found Frank "an appealing, potentially bright child whose mediocre language achievements suggest a turning away from academic learning." Her concluding remarks concerned evidence of "oral and anal regressive fixations, obsessive–compulsive features, phobic fears, acute castration anxiety, a symbiotic attachment to his mother, feelings of depression, loneliness and fatigue. . . . Frank's confabulatory fantasies suggest transient phobic distortions of reality. . . . Frank's need for help and his favorable therapeutic outlook are indicated."

Recommendation for Analysis

As Frank's parents and I discussed the psychological test findings, I emphasized how these provided an independent confirmation of my own impression: that Frank would be best served by an intensive therapeutic experience, preferably four times weekly in analysis. I added that the work so far on a twice weekly basis showed there was much for Frank and me to work on together, and that we would have every hope of accomplishing more in analysis. I recommended that I see his parents periodically so they could tell me what was happening in Frank's life. I suggested that I see his mother every week except when I saw his father, which was approximately every month.

Mr. and Mrs. Jay had developed a sufficiently positive connection with me by this time that they could accept the recommendation. Since the summer holiday was near, we agreed to begin four times weekly in September. The psychological testing also led to productive discussions of overstimulation at home, suggested by references to tickling in the psychologicals. During several interviews with Frank's mother, we clarified her tendency to withdraw into a self-involved state of mind, leaving Chris free to pick on Frank. At such times she provided little supervision or regulation. There was evidence of a fairly intense sadomasochistic relationship between the two brothers.

For the remaining months until the summer holiday Frank continued to come twice weekly. In these sessions, Frank's feminine identification became increasingly clear. He showed an excited interest in playing with a doll in the office, which he both warded off and which he expressed in sadistic games of killing. This was followed by expressions of anger, including wishes to kill the girl baby because it did not have a penis. Frank repeatedly confused the pronouns ''he'' and ''she.'' He also showed a tremendous preoccupation with what he received in his mouth: a tendency to put toys, guns, and bottles of soda into his mouth to suck them.

Mrs. Jay gradually told me about the concern she and her husband had about Frank's masculinity. The two boys often shared a bed, and Frank's brother tended to kiss him. In addition, Frank sometimes exhibited his body to his mother; he would wrap a towel around him and then drop the towel, saying that he was Miss America. He was also interested in dressing in his girl cousin's clothes.

In the therapy sessions, Frank repeatedly tried to outwit me. He played a robber who held me up. Or after I held him up, he would save himself with the help of a secret knife or gun. He initiated and played such games repeatedly with great excitement, while shying away from discussing fights with his brother in which he felt helpless. In his aggressive and tricky play with me he indicated the excitement, the sense of danger, and the seductiveness that must all play a part in the relationship with Chris, although little of this could be interpreted at this time. He brought up additional material that had to do with his envy of women and the diamond rings they might have. Meanwhile, Frank wished to drink up all the ginger ale that I would give him, and took pleasure in excitedly being wild and spilling it.

At the same time, I heard from his mother how he liked to act like the baby and sit on his mother's lap. There was a medley of regressive themes tied in with the aggressive ones, such as making chalk dust in the office, which would cause a person to choke to death. It turned out that his brother Chris had for years been quite preoccupied with violence and death, and with movies in general.

COURSE OF THE ANALYSIS

Following my August vacation, Frank began to come four times weekly. He was 7 years old and entering second grade. As had been true in the twice weekly sessions, the material spilled out in somewhat chaotic fashion. One salient focus was messing and spilling in the office. In this context, I interpreted Frank's wish to annoy his mother by making a mess and his worry that she would be mad at him.

An ambivalent transference appeared in Frank's frequently sticking me up or shooting me but also wanting to cuddle up on my lap. He introduced a game that was frequently repeated through the first year of analysis. He was a superbaby who could beat everybody up and fly around. There was a continuing intrusion of fears of injury to his body, such as losing his finger in a hole in a toy, which was then defended against with excited, sadistic fantasies of crunching ants or games of killing soldiers.

Frank's fantasies began to center on pregnancy and the birth process, following his mother's telling him about how babies are made. He could be cruel in the sessions, hammering on the penis of the baby boy. He developed a fear of being shot at a military organization for children called the Knickerbocker Greys, which he attended regularly. In play there were babies who survived persecutors who tried to destroy them all. Sometimes the persecutor shared Frank's characteristics.

Frank expressed gender confusion and bisexual fantasies involving his father and himself. He began to express a fear of being fat, which then led to the fantasy of an orange tree growing from a seed in his stomach, and then in turn to having a baby in the stomach; in this context Frank mentioned his father's large stomach. Maybe his father had a baby in there, he thought. What large doo-doos his father could make. Meanwhile there were many errors in the use of personal pronouns in which he confused the sexes. Frank's negative oedipal wishes and need for punishment were expressed in his tendency to provoke his brother, me or his father into an attack of a verbal or physical nature. (In fact his father *did* administer a spanking or a punch several times a year.) Frank's castration anxiety was expressed in his observation that women don't have ''a wiener'' because the baby has to come out there. An anal fantasy about birth was revealed in many jokes about doo-doo and how babies can make doo-doos, like mothers can make babies.

Interpretations were fairly limited during this time because of Frank's tendency continually to dismiss as unimportant anything I might say; he did not want any interference with his wild and exciting play. Frank's play in the hours paralleled his play with his brother and, later (when his brother seemed to settle down), with a friend and classmate who substituted for the brother. As Frank continued to belittle the value of any remarks I might make, he gradually brought out how dumb I must be to allow him to misbehave and be wild in the office.

Meanwhile material from Mrs. Jay indicated her great difficulty in setting limits. She allowed Frank to lie on her lap in public restaurants, for instance, and in many ways did not expect him to control himself or tolerate waiting. His father also acted somewhat helpless when challenged by his son. For instance, Frank told his father to kiss him on the behind, and called him fat. Frank was also excitedly interested in trying to peek and see his mother undressed.

I said that maybe Frank worried about being close to his father and therefore put his father down. Then Frank began to express wishes to be close to his father, and annoyance with his brother for being the one who is close to father. An incident occurred in which Frank acted out his wish for love from both his father and me. On the way home from my office Frank went off with a man who asked him if he would like to be a doctor's assistant. Although he finally left this man, Frank had strayed dangerously from his usual route home. As we explored this, he verbalized his temptation to be with this big man; associated with this was material about shooting people in the "ass." I interpreted that he wanted to be close to the man and was tempted to have something stuck in his ass. This led to his wish to be my assistant, to be able to look at naked people like doctors can. Simultaneously there was a representation in play of a fellatio fantasy. Frank wanted to poke a play sword into me but then put the sword into his own mouth.

After the New Year, he increasingly expressed his wishes to rob, first his brother, then me and, to a lesser extent, his father. He developed fantasies of a little person, a robber, who had a "maneuver mover" which was concretely represented by a protruding penislike object that could protect him from any danger. Frank's wish to rob his brother led to an interpretation of his fear his brother would kill him as punishment. There was much material pointing to excited, sadistic sexual fantasies and wishes to masturbate, and constant temptations to put forbidden objects in his mouth. At the same time Frank acted out his battle with me by frequently coming late and by accusing me of being a bandit if I had a wedding ring. This offered opportunities to interpret his envy of me. Usually the interpretations focused on Frank's anger at his father, but sometimes angry feelings at mother's rules emerged as well.

Jealousy of both mother and father and their intimacy with each other were evident, especially on Valentine's Day. This was accompanied by feelings about how it would be nice to be a "she" and receive father's gifts. Frank's urge to be the bad boy and do things he was not supposed to do increased. He attempted to take things he should not at the office, and expressed fantasies and play about superbaby beating up the father. An anal expression of defiance—the wish to make a doo-doo, or something messy—continued to color the material. Subsequently, considerable feelings of inadequacy, of being so small and of not being able to do many things he wanted to do, emerged. Then for a time Frank seemed to become more accepting of having to wait to grow up.

Frank expressed expectations that I would not help him to master things that he wanted to learn. This was the first direct expression of concerns about learning, as he approached his eighth birthday. Frank indicated how his mother keeps him a baby. After I interpreted how he wanted mother to keep him a baby but, in another way, he wasn't so happy about this, Frank verbalized for the first time the fun he sometimes had playing with his father. At this time Mrs. Jay began to complain that the boys were becoming more independent; it was evident that she wished to undermine this move away from her.

In the late spring Frank's tendency to take things that belonged to others became stronger; he told lies to cover his thefts. This urge was also related to Frank's wish to be a baby, in the sense that he acted like somebody who is so young that he does not know right from wrong. Frank was frightened by the consequences of his stealing sweet things: the cavities that he would get, the danger the dentist would pose.

During the same time interval Frank emphasized how boys love their mothers best. He returned to the view that he did not care for his father. He also explained he should not *want* to be close to father; that would be "sissy stuff." In play Frank continued to express wishes to be kissed by father. There were also people who were out of control and got hurt, and envy of those who had big water guns. Father manifested excitement and anxiety about holes that one man made in another by shooting him. Such fear and arousal were defended against by counterphobic play in which he was the one who was doing the damage.

Frank's emphasis on the pleasures of sucking and putting things in his mouth came into particular focus when he visited the dentist's office. As his anxiety about these pleasures was explored, Frank expressed his fantasy that he might bite the dentist's finger; acting like a baby protected him against danger from the dentist. Frank's oral regressive behavior sometimes became quite pronounced, for example, he once spilled ginger ale and then licked it off the table in my office.

Having survived the visit to his dentist, Frank brought out more clearly his envy of his father: the loud noises that his father's poo-poo made in the bathroom, how big his father's wiener and backside were. Frank attempted to make himself feel better by buying many objects he observed in my office. Interpretations were made of Frank's envy and fear of retaliation by father and me.

Once Frank's eighth birthday arrived, his parents started giving him a larger allowance to provide him with enough money to save for presents for family members. Instead he tried to get away with spending all the money on himself and went to considerable effort to conceal and dissimulate his disobedient behavior. At the same time he expressed a fear of adopting a more grown-up attitude toward controlling himself. Frank was also hesitant to admit that he might like his father, his brother, or me, especially as the summer interruption began to approach. Interpreting how he could not admit to liking men led to his explaining that he was afraid they would beat him up. Lonely feelings increased at the end of July, along with feelings of missing his mother when he was at home. Fantasies about the peaceful situation of being the baby in the womb were frequent, along with intensification of Frank's constant need to have a new toy.

Second Year of Analysis

After the summer interruption, and upon beginning the third grade, Frank's continuing tendency to take things that did not belong to him evolved into a widespread pattern. He was convinced that neither his parents nor his "feelings doctor" would recognize this; in this way he thought of himself as smarter than all the grown ups. A great capacity for lying, and for trying to pressure the analyst and his parents into accepting his specious explanations about how he had obtained certain stolen objects, came into full view. I often interpreted Frank's belief that he could fool the grown-ups and take all the things that he was not supposed to take.

I came to realize that I had failed to recognize the extent of Frank's delinquency. Frank had great difficulty saying "no" to himself. This was largely ego syntonic, and yet there was a part of him that also wanted to be good. However, he regarded the internal voice that said he should not do certain things as he regarded himself: small and unworthy of respect. Simultaneously Frank's pronounced fearfulness of standing up for himself, of his older brother, of many dangers that he feared from many sides, and his tendency to give in or run away if there were a confrontation—all came into focus. Frank felt himself to be helpless against the imagined power of a boy on a school bus who was not much older than he.

In his analytic hours, Frank regularly engaged in violent play involving a great deal of killing. In this way he expressed the excitement that he felt being in my presence. This homosexual aspect of the transference was not yet interpreted. Instead Frank's temptation to do things wrong was the main focus. He would give me clues to various thefts that he perpetrated, or other "wrong" actions. He tested whether I could set effective limits upon his subtly disruptive behavior in the office.

Some of Frank's play expressed his excitement at invading houses and killing babies. However, the sadistic, phallic meaning of these incidents was not sufficiently clear to allow adequate interpretation. His fear was that he himself could be out of control, like the out-of-control drivers of many of his play vehicles. Frank's infantile behavior was often a screen, a way of hiding his efforts to manipulate and control, playing dumb, so to say. For example, he forgot to bring in a bus token to repay me for the one that he had borrowed after losing his own token.

As Frank increasingly felt I understood his misbehavior and his tendencies to lie, the analysis took a more coherent form. He also began to directly express his longings for me.

He did not want to have his sessions end; he wanted me to wave at him through the window after his last session of the week. Eventually he also expressed disappointment that mother or father did not notice his wrongdoings.

Frank's tendency to provoke punishment seemed to be expressed more clearly in play, in which various criminals were so excited to be chased by the police that they ended up getting themselves killed. He also took money from another boy in the office and eventually had to pay it back. Then he opened up some of his presents before Christmas, inviting his parents to punish him. In this way Frank showed that the internalization of an effective superego was a process still incomplete. At the same time, he acknowledged in a more honest and straightforward way his own responsibility for these actions.

An important revelation by Mrs. Jay followed. She had regularly stolen from her parents and others and lied extensively during her own latency. Another part of her history gained additional significance. Frank's mother had the psychology of the exception. She had been, in effect, abandoned by her mother. However, she had also triumphed over her foster mother and had, in many respects, taken her place with foster father, including in bed. Frank's mother's twice weekly treatment was continuing. As these issues emerged, she made significant strides in becoming aware of the harmful effects of subtly encouraging her boys to disregard rules.

Frank continued to be determined to possess things which did not belong to him. He often showed cleverness in lying and presenting himself as an innocent. A turning point occurred when Mr. and Mrs. Jay discovered that he had stolen an airplane from a toy store and, after he committed a number of other infractions, decided not to let him accompany his mother and brother on a two-week ski trip abroad. Instead he stayed home with a babysitter. Frank struggled against admitting that he was upset and remorseful. Nevertheless he became more accessible to analytic work on his wish to ignore "the little man inside him" who told him when he should not do something. He made repeated efforts to dissociate himself from other boys in his school with delinquent trends. He felt rewarded when one of his erstwhile friends who had stolen from many people was publicly exposed and he (Frank) was spared the experience of embarrassment and punishment.

With increasing clarity, Frank's envy of the power and penis of his father, his wish to steal it and even bite it off, emerged. He defended against these wishes with a preoccupation with father's large doo-doos, and with getting pee in his own mouth which might make him have a baby. Frank then revealed incidents in which his brother had chased him and peed on him; his excitement at playing the part of the lady in the "husband–wife" game was evident. I explained that, no wonder he was afraid he would lose something precious; he wished to see what it would be like to be treated by big brother or father the way his mother is treated. In this context, Frank became more open about his attachment to me and expectation of missing me over the summer, especially after we had explored his reluctance to admit missing his brother who had left earlier for sleep-away camp.

As certain psychodynamic issues were worked on the previous spring, particularly the negative oedipal configuration of Frank's wishes and the associated symptomatic stealing and craving for what others had, Frank became more interested in what he could do for himself in school. Until now, he had not expressed (in any way that I could identify) feelings of envy about the academic accomplishments of others, or feelings of unhappiness about his difficulties in learning. In retrospect, the intensity of Frank's envious feelings, and his sense that he could not obtain what he wanted legitimately, but only through theft or deception, may very well have been consequences of early perceptions of his own difficulties in learning.

As Frank now made a much more active effort in school, Mrs. Jay had become more aware of his difficulty focusing and mastering academic material, both verbal and mathematical. She reported that he could read material ten times, and even then fail to comprehend its meaning. He skipped over words when writing, omitted punctuation marks, and reversed in math. In this context, Mrs. Jay requested another diagnostic testing evaluation by the learning specialist group to which she had taken Frank when he was 4 years, 8 months.

Third Psychological Testing Evaluation

Retesting was completed just before Frank's ninth birthday and as we approached the third year of his analysis. During the two testing sessions, Frank presented very much as he had several years before. He seemed young for his age, holding his tongue forward in his mouth and sucking his thumb on occasion. Frank took on each task willingly enough, although his effort was variable. For example, his investment in copying designs was greater than that in a reading comprehension test. At no time was he inattentive or poorly focused. However, he sometimes seemed caught in indecision, which contrasted with his typically impulsive approach to reading. An additional comment was that Frank "hasn't discovered yet that dreaming about some performance is not the same thing as carrying it out ... he goes through the motions rather than getting down to the task. Up to this point his difficulties with processing and his tendency to withdraw into fantasies interact."

The diagnostic impression was of difficulty with language processing, involving both spoken and written language. The evaluating psychologist concluded that Frank did not readily assimilate sounds, words, or syntactical units. He became confused on a task which required him to follow grammatically complex instructions. Problems with retention of auditory information were also noted. Frank's memory for sentences on the Stanford-Binet was at the 5-year level. On a test of auditory discrimination, he asked the examiner to repeat the stimulus eight times! She had the impression it took a long time for him to hold the information in his mind and process it. He passed the Binet Verbal Absurdities at the 12-year level, but in each case he asked that the examples be repeated. Then he was able to provide rather high order responses, so that it seemed clear he had difficulty processing spoken language.

Frank also evidenced a pronounced dysnomia and mild articulation problems. For example, it was by no means easy for him to recite the months of the year. He remembered his mother's birthday because "it was either a day after or before the uh ... (Frank proceeded to wave his hands) sparkling party," by which he meant the 4th of July. He was extremely dysnomic in conversation; for example, his account of a movie he saw was difficult to comprehend.

A weakness in graphomotor coordination persisted. Frank's figure drawings were somewhat primitive, and tinged with menacing qualities. Bender-Gestalt designs were less cohesive than expected for his age.

Frank's reading, while adequate, was below expectations for a child of his educational environment. On a test of paragraph reading he scored at grade level (which is actually below average for a student at the challenging school he attended), but did not read very accurately. He was noted to insert and omit words and to transpose letters within many words. On a self-administered test of reading for meaning and identifying words, he scored somewhat above grade level on both the vocabulary and comprehension portions. He tended to work overly fast, spending less than half the time allotted on each portion; when he was encouraged to use the full period of time allotted, his scores were not much improved.

Frank's written work was below age and grade expectations. He scored at the beginning of third grade level on a test of spelling individual words. In writing sentences he tended to omit punctuation marks, spelled poorly, and did not always convey his thoughts clearly. On an achievement test his mathematics computation score was slightly above national norm expectations (at the 4.3 grade level) which, however, is somewhat below private school levels.

On brief projective testing, Frank again expressed wishes for limitless opportunities, e.g., all the money in the world. In talking about the actor Paul Newman, Frank expressed his envy of his (imagined) capacity to float through life without frustration; he had "lots of luck" and "wins the lottery every time he plays."

On the basis of this evaluation, the psychologist thought Frank would profit from remedial help, which was subsequently arranged. She also suggested that Frank would benefit from repeating a grade at some point. The findings also raised new perspectives on the reasons for Frank's often observed imperviousness to interpretations: how much was he unwilling to listen because he was afraid of not comprehending? Was Frank's tendency (evident on many occasions) to fill in the gaps in his comprehension by creating an explanation of how certain facts fit together related to problems with receptive language? For example, when his teacher spoke about the last week of school and then mentioned (at about the same time) the date of June 22, Frank typically concluded that this date must be the last date of school. This was despite the fact that his teacher had not specified this, and it was not in fact the case. A consequence of Frank's creative effort to synthesize poorly assimilated information was his strong tendency to end up actually confused.

Third Year of Analysis

In view of the diagnostic test results, I made certain alterations in analytic technique during the course of the subsequent academic year when Frank was 9 and in the fourth grade. I became much more forthcoming in explaining actual facts or events in the world at large, whenever I suspected that Frank was actually confused about something he was describing or that we were discussing. This clarifying activity was frequently a first step. I often followed these preliminary statements with further interpretation of feelings and thought processes which might have led to Frank's confusion.

The same regressive trends of earlier years persisted and were repeatedly manifested in the analytic situation. Frank often turned repeatedly from some aspect of the analytic work to fantasies of a predominantly sadomasochistic nature with oral and anal elements, from which he derived considerable pleasure. He repeatedly expressed his dislike of all the restrictions which his mother placed upon him, while feeling his father to be his ally in promoting instinctual gratification. This view of father as the one promoting immediate gratification was a new aspect of the analytic material. It was possible to demonstrate, however, that Frank simultaneously had other feelings. He was disappointed that his father did not demand he learn to control himself, and he felt critical of his father's lack of self-control. Frank criticized his father's smoking and overeating, and sometimes explicitly telling the boys upon purchasing a treat the three of them would share, and that they should not tell their mother.

Nevertheless Frank's preponderant reaction was to repudiate the need for self-control or guidance of his own activities. His secret resentment of all rules was accompanied by efforts to persuade his family, analyst, and the adult world at large what a nice boy he was. The issue of Frank's being a "con man" had repeatedly to be addressed in treatment. This was particularly necessary because of Frank's considerable success in presenting himself in a favorable light. One salient example of his feeling that he could get away with sly expressions of his secret resentment was his writing an insulting and salacious variant of his teacher's name on one of the written assignments collected each day in class. School authorities threatened to expel the culprit. When Frank's handwriting was recognized, he was suspended. Deeply chagrined and remorseful about this experience, he seemed to turn further away from the tempting path of delinquency.

During this period, Frank's dishonesty with adults proved to be related to his learning difficulties. He felt a very considerable mistrust of adults, from whom he did not expect to get an honest or straight answer. In fact one enduring aspect of Frank's growing relationship with me was his increasing trust that I would not give him evasive or roundabout answers. He could rely on me to tell him as accurately as I could about many matters, from academic to sexual. Frank's effort to fool adults turned out to be a form of identification with the aggressor; he had experienced adults as thoroughly unreliable and inaccurate guides to the world he was attempting to master. Also pertinent was the fact that Frank's learning disability prevented him from fully understanding adults, and adults from understanding him well. This resulted in his misinterpreting their statements and instead thinking they were not telling the truth.

Indeed, I had changed my usual technique, based on my experience of working with Frank. It was clear that any evasions on my part in regard to information about myself, my family, or my history could be quite detrimental to him. Thus I had become quite straightforward and responsive in conversations which concerned my personal life. Some follow-up contacts in Frank's adult life revealed that his experience of me as straightforward made an enduring contribution to his sense of himself and his appreciation of the treatment. He had developed what proved to be a rather extensive identification with aspects of the way I functioned with him. These included valuing honesty in communications with others, a capacity for self-disclosure, and a trenchant self-reflectiveness.

Two events occurred at this time which resulted in an outpouring of castration fantasies, excitement, and anxiety. Frank attempted to master and discharge these via sadomasochistic preoccupations, fantasies, and play. His best friend's urethra was injured when he jumped on his bike in a wild way. Surgery was required, following which his friend had to be absent from school for the balance of the year. The second event was his mother's minor gynecological surgical procedure. Both Frank and his father evidenced extensive avoidance, and then confusion, regarding the meaning of this event.

During this period of the analysis there was considerable interpretive work on Frank's anxiety, confusion, and fantasies about girls having a penis, and the excitement and danger of losing his. As in the past he tended to turn away from sustained awareness or further work with this material as soon as the immediate event had passed. His tendency not to take himself seriously turned out to have an important defensive significance; Frank had a strong wish to exhibit himself (in all senses) but felt it was a lot safer to clown around. If he revealed that he wished to be genuinely admired, he imagined that he would be much more vulnerable and stimulate fearsome attacks.

In retrospect, this might have provided a good opportunity to focus more specifically on the way Frank dealt with his experience of not being able to function in school as well as the other kids. This might, in turn, have led into a discussion of the particular areas in which he had difficulty processing information. The first part of this—feeling not as smart as the other kids, as he saw himself struggling to get the right answers—*was* discussed with Frank on several occasions. However, I do not recall introducing his information processing difficulties, and their relationship to the tutoring. The connection that *was* meaningful for Frank was his wish to find an easier way when he encountered difficulty with academic work. He often wanted a pleasurable treat to be bestowed upon him as compensation for the bad feeling he got from having trouble understanding the material. I spoke to Frank's tutor (whom he was seeing two or three times a week) a few times during these years, and we both agreed that he continued to make very good progress. However, I did not recognize at the time that Frank's failure to discuss the tutoring in his analytic hours was an expression of his denial of distress about his (relative) disabilities. Looking back at this now, there would have been an advantage in approaching this omission as a manifestation of his wish to forget about the areas of difficulty. Similarly, in retrospect, some of the details of the test results could have served as a springboard for discussions with Frank about his specific learning problems. At the time it did not occur to me that I would be able to initiate such discussions without causing him to feel too self-conscious and ashamed. In other words, to some extent I joined unwittingly in Frank's attitude of avoidance of full acknowledgment of his learning difficulties.

Frank did nicely at sleep-away camp during the summer of his tenth birthday, before fifth grade. He won an award, but had to minimize his pleasure about this in order to avoid showing off. He was envious of two wealthy boys at camp who frequently called home; Frank did not call home very often because he felt he had nothing to tell.

Fourth Year of Analysis

During the fall of Frank's fifth grade year, when he was 10, there was a diminution of the directly charged sexual material described above, as he struggled with schoolwork and his sense of being intensely burdened by the demands placed upon him. This change no doubt reflected Frank's maturation, but also the impact of the greater challenge of fifth grade work. His continuing tutoring helped to prevent him from simply shutting out his school difficulties.

As Frank emphasized success in schoolwork now, I had the opportunity to explore with him ways he kept from feeling bad about his less than outstanding academic performance. We discussed his tendency to make assumptions about things he did not understand completely, and to avoid asking those who might know because it made him feel bad to admit that someone knew more than he did. Additionally, there were repeated opportunities to clarify how and why he could not make sense of what he studied. When he had trouble understanding things, Frank frequently said there was no need to try. For example, he thought the symbols on the buttons of a complicated calculator might not mean anything at all! If the buttons did not mean anything, Frank did not have to feel bad about not knowing what they meant.

It was interesting to note the parallel with his mother in this regard. She tended to have trouble understanding verbal instructions and lacked a belief that clear explanations would be helpful. Indeed both of Frank's parents had difficulty comprehending written instructions. His mother also had difficulty in finding the right word to express herself. Yet the game of bridge intrigued her, and she devoted great effort to it, winning several significant championships. Like Frank, she was able to figure things out when verbal decoding skills were not the primary modality.

Often the analytic material would appear to point in a certain direction. However, efforts to discuss this with Frank led him to change the subject, to complain of being bored, feeling (or looking) blank. All of these were his defensive reactions to not understanding what I said. Additionally, Frank sometimes got things mixed up because he changed them around to fit his preconceptions. For example, he had the idea that street numbers (such as 79th Street) applied to the particular block, not to the entire length of the street, despite his own experiences to the contrary. It seemed that often he adhered to such mistaken ideas because *he* had thought of them; he hated to have to give up *his* ideas for what everyone else thought was right.

Another contributory element to Frank's confusion was his not making a sufficient effort to get exactly the right word or right mathematical concept. This was an expression of his pessimism about his own ability, his resentment that so many others knew so much more than he did, and his wish to defy all the rule-giving adults.

I could often point out how he often insisted on a lack of interest in a subject so that he would not feel sad or unhappy about tasks that were hard for him. His unhappiness as he realized he would have to work extremely hard to obtain results that others could achieve much more easily became a frequent focus. This was in contrast to Frank's earlier tendency to hide his distress about this, particularly with a combination of regressive behavior and avoidance of academic effort. He had acted as if school success were of no interest to him.

Frank's failure to actively attempt to understand things also served as a defense against other anxieties. For example, when his father developed a cardiac arrhythmia requiring medication, Frank initially reacted as if he had no understanding whatever of his father's condition or what the consequences of the condition might be. His parents also avoided giving direct explanations, and were vague and confusing. Frank and I discussed how he attempted to avoid anxiety about something going wrong with his father's body by not understanding what was really going on. Self-punitive trends were evident in his forgetting to bring his homework home, getting instructions confused about where to meet people in his family, and letting himself get into trouble. This masochistic trend could not be directly linked with fantasies about his father's health, although this appeared to be a likely connection. Frank had other ways of being self-defeating as well. He failed to lock his locker, lost precious possessions, and forgot assignments or left books in school that were necessary for homework.

In his analytic hours Frank still displayed considerable difficulty getting things straight and an inclination to avoid concentrated mental effort. He treated this as if it were assigned work that he might have trouble accomplishing. This had a major effect upon the treatment and was interpreted. For example, if I posed a question about his feelings or motivations, which implicitly or explicitly called for a response, Frank would often act as if he had not heard the question.

Another important focus of the work during this year was Frank's wish to receive treats of one kind or another whenever he encountered difficult situations. These required him to struggle to learn something he had not previously understood. His school nickname Milky reflected the strong oral coloration of these defensive trends, and also referred to his habit of opening his mouth and closing his eyes at a teacher's suggestion. The teacher popped chalk (instead of the M&Ms he had promised) into his mouth, but Frank did not mind because he liked the teacher.

There were many expressions of Frank's difficulties with his impulses, such as hating to wait, rushing through homework, and being bored with having to walk home. The latter was also associated with envy of mother who traveled by taxi. Frank had doubts about his own determination to be strong in saying "no" to himself, especially about saving money. He failed to take advantage of his father's offer to double his savings at Christmas time, and thus kept on undermining the possibility of receiving money from his father in this way. Frank resented many limitations on his pleasure, particularly those placed by mother upon candy eating.

Following discussion of the ways in which he undermined himself, Frank became more directly competitive. In school and in the consulting room he was more interested in doing his work carefully and was proud of the results. For the first time he seriously considered that, if I won competitive games with him, perhaps I understood things about how to play which he had yet to learn.

Gradually and repeatedly, sad and other discomfiting feelings appeared when Frank did not understand something, or when he could not find the words he wished. Frank's tendency was to minimize the unhappiness this caused him and to look for some gift or some supply of money to make him feel better. I could show him how he often felt bored and unhappy because he had trouble doing something; that was when he tried to find solace in a treat. Frank told me more directly how he felt that he could not do certain things as well as others and how badly this made him feel. He also felt encouraged when I kept pointing out that he needed to spend more time than other kids to get a good result with his homework or other studies. It was as if he had not allowed himself to recognize this need because it made him feel too bad to be disadvantaged in any way.

Frank's actual efforts improved as I clarified these various defensive maneuvers. Simultaneously we discussed how he felt he had a harder time getting things straight and remembering words than other children did.

Frank's tutoring added to his awareness of his specific cognitive problems, and he more readily recognized his difficulty getting things straight, both academically and in the ordinary circumstances of life. It was often possible to show him the influence of his wishes. For instance, Frank wishfully imagined that a certain order form he noticed on his mother's desk before Christmastime meant he would get six Star Wars figures (instead of one).

As the Christmas holiday approached, his mother became depressed and sad as she often did at this season. This time he, too, became sad and discontented, complaining of having no one to do things with and of his mother's neglect of him. Frank's angry, hurtful feelings toward his mother and his fantasies of retaliation for them (especially at the hands of father) frightened him. When he felt disappointed by his mother's inconsistent attention, he wanted to be the one who did the disappointing; he forgot things that he had undertaken to do. He also connected this urge to get things mixed up, or not to get them straight, with the devil in him who hated all rules and expectations.

After the New Year, Frank started collecting Whacky Pack cards with an ever-increasing intensity. At first he viewed his own collection as so inadequate that he had to rely upon the strength of others. He wished to share the collections of his brother and then of a slightly older child known to be a cheat and a thief. As I interpreted his feelings of envy, which served as a basis for this particular arrangement, Frank chose to pursue a collection in his own right. This was despite his long-standing experience of vulnerability to any comparison with another boy who might have more. Such comparisons were associated with wishes for lots of money to buy a really big collection. Gradually

Frank built an impressive collection due to his shrewdness in bargaining.

Frank ultimately revealed how much his brother picked on him and injured him when their parents left them alone. Chris twisted his nose, scratched his face, and possibly hurt him in the genitals. He explained that he did not tell his parents about this because he did not want to lose the money that he and his brother received for babysitting each other. I repeatedly interpreted Frank's excitement in being hurt, as he presented many examples of his tendency to take chances that caused him to lose things or to be hurt. For example, he risked his treasured Whacky Pack collection by bringing it to school where it could be confiscated. In sessions Frank sometimes responded by sitting in his chair so that he could bang himself on his rear end with his foot. I connected this behavior with the feeling that he might, strangely enough, have liked to be spanked by his father as used to happen.

During this period I also interpreted the connection between Frank's wish to be taken advantage of and his continuing excitement in fighting with his brother. There were many expressions of this. Chris shot a rubber BB into Frank's eye and then paid him not to tell, to which Frank agreed. Frank made up or recounted stories of exciting killing games. In watching a recording of a football game, he became excited by the grunts and groans indicating the players had been injured.

Frank expressed his strong investment in overpowering or fooling anyone bigger than himself; this was something he doubted he could do. He wished to accumulate enough money, partly by cheating Chris, to buy a gun more powerful than his. Frank often referred to the story of David and Goliath. He frequently told people things that were not true, to obtain a better deal. Also he expressed a belief that one's success in life was simply a matter of luck and harbored an urgent wish to have good luck himself. When things did not go his way, Frank became enraged. For example, once when he lost a series of flips of his Whacky Pack cards, he gave away his whole pack in a temper. When he lost games to me, he loathed admitting that I was a serious contender who had learned how to play well. He did sometimes observe that his performance improved when he paid more attention to aspects of the game he had not previously known. However, he was still unhappy about not winning and had trouble experiencing satisfaction in his increased skill in playing.

Frank's sadistic pleasure regarding his mother emerged, causing him to fear her retaliation. He loved to break her rules. For instance, he cleaned his nails by rubbing them on his teeth, maintaining that this was all right because he had not gotten sick from doing it yet. He elaborated fantasies of killing me when he beat me in blackjack, thus expressing in the transference his pleasure in killing and being the one who survives.

Before the summer interruption, Frank's feelings about his brother took a different focus. Chris was going away to sleep-away camp, and then to boarding school in the fall. This offered us an opportunity to see how much Frank liked and would miss his brother, although he hated to admit it. This loss was also associated with feelings of insufficiency as a male and castration fears. The visit of Frank's female cousin led to the elaboration of his fantasy that they were somehow alike. As we discussed this he denied the difference between boys and girls by explaining that boys can have a sex change operation.

He expressed shame about another aspect of his play with his brother; his brother had been the boy and Frank the girl in their aggressive, excited play together. I interpreted Frank's wanting so much to take cards and other objects from friends because he was uncertain whether he was enough of a boy . It scared him to be so willing to lose precious things of his own, including his Whacky Pack, his penis and balls. He was then able to verbalize fears of being attacked and injured in camp, which included a fear of genital injury. Frank wanted to take a special electronic football game with him so that boys would be on his good side and protect him. He said that there was nothing scarier than the idea of losing his penis and balls.

Fifth Year of Analysis

In the fall of Frank's sixth grade year, when he was 11, school problems were again in focus. He frequently turned away from difficulties in understanding things. Feeling angry and disappointed in himself, he sought comfort in indulgences such as a bar of chocolate, which he preferred to a question that was hard to answer. There were many occasions when we discussed Frank's resentment about being expected to act in a grown-up way. Much of this anger, which he directed toward his mother, made him feel that he was a bad boy and that he had to keep his feelings hidden or be badly punished. We discussed previous occasions when such resentful feelings had emerged; for example, the incident with the teacher whom Frank secretly cursed on his writing tablet. He revealed that he also hated to have to flush the toilet, and frequently "forgot."

Frank often had similar responses to discussing his feelings; he laid his head down, turned away, expressed boredom, and found some way of playing with something that would make him feel better, including his mouth, eyelids, or other parts of his body. This was how he tried to shut out unpleasant subjects that angered him when I mentioned them. In some respects he was more able to give direct expression to his angry feelings, as when he delighted in having kicked a ball that hit the gym teacher in the testicles. He extolled the power of evil, and exulted in his weapon collection in *Dungeons and Dragons*. I emphasized how he enjoyed the feeling that he had evil powers, particularly when he found it hard to learn things in school. Often he talked about his reluctance to think when he was at school and during analytic sessions. He hoped that just coming to his analytic hours would be sufficient, that he did not have to work or think during our meetings. He could also avoid thinking by missing sessions because he overslept or forgot.

There was another side to Frank's preoccupation with aggression: fantasies of bad things happening to him. For example, he had seen the movie *Dressed to Kill*, in which a psychiatrist has to cut people when they mention sexual matters. Frank revealed that whenever the elevator door opened as he came to see me, he had the fantasy he might get cut, a clear expression of a masochistic fantasy. At the same time, he denied sexual knowledge or knowing the meaning of the word *masturbation*.

In sum, there were many expressions of Frank's anxiety

about being grown-up, which were repeatedly interpreted. Gradually there was more of a feeling of a collaborative effort. Frank began to refer spontaneously to his use of the "baby voice," which I had repeatedly commented upon in the past. This baby voice gradually dropped out of the treatment sessions. Frank often elaborated fantasies of harm befalling others. Many times it was possible to show how these fantasies reflected disappointment with and anger toward people in his life. Regressions had previously served to ward off awareness of these fantasies.

I discussed many situations in which there was something ambiguous, or in which Frank had trouble getting the facts straight. These included various sports situations, mathematics and English problems, questions of general information, geography, and history. He gradually developed, and specifically referred to, a greater interest in getting things straight. There were occasional he/she confusions when Frank felt particularly upset or angry.

Interpretive work focused on several major interrelated issues: Frank's distress at being challenged to do something he felt he could not do, anger at the rules of the grown-up world, and the conflict that he experienced between his wish to be well accepted, admired, appreciated, and proud of his own work and his wish to defy the requirements of the school, home, and the analytic situation. These called for relinquishment of more childish gratifications in favor of developing skills and knowledge. Frank's conflict over purposeful, mature, and admirable actions aimed at success was of course exacerbated by the extra difficulty he encountered in succeeding academically because of his learning difficulties. The analytic work, typical of a working through process, was a continuation of the previous years, but with the transformations and extensions that Frank's increasing maturity and self-awareness made possible.

Sixth Year of Analysis

Frank's seventh grade year, when he was 12, turned out to be his final year of treatment. Frank's mother had been puzzled about his continuing lack of ambition in school and failure in spelling, and his lackluster final report the previous June. She decided that a reevaluation specifically focused on his school difficulties might be helpful. She was also considering whether he might benefit from a special boarding school experience, which was proving very helpful to his brother.

Fourth Psychological Testing Evaluation

Another testing evaluation took place when Frank was 12 years, 4 months in the fall of his seventh grade year. Frank's teachers were generally pleased with his work. His tutor felt he had developed beautifully and was making excellent strides in dealing with the earlier diagnosed language problems. In her view, Frank could manage reading well and had worked hard on a research report required of him the previous year. However, Mrs. Jay continued to feel that she did not understand why Frank was not more ambitious about his schoolwork. Furthermore, she was concerned about his persistent spelling problems. Frank had received C's and B's for his final grades the year before.

The same psychologist tested Frank at the beginning of fourth grade and before Kindergarten. He was seen for two testing sessions, during which a partial battery was given including the Grays Oral Reading Test (which examines accuracy, speed, and comprehension in reading paragraphs), a test of spelling, the Bender-Gestalt, Figure Drawings, the Sentences and Verbal Absurdities portions of the Stanford-Binet, an informal writing composition, and brief projective testing (a request for three wishes and some type of story-telling exercise). The psychologist described Frank as agreeable and cooperative, focused and feeling good about himself. At the same time, she commented that "he did not catch fire about anything."

In her view, Frank continued to manifest problems with expressive oral and written language and with auditory processing. In contrast to solid abilities in naming, Frank's sentence formation was sometimes awkward and ungrammatical as in, "Meanwhile James Bond from information had found out where the hideout was of the people." Gestures sometimes replaced verbal communication. Frank could become lost in details as he recounted the story of a movie. An essay he produced was disorganized, as was a speech he wrote which resembled the work of a considerably younger child.

Frank performed adequately, although below the level of his private school peers, on a test of paragraph reading. His score on comprehension of passages (between the 54th and 63rd percentiles) was higher than that on word decoding and recognition (between the 32nd and 45th percentiles). More generally, Frank's language comprehension was stronger. However, his immediate retention of orally presented material was marginal; he scored at the 11-year level on the Stanford-Binet Sentences portion.

Frank scored somewhat above grade level on a test of math computation. However, the examiner commented that there were "worlds he does not know," including his uncertain grasp of aspects of division, multiplication, decimals, and fractions.

Frank's weaknesses in graphomotor coordination persisted. Bender-Gestalt designs were awkwardly reproduced, revealing difficulties with angulation and integration. Figure drawings were detailed and nicely elaborated, although there were difficulties with execution. The two sides of the body were asymmetric, the fingers attached directly to the wrists and the mouth was off to one side of the face.

Brief projective testing revealed Frank's worries about finding a decent job and having enough money. "The shadow of bad fortune" haunted some of the protagonists. People were sad because they were left by others who were important to them.

The examiner felt that Frank was doing reasonably well in spite of residual problems. She encouraged Mr. and Mrs. Jay not to be too discouraged by momentary lapses, commenting "one reason why he is not a more enthusiastic worker is that it is still harder for him than for others—his feeling about schoolwork is about as good as could be expected." She recommended that Frank continue in twice weekly tutoring.

Following this evaluation, Frank brought up several matters. He opened the subject of termination several times. This
led to discussion of his continuing inconsistent school performance. Frank asked me whether he had a good mind, and
whether his school was a good school compared to others. This
exemplified his increasingly direct communication about aspects of his self-appraisal, and his efforts to compare himself
to others. The "goodness" of the school was a measure in his
mind (as well as that of others) of his adequacy and status.
The tone of these inquiries was one of greater maturity and
reflectiveness than before. At this point there was ongoing discussion of termination with Frank's parents as well. Mrs. Jay
still came to see me every couple of weeks and his father once
every month or two.

The above-described themes were often revisited, now with
a particular emphasis upon Frank's mixed feelings about ending treatment. One important elaboration was his pleasure in
being taken care of in one way or another, rather than developing more actively his own sense of achievement in school
and other arenas of life. Frank and I discussed how these wishes
sometimes made him feel inclined to undermine his greater
success in school; if he did well, there would be no further
reason for him to continue in treatment, and who knew what
would happen then? He was not at all sure that he could handle
things well on his own. He also felt conflict about relinquishing
his habit of not spending time and energy to think things
through.

As Frank's more infantile behavior kept coming under
scrutiny, he took a more active interest in how I had handled
various challenges and issues in my own development, both
academic and in sports. He also found other men to identify
with, so that his continuing awareness of his father's difficulties
with impulse control no longer exerted as great an impact on
his self-esteem and motivation for performance. There was a
gradual alteration of Frank's masculine identification and his
sense of purpose in working toward satisfactory performance
in school.

The analytic work focused with great regularity on academic and homework issues. I became increasingly adept at

picking up indirect indicators of Frank's difficulty with school-work. He responded by gaining interest in what he could accomplish if he tried to master material, even if it took him longer. Although I rarely spoke with Frank's tutor, there was a useful mutual potentiation of each of our efforts. Frank's tutor helped him recognize details of his disability and taught him new and adaptive ways of dealing with it. We both showed him how he dealt with his cognitive difficulties. My focus, of course, was on the psychological issues, especially inner conflicts, reflected in Frank's problems with academic material.

A description of one session and its sequels may convey the flavor of the work during this period. In the previous session Frank had expressed the idea that, if he tried hard in a subject, he should get good grades, no matter whether he learned anything or not. In the subsequent hour Frank and I discussed his irritation with his father for trying to teach him how to tie a tie. He felt angry that he was being asked to attend to the way his father wanted him to do it. Then he mentioned his fear that perhaps his brain was not that good; even if he tried, he would not do well. Frank attempted to tie his tie in the office. When it came out badly, he explained that he did not care what it looked like. As I showed him how to do it, I said that his Dad surely wanted him to look good. (There was a dance Frank was going to attend, one reason Mr. Jay was teaching Frank to tie his tie.) Frank replied that *he* did not want to look good; he then wrapped the tie around his neck and said "this is how you get hung." I interpreted that he sure felt it was dangerous to try to look good. He might end up getting hung!

Fantasies of the dangers Frank associated with his father and with me were elaborated in a dream that occurred after he attended the dance. In the dream he was in danger from a certain tall army officer (a reference to me). Exploring the dream led to the idea that I could keep him in treatment forever since I had his mother's confidence, and that I might well do this for money. At this time, Frank discussed fears of being raped by men at greater length. Following exploration of this fantasy, he became more actively determined to get in shape and to slim down. He allowed himself to be actively interested in a part in a play, after exploring his fear of being unable to learn the lines, and was pleasantly surprised a girl remembered him from summer camp some time before. At this time boarding school was being actively considered for the following year.

In the final months of Frank's treatment, there was a fluctuation between his new self-assertiveness (including an interest in sexual matters) and his feeling that his mother would not be happy if he were interested in penises and what they could do (for instance in ejaculation). Frank attempted to prove this to me by saying that *my* (Dr. Waldron's) mother would not think I should talk about masturbation either. In this statement he made a slip that he corrected. He meant to say Dr. Waldron's "wife" but said "mother."

It became clearer during this time that, in part, Frank's wish to get away with things had to do with his fantasies of the repressive nature of parental authority and of the adult world. After his visit to the boarding school being considered for the following academic year, Frank told me that he liked the possibility of getting a room where you could see the teacher coming, and so get away with things.

Meanwhile, Frank continued to fluctuate concerning whether he really wanted to learn things. He was uncomfortable with intentionally aiming to do well; he liked the easy life and wished for the good old days when he did not work. Some degree of ongoing instability in superego formation was suggested, for instance, when Frank explained that if he ran the government he would make sure he made money by selling arms to both sides in a conflict. Frank's conflicts about aggression were epitomized in his explanation that everyone might reject him if he fought with anyone: "If everyone stood up for themselves there would be a lot of killers around." He asked if I would punch *my* mother? In this context, Frank retreated to gratifications of a different kind, telling me: "My mouth is my favorite place."

The decision to attend boarding school was completed over the summer, at a time when termination was already planned for the early fall. Consequently, Frank and I had two weeks before he went off to school. During this time we reviewed much of what has already been described. He ended treatment at the age of 13, after $6^3/_4$ years of analysis and 1170 sessions.

FOLLOW-UP CONTACTS

Initial Follow-Up

When Frank was $14^1/_2$, I received a letter and telephone call from his mother. She was brimming with pride because he scored at the 89th percentile on a standardized test required by his boarding school; this compared quite favorably to his 33rd percentile score when he first took the test some years before. Frank had also been doing well academically. Mrs. Jay sent me a copy of a story he had written in school describing "an unforgettable person," in which Frank named me, but thinly disguised my relationship to him as a camp counselor. He emphasized in the text how I had helped him to deal with feeling so unsure of himself when he was alone, to use his time productively, and to be more responsible for himself. Frank mentioned that the most important thing he had learned from me was how to learn.

Second Follow-Up

The next communication was 14 months later, when Frank was nearly 16 years old. His parents wanted him to see me after they found him passed out from drinking at home. He agreed. We met for five visits, during which he told me he had been aware he was using alcohol to excess, and that part of his problem was that he could get away with it in school. Frank did not mention girls in these sessions and, when I asked him about this, explained that he believed if he tried to kiss a girl whom he liked, he would lose her friendship. As during the analysis, he talked about his longing to get things for nothing, to "beat the system." It was hard to tell whether Frank's obtuseness in discussing things with me at this time was due to his way of

processing information, defensive obfuscation, or both. I remembered how he had looked forward to having a special room
in boarding school that allowed him to see in advance if the
teacher was coming, and thus to avoid detection of any mis-
deed. And I wondered if his obfuscation reflected his feeling
that he needed to hide from me what he was up to. The visits
stopped at the end of school vacation, and I subsequently received indirect reports that Frank had resumed doing well at
school.

Third Follow-Up

I initiated the next contact shortly after Frank graduated from
college. I had become interested in the possibilities of systematic follow-up based on my experience of follow-up with another of my former child analytic patients. I called Frank and
explained that I was interested in finding out how life had
developed for him, and asked if he would be willing to come
in to see me. He readily assented.

The picture that emerged during a series of sessions was
of a tall, handsome, engaging young man who was moderately
self-assured. He was very reflective about himself, his life, and
his learning difficulties and how they had affected him. It
turned out that he had a long-standing relationship with a
young woman, whose very considerable intellectual powers
he admired.

As the end of each interview approached, I sensed Frank's
reluctance to stop. We continued to make additional appointments until he finally divulged what he was most worried about:
his father's excessive consumption of alcohol. When I responded by discussing courses of action he could take, such as
talking with his mother about the problem, and perhaps helping to arrange a family intervention for his father by a substance
abuse specialist, he became uncomfortable and did not pursue
the subject further. Nevertheless what was striking to me was
the way in which Frank used self-reflection in the service of self-
management in ways that appeared to considerably enhance his
effectiveness and satisfaction.

Fourth Follow-Up

A year later, just before his twenty-third birthday, Frank contacted me seeking support to take the LSATs untimed, in view of his learning difficulties. Following a new psychological testing evaluation in order to determine the appropriateness of this request, I wrote a supporting letter. The psychologist found Frank to have a dysnomia with marked word-retrieval problems, residual dyslexia involving word omissions, substitutions, and transpositions, and a mild Attention Deficit Disorder that slowed his rate of processing. The dysnomia was quite pronounced, and there was a tendency in reading to omit small connectives and prepositions that change the meaning of a sentence. Frank labored over the Woodcock-Johnson passage comprehension subtest in a way that showed he needed two to four repetitions to derive the intended meaning. Similarly, on a test of reading vocabulary he had to self-correct between one-third and one-half of his responses. Fluctuations in attention were seen in that his scores on the Digit Symbol and Digit Span subtests of the Wechsler were only at the 50th percentile, whereas measures of his analytic thinking were at the 84th and 91st percentiles. Frank was allowed to take the LSAT untimed, and achieved a 98.4 percentile score.

Fifth Follow-Up

I saw Frank five times $1^1/_2$ years later, at the age of 24, concerning the breakup of his relationship with the girl friend he had previously told me about, and some self-doubts that emerged about this. I found out that he had been accepted at an outstanding law school. However, he had deferred beginning for a year, since he was working in a prestigious industry where he was very well regarded. Frank also found satisfaction at his job because of the women he was meeting. His assertiveness and poise had noticeably increased during the previous few years. His struggle with his old girl friend seemed to revolve around his wish to leave her, and associated feelings of guilt about pursuing his own path without her.

Chapter 10

Discussion of Frank's Analysis

Dr. Waldron's account of the analysis of Frank vividly illumi-
nates several matters of crucial importance in working with
patients who are learning disabled: (1) the analyzability of most
of these patients, even when there is a disability in cognitive
capacities central to analytic work (in Frank's case expressive
and receptive language); (2) the enlarged perspective of the
analytic work when a previously undiagnosed learning disability
is discovered; (3) alterations in technique which may sometimes be necessary; and (4) the problems and limitations which
may result when the diagnostic testing evaluations performed
are of insufficient scope to permit an optimal integration of
neurospychological and psychodynamic considerations. Had
the diagnostic evaluations of Dr. Waldron's patient been
broader in scope and more integrative, it is likely that his attention would have been drawn to the central significance of
Frank's learning disabilities earlier in the analysis.

When Mr. and Mrs. Jay brought their $6^3/_4$-year-old son
Frank for consultation, their focus was on his fearfulness and
angry demandingness. Problems in learning did not seem to
be at issue. In his account of Frank's analysis, Dr. Waldron
sensitively conveys the gradual unfolding of his awareness of
the salience of Frank's painful concerns about his difficulties
in learning in general, and his problems in receptive and expressive language in particular.

During the consultation Dr. Waldron's observations suggested that his patient did have cognitive difficulties. He noted

that Frank "had a limited capacity to grasp or respond productively to [his] comments" and "a certain obtuseness." These
observations made him reluctant to take Frank into analysis,
but his supervisor felt "the disturbance in communication
might yield to analysis." Paradoxically, one gets the impression
that, had the psychologist who tested Frank when he was 4
years, 8 months been more forceful in pointing out suggestions
of a neuropsychological disturbance, there was some possibility
that Frank would not have been analyzed, and hence received
the benefits he clearly did from intensive treatment. We believe
that Dr. Waldron's account of Frank's analysis demonstrates
that his learning disability was not a contraindication to analysis
as is true in most cases.

As Dr. Waldron came to appreciate the significance of
these aspects of Frank's functioning, his analytic work with
Frank was amended. The scope of his interventions was broadened to include the interweaving of these disabilities in the
development of Frank's personality. In addition, Dr. Waldron
(to some degree) modified the form of his interpretations, in
view of Frank's problems in processing language. In writing up
this analysis many years after its termination, Dr. Waldron can
see oversights, as any of us would when we look back over our
own work with a patient. In this case, he feels that it was not
until the third year of the analysis that he began to clearly
appreciate the significance of Frank's neuropsychological dysfunction, contributing to his learning disabilities.

Up until that time Dr. Waldron and Frank had productively worked on many central conflictual issues. The first two
years of the analysis were replete with Frank's repetition with
the analyst of wild, sadistic erotic games. These expressed many
things. Among them were Frank's actual exciting and frightening experiences with his brother, his fantasies of his parents'
sexual life, and his wishes for his parents to set limits on the
tendency of all members of the family to act on their impulses.

There were many factors in Frank's history which would
contribute to his presenting problems of fearfulness and angry
demandingness and to his investment in these games. Overstimulation was an ongoing experience in Frank's life. He was
involved in an exciting sadomasochistic relationship with his

older brother. He was also exposed to inappropriate TV programs and encouraged to crawl into mother's bed.

In other respects as well, Mr. and Mrs. Jay were people who had significant difficulties in being close to others (including their children) and in setting limits for themselves and for their sons. Frank may have turned to his brother, in part, for the tenderness he could not easily find with his parents. However, this too became a source of many conflicts: homosexual anxiety, fear of the unprotected, exciting, and terrifying satisfaction of sexual and aggressive wishes, and conflicts about knowing, and being active. Furthermore, Frank's natural loving feelings for his father and brother posed an unconscious threat to mother who, because of her own traumatic past, envied the closeness of others which she experienced as a rejection. Being her baby was a way for Frank to get close to mother, *and* spare himself the dangerous fantasied consequences of competing with father and brother, and mother's displeasure at his independent activity.

Frank dismissed Dr. Waldron's interpretations of many of these ideas during the first years of the analysis. He thought they were "unimportant" and the analyst was "dumb" for saying these things. Dr. Waldron understood this as Frank's way of preventing the interruption of the gratification his play provided. He did not consider as well the difficulties Frank was having in processing language and in expressing himself. Nor did Dr. Waldron initially view Frank's "considerable feelings of inadequacy, of being so small and of not being able to do many things he wanted to do" from the standpoint of his experience of other cognitive and specifically academic disabilities. Comparisons with his father, brother, and mother were no doubt extremely disturbing too. Frank expressed a fantasy that Dr. Waldron would not help him to master the many things he wanted to learn, as Frank approached his eighth birthday. Dr. Waldron understood this as a repetition in the transference of Frank's experience of his mother's intolerance and her undermining of his (and his brother's) increasing capacity for independence.

It is useful to consider the impact of Frank's significant language difficulties upon a host of aspects of development which are heavily reliant upon the acquisition of language: self–object differentiation, reality testing, secondary process thinking, concept formation, modulation of drives, and frustration tolerance. Some of these were central problems for Frank, a boy who could not fully profit from the structuralizing possibilities afforded by language in the course of normal development, which we will sketch briefly. The compromising of Frank's development by language problems of course combined with many other factors.

With increasing linguistic and cognitive capacities, the child is gradually able to tolerate greater periods of delay and dosages of frustration. This is, in part, related to caretakers' explanations first that there is a "later," and ultimately their identification of time sequences in the past and future: "before," "yesterday," "after," "tomorrow." Verbalization of the baby's experience and feelings contributes to drive and affect modulation (Katan, 1961) and the curbing of their expression through motor channels. Weil (1971) comments on the miscarriage of this process in the form of exacerbation of motor activity in the constitutionally hyperactive child who additionally suffers from a language disorder: "Dysfunctions in the areas of language and speech will further spur such trends toward hyperactiveness. Dysnomias and language difficulties foster discharge in action (at an age when verbalization would usually take over) and this tendency toward action then interacts unfavorably with the child's general basic hyperkinetic drivenness" (p. 85). These features are also characteristic of the dysnomic child without neuropsychologically based hyperactivity.

Simultaneously, parents expand the baby's knowledge of the world as they supply information, point out interesting events, and answer questions. The child's reality testing is fostered as he can express his observations and feelings and, therefore, make them available for parents to correct and elaborate (Katan, 1961). Language development coincides with the discovery of sexual differences to which there is an unavoidably disturbing reaction due to the conclusion that to not have externally visible genitalia is equivalent to castration. Through language caretakers can correct this theory by providing information that the child is like his (her) mother or father, thus fostering pride in likenesses to loved and admired parents. Other magical and omnipotent beliefs and fears about the child's and parents' powers can similarly be corrected as language permits distancing from the immediacy of the situation.

Not only do caretakers expand the child's horizon and better adjust his beliefs to the bounds of reality, but they utilize language to organize and integrate his experience into meaningful segments. In the absence of language, much as in the presence of hyperactivity, the child's taking in of his surroundings is more fragmented and diffuse. Verbalizations of time sequences, spatial relationships, and causal relationships contribute to the stabilization of experience and the establishment of secondary process thinking. Furthermore, concept formation and symbolic thinking is stimulated by parents' identification of connections between like objects, events, and people in the environment.

All of the above ego functions so heavily reliant upon language are essential for the tasks of learning expected from latency onward, which in turn further contribute to ego development. A specific example is the contribution of reading to reality mastery. The ability to grasp conditional concepts is one of the many higher level organizing principles which may be recognized as deficient in some neuropsychologically impaired children somewhat later in their lives. Weil (1978) regards this as one of the "organizing faculties" that are required, beginning in the second half of elementary school, when learning is no longer predominantly rote, but instead requires conceptualization, reasoning, and organization of various sorts.

The superego's contribution to organization also depends on receptive language. Dr. Waldron observed that Frank's superego deficiency depended in part on his misunderstanding his parents. Without accurately understanding their stated standards, he could not internalize them.

Given the many psychodynamic factors involved in Frank's clinical picture, in combination with the problems related to his language disability in particular and learning disability in general, it is easy to understand how these disabilities could have been missed for a period of time. Also contributory was the failure of the multiple diagnostic evaluations carried out with Frank to clearly define the nature of his cognitive problems.

We will first discuss the nature of these evaluations in detail, to define both what they offered and in which respects opportunities for clarification were missed. This case offers an unusual chance to examine the possibilities and potential pitfalls in diagnostic work. Then we will explore the analysis of Frank in terms of the role of his learning disability in the development of his personality and some resulting technical considerations.

DIAGNOSTIC TESTING EVALUATIONS

This case is remarkable in permitting us to follow Frank over a period of many years and a series of evaluations carried out from varying perspectives. The need for psychological testing was by no means overlooked. Indeed Frank was reevaluated five times, at important points in his development. Both Mrs. Jay and the analyst viewed diagnostic evaluation as a source of valuable information in their efforts to help Frank. However, an optimal degree of clarity was not achieved through this process.

The psychologists to whom Frank was taken had different emphases and did what we would consider only partial evaluations. This was evident in the nature of the test batteries they administered, and in their approach to interpretation of their findings. Indeed Frank's mother implicitly discerned this. For example, at the time of the second evaluation during the consultation with Dr. Waldron (when Frank was 6 years, 9 months and in first grade), she stated ''her wish to consult a psychologist who did not have a particular bias toward learning difficulties.''

She believed the psychologist to whom she had taken her son (when he was 4 years, 8 months) did have such a slant. At that earlier time, Mrs. Jay consulted a psychologist noted to be a specialist in the diagnosis of learning disabilities to better understand the reasons Frank had not been accepted for kindergarten by the private school of her first choice. She also hoped that, in view of her older son's difficulties (for which he was being treated by both an analyst and a learning specialist), testing might reveal whether Frank shared any of his brother's problems. The family history included Frank's older brother's major behavioral disturbances in school which were thought to be related to "developmental lags" and graphomotor problems, and the possibility that Frank's father had been an undiagnosed dyslexic. By this time in Frank's life Mrs. Jay felt her son's speech "left something to be desired," although it was better than that of his older brother.

This first test evaluation performed several years prior to consultation with the analyst strongly suggested problems in expressive language, fine motor coordination, and possibly immediate auditory memory. However, these diagnostic impressions were not made clear. Curiously, while the composition of the battery was more heavily weighted toward tests of cognitive skills, the diagnostic conclusions emphasized Frank's anxiety as the major interference in his performance and behavior.

The psychologist at this time reported that Frank confused pronouns, misnamed animals when telling stories, had trouble formulating what he wanted to say, and evidenced language constructions which often took "immature" forms. She also commented that he was "fairly silent" (which she attributed to his not knowing her) and "not terribly informative" in the context of his stories and responses to questions. She viewed this as one manifestation of his being a "somewhat anxious child for whom pleasing the adult has high priority." She also felt that, appropriate to his age, he was "finding his way out of primary process material" and wondered what he did with his aggression. The tester further reported that Frank had some coordination problems: in his throwing and catching a ball, his use of a pencil in executing figure drawings and Bender-Gestalt designs, and his slight lisp.

The battery administered to Frank was partial, and was completed in only one session. Frank was given tests of graphomotor functioning (the Bender-Gestalt, Figure Drawings) and several tests of language (a formal naming test, a syntax screening test, word matching, pattern matching, sentence memory).

Projective testing included telling stories, as well as the above-mentioned figure drawings. In addition Frank's ability to blend discrete sounds together to form words, to make auditory discriminations, and to imitate tapped sound patterns was examined.

While it is true that some aspects of functioning may be difficult to examine conclusively in someone of preschool age, there are many areas which it is entirely possible to examine—ones that were omitted in this evaluation. In this sense, it might more accurately be viewed as a screening, rather than a comprehensive assessment. An IQ test was not administered, perhaps because Frank had recently taken the standard preschool intelligence test as part of his parents' application for kindergarten. However, even if these scores were available, it would have been optimal to administer an alternate intelligence test, in order to be able to examine qualitative features of his performance. Nor were tests of prereading and premath skills, or of the array of memory, sequencing, and visual processing skills, included. Projective testing should also have included the Rorschach, to assess both psychic structure and the ability to organize visuospatially.

The psychologist concluded that Frank was a "very nice little boy" who was experiencing a great deal of anxiety, and probably suppressing and projecting his aggression extensively. If things did not improve (she did not specify which things), he should come for help in the fall (she did not specify what sort of help). At any rate, she suggested reevaluation in six months' time, which was not done.

A valuable opportunity was missed. The manner in which Frank's problems in language might have compromised and shaped development was not put in focus. Instead, findings of a psychological nature were presented side-by-side with selected aspects of cognitive functioning, without an effort to grapple with their interplay. For example, the psychologist commented that the projective material highlighted Frank's "immaturity" and his "tendency to flight of ideas with a loosening of secondary process thinking" and "omnipotence." It would have been useful to consider the possibility that limitations in language might be interfering with the normal curbing of omnipotence and strengthening of secondary process thinking. Nor was the likelihood that Frank's confusion of pronouns was one manifestation of his language difficulties given consideration. Similarly, Frank's figure drawings were described exclusively in psychological terms, as reflecting a confused body image. However, Frank's graphomotor problems were likely to have contributed as well.

The results of the second diagnostic evaluation done by another psychologist in the course of the consultation with Dr. Waldron (when Frank was 6 years, 9 months) were again strongly suggestive of language problems. However, their significance in Frank's overall functioning was again not adequately emphasized. The tester seemed to opt for a primarily psychogenic explanation of his clinical picture.

The diagnostic conclusion was of a bright boy whose "mediocre language achievements suggest a turning away from academic learning." Sadomasochistic preoccupation, related to overstimulation at home, was highlighted, as was Frank's tendency to regression, phobic fears, depressive feelings, and obsessive–compulsive features. His immaturity was primarily viewed as a retreat from competition associated with castration anxiety. So-called "developmental lags" were thought to exist, but not to meaningfully account for Frank's immature presentation. Thus he was thought to require, and to be able to profit from, intensive psychotherapeutic treatment.

This battery was also partial, but of different composition. It included an IQ test, a test of graphomotor functioning (the Bender-Gestalt) and standard projective tests (the Rorschach, CAT, and figure drawings). Examination of academic performance, and the individual building blocks for the mastery of these functions, was not carried out. Frank's Verbal IQ was remarkably below his Performance IQ, with a discrepancy of 21 points. Most pronounced was Frank's weakness in general factual information and number skills. This was attributed to his "selectivity about what he wanted to know and not to know" and his "passive negativism rooted in conflicts over sexual and aggressive wishes." The catastrophic content, and the tendency toward passivity and helplessness evident in Frank's responses on the verbal portions of the IQ test was emphasized. The fact that he was successful in sequencing visual narrative materials and manifested "a good understanding of social relationships that was at odds with his surface immaturity" (on a test where use of language was not at issue) was not viewed as a matter of curiosity. Qualitative features of Frank's use of syntax and other aspects of language were exemplified, but not commented upon. Frank's tendency to make errors in his use of pronouns was described. Again, psychodynamic aspects of his figure drawings were interpreted, but the intactness of the fine motor skill with which they were carried out did not receive mention.

Once again an important opportunity was missed to bring to Dr. Waldron's attention the existence of Frank's later appreciated learning disabilities (affecting reading, writing, and the use of language), and the way in which the specific nature of Frank's cognitive problems would impact upon the analysis, and had already shaped, and been shaped by, his developmental experience.

The third diagnostic testing evaluation was performed just prior to Frank's ninth birthday and at the end of his third grade year and his second year of analysis. This was prompted by Mrs. Jay's concerns about Frank's difficulty focusing upon, retaining and/or grasping academic material (both verbal and mathematical), despite his greater ability to make an active effort in school. This ability had presumably strengthened through the analytic work. Probably because of the nature of her questions, Mrs. Jay returned to seek the help of the psychologist whom she thought of as a learning specialist (the one who had evaluated Frank as a preschooler).

Another partial assessment was made. The psychologist administered some tests of specific language functions (memory for sentences, word finding), graphomotor coordination (Figure Drawings, Bender-Gestalt), auditory discrimination, and of achievement (including tests of reading single words and brief passages, writing single words and sentences and written mathematical computation). Brief projective testing included being asked to express three wishes. Intelligence testing, comprehensive projective testing, and specialized tests of specific neuropsychological functions were omitted.

This evaluation revealed that Frank had a host of problems in expressive and receptive language (in word finding, syntax, assimilation of sounds, words and syntactical units, auditory discrimination), in speech (mild articulation problems), and in at least some memory functions (retention of auditory information). The psychologist accounted for not having previously diagnosed Frank's specific deficits in language on the basis that these problems were now more striking in view of increased demands for processing. Furthermore, academic problems were revealed. Frank's performance of achievement tests of reading and math was just on (or in some instances slightly above) grade expectations. However, given his educational environment, this was below the expected level. His written work was below age and grade expectations, and even more deficient when he was compared with his classmates. The latter included all aspects: spelling, punctuation, and grammar. The specific components of difficulty in these academic skills (for example, those resulting from problems in right–left discrimination or other types of problems in visuospatial reasoning, sequencing, and visual processing) were not specified, and apparently not examined.

One of the presenting issues, Frank's problems focusing, was not definitively addressed in the conclusions of this evaluation. The possibility that he had an Attention Deficit/Hyperactivity Disorder was neither ruled in, nor ruled out. Perhaps this is, in part, because it was not as common at that time to consider this diagnostic possibility. In addition, the psychologist did not perceive Frank as inattentive or poorly focused. She *did* observe that he skipped words when writing and misread many small words. Instead she understood these matters in terms of a combination of language processing difficulties and characterological issues. Frank's tendency to withdraw into fantasies was related to his processing problems. Furthermore, in her view, Frank "does not realize that dreaming about performing is not the same thing as carrying it out."

The psychologist recommended that Frank would probably benefit from tutoring. She did not specify the focal areas, or the specific aspects of neuropsychological dysfunction which would need to be taken into account in developing an approach to remediation.

This evaluation clearly offered additional perspectives on Frank's previously noted imperviousness to interpretation, and his tendency to confabulation. In his effort to synthesize poorly understood (and/or retained) information, he had made some sense of what he heard, even if this was not guided by entirely realistic considerations.

Now, presented with a clearer definition of Frank's problems in receptive and expressive language, Dr. Waldron made some alterations in his technique in the analytic hours. He more carefully explained facts and events, in the service of reducing Frank's confusion and further clarifying which feelings and thoughts contributed to this confusion. He did not seem to pay equally explicit attention to the weakness in retention of auditory material which the testing revealed but did not underscore. Dr. Waldron also considered that Frank might have been unwilling to listen to interpretations because he anticipated his inability to comprehend.

The final testing evaluation during the course of the analysis was undertaken when Frank was 12 years, 4 months and at the beginning of the seventh grade and the sixth year of his analysis. This was again at the initiative of Mrs. Jay who found Frank much easier to live with, but had lingering concerns about his lack of ambition about school and his continuing failure in spelling. During the previous school year Frank had received mostly C's and some B's. His teachers and tutor were pleased with his progress, but Mrs. Jay was disappointed. Although Frank's reading was solid by this time, he still struggled with organizing and executing his writing. Mrs. Jay again took her son to the psychologist whom she regarded as a learning specialist.

Frank was once again given what was in our view a partial testing battery which examined some aspects of his academic work (a silent reading test of word identification and reading of brief passages followed by an assessment of comprehension, and written mathematical computation), his graphomotor functioning (Bender-Gestalt, Figure Drawings) and his language (naming, sentence repetition). Intelligence testing, comprehensive projective testing, a detailed examination of the building blocks for basic academic skills and the like were omitted.

The diagnostic impression was that Frank was managing reasonably well despite "soft signs" (in graphomotor functioning, grammar, organizing what he says and writes, and vocabulary). His expressive language had improved (in the sense of his capacity for word finding) with continued problems with grammar and syntax, and his general language comprehension seemed proficient. In the psychologist's view he had done about as well as could be expected. She noted that it was harder for Frank than others, about which he clearly had feelings. Achievement test scores were acceptable, although clearly below the level of his peers.

Several important features of Frank's functioning were mentioned but their implications were not sufficiently emphasized. The psychologist noted the interrelationship between his "obsessionalism" and his organizational difficulties: "he finds it hard to impose structure on a body of verbal information." Although the psychologist made an excellent case for Frank's pronounced problems in writing, she did not specifically diagnose him as dysgraphic. While she reported that his immediate memory for sentences was well below age expectations, she did not underline that he had a specific difficulty in this area.

Thus despite many well-intentioned efforts to clarify the nature of Frank's difficulties in learning and his psychodynamic constellation throughout his childhood and preadolescence, the specific nature of his problems was not carefully delineated. An integration of the varying perspectives of the multiple professionals who evaluated him was not offered. As a consequence the picture that emerged was more vague than needed to be the case, and the required focus and scope of his needs for remedial intervention were not well-defined.

THE ANALYTIC WORK FROM THE PERSPECTIVE OF COMPROMISE FORMATION THEORY

Dr. Waldron notes that it was near the end of Frank's first year of analysis, as he approached his eighth birthday and the end of second grade, that Frank first directly expressed his concerns about learning. Frank had an organizing unconscious fantasy that his analyst was not willing to help him with mastery, which was associatively linked with his feeling that mother could not tolerate his (or his brother's) growing independence, including his (Frank's) initial expression of feeling that father was "fun." A corollary was Frank's difficulty tolerating his parents' intimacy (such as Valentine's Day) and the analyst's intimacy with his wife (he accused Dr. Waldron of being "a bandit" if he had a wedding ring). Intimacy, along with independent activity, was experienced as "criminal."

Frank began to engage in other types of "criminal" behavior, the incidence and extent of which grew over time. He took things, spent money on purchases which were not allowed, and told lies to justify his actions. Frank thought no one would be smart enough to figure this out. After many months Dr. Waldron began to recognize the seriousness of Frank's delinquency. At the same time Frank's envy of his father's and analyst's power and penis emerged. Frank felt weak and defective; he believed he had to cheat to retain his masculinity.

While he and Dr. Waldron were analyzing his negative oedipal complex, in the context of his parents' being firmer in discouraging his antisocial behavior, Frank started to become interested in what he *could* do for himself in school. This interest in schoolwork emerged without Dr. Waldron's directly interpreting the effect of Frank's academic disabilities on his feelings of weakness and defectiveness. It grew out of the analytic work on Frank's conflicts and led to his revealing, and his mother's observing, his academic difficulties; further testing was then arranged. We heartily agree with Dr. Waldron's retrospective thought that the intensity of Frank's envy, and his depressive sense he could only get what he wanted through dishonest means, "may very well have been consequences of his early perceptions of his own difficulties in learning" which had not yet been diagnosed.

Frank was not without conflict about his "crimes"; he did not want to be left to commit them—exemplified by his provoking punishment. Furthermore, Frank experienced himself as unequal to the task of regulating his impulses; the "no" voice in him which was "relatively small and unworthy of respect" could not stand up to the more powerful urge to be "bad." Looking back, Dr. Waldron considered the additional contribution of Frank's still undiagnosed learning disability to his tendency to depressive affect: "[his] considerable feelings of inadequacy, of being so small, and of not being able to do many things he wanted to do." As Frank increasingly felt the analyst understood his struggle with being "bad," he more directly expressed his longings for the analyst and his disappointment that his parents did not appreciate this. His negative oedipal wishes to be loved as a woman by father and by the analyst came into focus. His guilt over such wishes, and his need to seek punishment for this was seen in his taking things in the office. He felt this was wrong and had superbaby beat up the father. Thus Frank's reactions to his learning disability dovetailed with other determinants of his feelings of castration and deficiency.

As Dr. Waldron interpreted Frank's cravings for what others had, Frank's effort to perform in school increased. He became more interested in what he could do for himself. However, this did not yield much success. This was the point at which Mrs. Jay arranged for the third diagnostic testing evaluation, which led Dr. Waldron to begin to consider that Frank's "imperviousness to interpretations" might be, among other things, an expression of his problems with language. As Dr. Waldron began to take this into account, he more carefully worded his interpretations, and more specifically explained actual facts and events. He came to think that failing to answer Frank's requests for personal information was detrimental. Answering straightforwardly was important. Tutoring was also instituted.

In addition to technical modifications, new conceptual, exploratory and interpretive emphases were opened up by the results of this evaluation. This was despite the fact that it was considerably less comprehensive, specific, and integrative than could have been the case. In the third year of the analysis, Dr. Waldron began to examine cognitive contributions to Frank's confusion in the analytic hours. In turn, he and Frank explored the ways in which his disability was put to defensive purposes. This process went on over the course of many years.

Frank was a boy who had trouble getting the facts straight (processing language and, we might add, retaining it in view of the findings of a deficit in immediate auditory memory). At times he did not invest sufficient effort in comprehending because of his expectation of failure, and/or of having to work harder than others to succeed. His penchant for idiosyncratic interpretations of information, his "changing things around," could also be seen as one of his attempts to organize what he did *not* understand in accordance with ideas already familiar to him (his preconceptions). It was Dr. Waldron's experience with Frank that, while the material in an hour appeared to point in one direction, his efforts to capture that direction interpretively often met with failure or frustration. Frank frequently changed the subject, expressed a sense of boredom, or looked blank. These clinical manifestations could now also be understood in terms of Frank's efforts to grapple with receptive and expressive language problems.

Such an understanding did not eliminate or diminish the significance of the psychodynamic aspects of such responses. Frank still needed to be approached as a child for whom knowing was conflicted, since it was associated with anxiety about discovering frightening things, about committing the "crime" of being more independent, of competing with father, mother, brother, and the analyst. Furthermore, not knowing, being confused and/or forgetting satisfied superego demands for punishment for these "crimes"; for example, if Frank forgot or remained confused, and did not produce his homework, he could get into trouble.

Similarly, Frank's tendency to confuse the pronouns "he" and "she" were manifestations of his neuropsychologically based language disability, which was also interwoven with, and expressive of, a host of elements of conflict over his sexual identity. Frank wished to be a boy who was a girl. This was an expression of his oedipal longings for mother (he exhibited himself as Miss America, disguised as a girl in a towel, and by dressing up as a girl). He also expressed his negative oedipal wish to be loved by father as mother was in this way. There was also evidence that Frank perceived his father as having a feminine identification: his big stomach, his passive oral wishes, his lack of assertiveness. Frank's feminine identification was also an effort to defend himself against his intense castration anxiety (as seen in his play early in the analysis in which the baby's penis was sadistically hammered, and his greatest fear was of losing his penis and balls). In dressing like a girl, Frank appeared to have already lost his penis. Thus he attempted to render himself invulnerable to the attacker. This, like his "baby behavior," could be understood as a defense against castration anxiety and an effort to make himself more lovable to his mother. Although not mentioned in Dr. Waldron's account, one wonders whether mother preferred that her second child be a girl, since she already had a boy.

Frank probably experienced himself as defective, ill-equipped, and castrated, given his significant cognitive weaknesses (in language, immediate auditory memory, all academic subjects, and graphomotor coordination). This no doubt contributed to his envy of others and his urges to rob what he felt they had, which he felt himself to be missing. A sense of damage could well have been elaborated by Frank in fantasy as a punishment for his "crimes." Frank's efforts to fool and to lie, for which he appreciated being caught, and for which he felt he should be punished, were also likely to have been expressions of unconscious fantasies about others not noticing his pronounced difficulty at school and elsewhere in his life. Perhaps he felt he had "fooled" them, since he knew his brother to have been receiving tutorial help for years.

This may have been an opportunity Frank envied. Dr. Waldron emphasizes Frank's intense envy of others, as seen, for example, in his voracious appetite for Whacky Pack cards. He never felt he had enough of them, and never felt his collection to be as good as that of others. Frank's depressive feeling of hopelessness about never having enough may also have contributed to his attraction to the exciting sadomasochistic relationship with his brother, and, when this became less possible, to enacting this type of play with friends as well as with the analyst for a period of time.

Dr. Waldron commented that Frank engaged in less directly sexual material in his hours as he began to struggle with his schoolwork. One way of looking at this is that Frank found something salutory in his beginning efforts to control these problems and in discovering that others understood the extent of his academic difficulties. He consequently felt more hopeful, less depressed, and found it less necessary to attempt to relieve his depression via sexual, especially sadomasochistic, activity. He now had his analyst and a tutor willing to help him with mastery.

Dr. Waldron noted that Frank expressed a lot of anger toward his mother during the period of the analysis when with great difficulty he began to more actively attempt to engage in schoolwork. This coincided with his wondering if he were "enough of a boy" and his taking chances losing things, followed by reassurances that they could be recovered. Like many learning disabled children, Frank's rage may have related to the fantasy that mother intentionally had not given him everything he needed (genitals, a well-functioning brain, and the like).

During the last years of the analysis Dr. Waldron's awareness that Frank had substantial learning disabilities was sharpened by the diagnostic work performed when Frank was nearly 9 and completing the third grade. His cognitive problems affected not only expressive and receptive language but also many academic subjects. In view of these findings, Dr. Waldron and Frank gave more consistent attention to the many aspects of his learning problems: his tendency to deny their existence, the nature of his feelings about them, his panoply of defenses against admitting that he had these feelings, and against addressing his difficulties more adaptively. The evaluation performed when Frank was 12 years, 4 months and at the beginning of the seventh grade further highlighted these problems.

Denial played an important role in Frank's life. His belief that he became strong through sucking like a baby, stealing, and keeping his allowance (rather than purchasing presents for others as he was expected to do) involved denial in fantasy.

He also denied that his parents could catch him at his misdemeanors because, he asserted, he was smarter than they. In addition, by avoiding talking about his tutoring in his analysis, he hid from himself and his analyst the painful feelings he experienced when he tried to master academic work.

As was suggested in our discussion of Mrs. Barrett's case of Leah in chapter 4, it would appear that Frank's learning disability played an important role in his use of denial. Misperceiving, poorly perceiving, or failing to perceive the environment is the essence of denial. Frank's denial was supported by his environment. To a great degree Frank's use of denial resulted from his identification with his parents. For example, his insistence that the symbols on his computer's buttons were devoid of meaning was similar to his mother's "difficulty comprehending written instructions." The fact that his parents often failed to tell the truth also contributed to his denial. So too did his ability to hide the pervasiveness of his dishonesty from his parents and his analyst for quite a while. Similarly, his mother and his analyst were able to hide from themselves the fact that he had cognitive difficulties despite recognizing manifestations of such difficulties. Dr. Waldron and his supervisor discussed Frank's obtuseness, but initially decided it was psychogenic. His mother repeatedly sought tests that eventually revealed his learning disability. For many years, however, the psychologists who tested Frank neither emphasized the evidence they had for learning difficulties nor tried to ferret out further evidence.

Interpretation helped Frank overcome some of the ill effects of his denial. For instance, Dr. Waldron showed Frank how he tried to avoid anxiety by failing to understand what was happening when his father developed a cardiac arhythmia. Interpretation also enabled Frank to better attend to his tutor's concerted efforts to draw his attention to and remediation of his academic difficulties, thus furthering the analytic achievement.

Frank's reliance upon "clowning" was viewed as an expression of his strong wish to exhibit himself, camouflaged by an outward appearance of self-mockery. It no doubt also reflected Frank's feelings that he could not be taken seriously. We believe (as does Dr. Waldron) that this was in part related to his inability to perform like his peers, for which he feared being ridiculed. Dr. Waldron appreciated this in retrospect. He and Frank had spoken of Frank's feeling not as smart as the others, but not specifically about his information processing difficulties and about his need to be tutored for this. In retrospect, Dr. Waldron also considered that it would have been optimal to have interpreted Frank's failure to discuss his tutor as one manifestation of his effort to deny his distress about his disabilities.

A number of other defenses were effectively explored in the analysis. Frank's tendency to make assumptions about things he did not understand fully, and to not ask for help in doing so, was viewed as an attempt to avoid feeling bad about not knowing and about the fact that someone else *did* know. Similarly Frank's insistence on being "disinterested" in school was understood as a defense against feeling sad or unhappy about finding academic material difficult. In the analytic hours Dr. Waldron observed with Frank that when he could not "get things straight," he avoided concentrated mental effort and wished for "treats." He approached the hours themselves as assignments which he could not successfully carry out. (This was also an important component of the analysis reported by Dr. Wyszynski of her adult patient Mr. G in chapter 19.) In his play in analytic hours Frank expressed fantasies of his extraordinary "evil" powers, which were interpreted as a defense against his sense of inadequacy in doing what comes so easily to others.

Again, clarification of these defenses was accompanied by Frank's more direct competitive efforts in school and with the analyst. Frank became more interested in doing his work carefully. In this context, Dr. Waldron pointed out that Frank *did* have to spend more time than his peers to complete the same work successfully. Up until that point Frank had not let himself recognize this. Once he did he was encouraged; schoolwork was something he *could* do. It would have been even more helpful—if Dr. Waldron had had access to a clear and detailed picture of what exactly was the nature of his difficulties (and what was not difficult)—to assist Frank in becoming acquainted with these specific features of his functioning. Frank clearly wished to face reality. With poignancy, he posed frank questions to Dr. Waldron. Was his (Frank's) a good mind? Was his school a good school? When he returned to see Dr. Waldron many years later, Frank said it was Dr. Waldron's honesty that he most cherished.

Dr. Waldron also understood Frank's anxiety about claiming responsibility for (intentionally) aiming to do well in school. This anxiety arose with similar intensity in the context of setting himself the goal of losing weight (at which his father had failed). Frank experienced associated fantasies of being punished, hung, and raped.

During termination Frank was concerned that, in Dr. Waldron's absence, he would not spend time and energy thinking things through, and working to achieve, no matter how much effort it took. Fear of mother's disapproval for his rewarding efforts to find romantic and sexual satisfaction was also prominent. In this regard, it was noteworthy that Dr. Waldron's later contacts with Frank highlight his success in struggling with his conflicts over wishes for romantic partners who were intelligent, and his efforts to balance his intellectual and romantic pursuits.

Chapter 11

Eric's Analysis

Judith Yanof, M.D.

PRESENTING PROBLEMS

Eric was brought to see me by his parents at the end of his kindergarten year, when he had just turned 6. Kindergarten had been difficult for Eric. He had repeated conflicts with his teacher because he was disobedient, angry, and out of control in the classroom. On several occasions he kicked his teacher during a tantrum. Eric also had trouble doing his schoolwork. He had difficulty writing and could not sit still long enough to draw. At home, too, he was easily upset by small incidents "which sent him off the deep end." He would fall down on the ground screeching verbal abuse at the top of his lungs, completely oblivious to where he was, even if in a public place. His parents felt desperate as they tried to exert control over his behavior. Instead, he drove them to lose control of their own tempers. They loved him, but his difficulties made them feel like failures.

Their concern about Eric was not new. They had been worried about him since he was a small boy. He seemed to them to be "hyperactive since he began to walk," always on the move and always courting danger. They felt unable to protect or control him. As a toddler he had had several serious injuries from tricycle accidents and falls. As he grew older he had become withdrawn and sullen. He seemed to take little pleasure in any activity or relationship.

Eric's situation stood out in stark contrast to that of his two older sisters, who were 10 and 12 years old. They were good students and seemed happy. Eric predictably was consumed by jealousy of his sisters, particularly the one closest in age to himself, with whom he fought bitterly. His only playmates were some older neighborhood boys who tended to tease him.

In the last weeks of kindergarten, Eric's parents consulted a psychologist who said that Eric had an Attention Deficit Disorder (ADD) and told his parents that he might have a specific learning disability as well. Before my evaluation, Eric's parents, the school, and the psychologist had made a joint decision for Eric to repeat kindergarten.

PSYCHOLOGICAL TESTING

Before seeing me, Eric had had psychological testing. The psychologist noted that Eric was restless throughout the testing. Although he could be persuaded to complete most tasks, his squirming and persistently asking when the test would be over interfered with his performance. The psychologist also reported that Eric was unusually aware of outside sounds and was easily distracted by them.

Eric performed better on the structured tests than on the unstructured ones. On the WISC-R he scored a Full Scale IQ of 111 with a Verbal IQ of 115 and a Performance IQ of 104. There was not much scatter on the subtest scores, but verbal tasks were generally stronger than visual-perceptual, visual-motor, and visual-spatial tests. More generally, he had poor fine motor coordination, including labored handwriting with some directional confusion. Eric became very uneasy with the projective tests and produced very few responses to them. What he did say indicated that he had many fears of bodily injury. He saw himself as vulnerable because of his behavior, which he could not control.

The psychologist felt that on the basis of the history and her observations, Eric should be diagnosed with ADD. She felt his mild to moderate difficulty with all perceptual-motor tasks might contribute to a future learning disability. She recommended that Eric repeat kindergarten, have a trial of medication for ADD, and begin psychotherapy to help him with his poor self-esteem.

CONSULTATION

When I first met Eric, he was a handsome, active 6-year-old boy with a "macho" facade that barely disguised a great deal of anxiety. He was well-related and eager to please, but tense. In our first sessions together he drew pictures and built with blocks quite creatively. He also sustained a somewhat stereotypical play, a war game, in which he repeatedly set up soldiers, mine and his, and knocked them down. Although there were times when he moved from one toy to another in rapid succession, there were other times when he concentrated for long periods on one particular task. In my office he was not restless or fidgety. He did not make extraneous noises, hum, tap, or interrupt. In fact, he was not the hyperactive boy described at home and at school. His speech articulation and fine motor coordination were somewhat immature.

As his parents had mentioned, Eric seemed to take little pleasure in himself or his play, frequently making disparaging remarks about what he had done. However, he had an impressive ability to articulate his concerns verbally in a direct way. He referred to himself as "dumb" because he had been left back in the "easiest grade of all." He said that he had been left back because his teacher had punished him for his "naughty" behavior. He used the words *dumb* and *naughty* interchangeably. He said rather desperately that he hoped I could help him "get smart."

Family Background

Eric's mother and father had had marital difficulties for many years and had been intermittently in couples' therapy without substantially improving their relationship. One point of disagreement was how to manage Eric's behavior.

Eric's father was an accountant in what he considered a pleasureless and underpaid job. In spite of this he "worked all the time." He felt very identified with Eric, who reminded him of himself as a child. He was eager to get help for his son, but in the heat of anger he said things he did not mean.

Eric's mother was a musician. She worked part-time and was the parent with the major responsibility for the children's care. She was angry at her husband's "unavailability." As with Eric, she felt helpless to effect any change in him and retaliated by criticizing her husband in front of the children. With some insight, she recognized that her intense involvement with Eric may have been in part a reaction to her wanting more from her husband. She also associated to her childhood experience of being left in full charge of her younger brother when her mother worked during the day. This was a duty she found overwhelming because she could not control him.

Developmental History

Eric was a much wanted child and was the product of a normal pregnancy and an uncomplicated delivery by planned C-section. There were no difficulties at birth. He was a well-regulated infant who slept well and ate without problems. His developmental milestones were all within normal limits. He smiled at 4 weeks, sat at 6 months, stood at 10 months, walked at 14 months, and said single words at 16 months. He was toilet trained at 3 years, 3 months. At the time he began to walk, his activity increased and he became oppositional. His parents indicated that it was at this point that things seemed to become difficult with Eric. In preschool he was unable to function in the group and retreated to his cubby.

Decision for Analysis

I had begun to see Eric in the aftermath of the above-described diagnostic testing consultation with the expectation that we would begin psychotherapy. At the conclusion of my consultation with Eric, I recommended psychoanalysis. Certainly his development was in jeopardy. He had serious trouble at home and at school because of his conduct. The other prominent feature of the clinical picture was Eric's low opinion of himself. Here was a youngster with many assets who was distraught. I recommended psychoanalysis because I thought it was the treatment of choice for Eric's conduct disorder, anxiety, and low self-esteem. Nevertheless, I had many diagnostic questions.

Eric's parents presented a picture of a boy having chronic difficulties with overactivity and impulsivity. The psychologist observed distractibility, and Eric's teacher corroborated this finding (although his second kindergarten teacher did not). However, Eric was not hyperactive or distracted in my office. This caused me to wonder about, but not rule out ADD (Attention Deficit Disorder) or ADHD (Attention Deficit/Hyperactivity Disorder). The one-on-one, unstructured situation with me had few demands. It could not be equated with home or school where repetitive or difficult tasks were required on demand and had to be carried out without close supervision. Moreover, children with ADD or ADHD frequently have variable activity levels as part of the clinical picture (Barkley, 1990).

I found myself wondering: Was Eric's hyperactivity a defense against anxiety or depression? Or was his anxiety and sense of defeat a response to some neuropsychological inability to control his impulses? Was Eric's disinhibition and oppositional behavior his way of dealing with a stressful family situation? Or was the tension in the family a consequence of dealing with a child who was having difficulty responding to an appropriate set of expectations? Were we dealing with something that was basically physiological or psychological?

Although hyperactivity was never a large component of Eric's behavior in my office, once the treatment began I quickly became aware of Eric's impulsivity and behavioral disinhibition. Eric was heedless at times, acting quickly, and not being able to consider fully the potentially negative, destructive, or dangerous consequences of his behavior. He could be careless, fly off the handle, or regress rapidly. He was oppositional. At the same time Eric's new kindergarten teacher did not see signs of distractibility or hyperactivity in the classroom. I was not sure to what extent Eric's problems were exacerbated by, or originated from, a constitutionally based neuropsychological problem, such as ADD or ADHD. I hypothesized that there was a complex interplay of both constitutional and environmental factors that contributed to the clinical picture I now observed.

When I began to treat Eric, I was not certain if his symptoms would interfere with establishing an analytic process. While a diagnosis of ADD or ADHD does not contraindicate an analysis, the core symptoms of ADD—hyperactivity, impulsivity, and distractibility—might well make psychoanalytic work more difficult. Ideally, analytic work requires that the analyst be able to communicate with the child in words or play, and that she has the freedom to take an analytic stance toward what happens in the analytic hours. When a child is driven by activity and impulsivity, limit-setting can become the main feature of treatment, postponing any other kind of therapeutic intervention. Moreover, the child in analysis needs to be able to focus cognitively in order to play coherently and to use interpretation and verbal interventions for insight. This, too, is more difficult for children with ADD or ADHD.

In Eric's case, however, I thought his motivation, intelligence, ability to verbalize feelings, and good object-relatedness would be assets in an analysis. Moreover, I thought that his family was stable, caring, and very committed to getting him help.

I did not begin by prescribing Ritalin or any other stimulant medication. First, I wanted to see what impact the analytic treatment alone would have on Eric's behavior. Second, I use stimulant medication very judiciously in my treatment of children. While there is ample evidence that stimulant medication effectively "normalizes" the clinical symptoms of ADHD (hyperactivity, distractibility, and impulsivity), there is no substantial scientific evidence that such medication is therapeutically effective for any of the long-term academic deficits or comorbid emotional symptoms of these patients (Richters, Arnold, Jensen et al., 1995, p. 993). Medication, however, becomes particularly important when the symptoms make an analytic process too difficult to engage in, or when analysis cannot affect the symptoms quickly enough to stop an increasingly negative cycle at home or at school, or when the analysis has little impact on the symptoms over time. Let me emphasize that medication is in no way a contraindication to psychoanalysis.

Several other factors, in this case, contributed to my decision to wait and see before prescribing medication. First, Eric's parents were not eager to medicate their young child. Second, because the decision to repeat kindergarten already had been made, the pressure to perform well in school was much less of an immediate issue. A third factor was that Eric's new kindergarten teacher was an excellent match for him. She was easygoing, yet consistent and clear about her expectations, and she liked Eric very much. She did not see his classroom behavior as symptomatic. As it turned out, medication was never necessary, because as the analysis took hold Eric's behavior outside the treatment situation improved dramatically.

I arranged to see Eric four times a week and referred his parents for weekly sessions to a social worker with whom I work closely. I thought that Eric's parents would need a lot of support and guidance in managing Eric's behavior, as would any parents in a similar situation. I also hoped that as time went on Eric's parents could use these sessions to address their marital issues. I saw Eric's parents on a monthly basis. My primary goal in seeing them was to exchange information and to keep the lines of communication open between us. I knew that without a good analyst–parent alliance it would be almost impossible to prevent a prematurely interrupted child analysis.

COURSE OF THE ANALYSIS

The Opening Phase: Transformations

Eric's lack of control at home and at school became a problem in my office within a matter of weeks. This usually took the form of his shouting verbal abuse at me and running out of my office. Of necessity our analytic work began by addressing

this issue. I decided to analyze this behavior rather than prohibit it (which I must admit I felt inclined to do). My interventions were of several types. I verbalized what he was doing in a
nonpejorative way; I imagined what he might be feeling; I im-
parted my belief that there was a reason for this behavior; and
I defined myself as a person who would help him figure out its
meaning. I allowed Eric to leave the office when necessary,
encouraging him to use the waiting room to regain his compo-
sure and to return at will.

Sometimes Eric tried to destroy objects in my office, write
on the walls, or throw things at me. When his behavior was
dangerous or damaging, as in these cases, I did prohibit it out-
right, saying to him that my office had to be a place for both
of us to feel safe or we could not do our work of figuring things
out. I tried to convey to him that I wanted to know about his
feelings in order to understand them. However, I needed him
to show me his feelings in a way that would make neither of us
feel too bad. Obviously this was more easily said than done. In
practice, there were times when I became too controlling and
times when I did not act quickly enough and something was
broken. We then tried to talk about what had happened.

At first these outbursts seemed entirely unpredictable to
me, but over time it became clear that Eric was sensitive to any
real or imagined rebuff on my part. Even when I recognized
the precipitant, the transition to this out-of-control state was so
rapid that Eric himself was hardly aware of what had happened.

I learned that Eric was fascinated with transformer toys
that he brought to his sessions. On several occasions he drew
monsters that had "transformed" into armored tanks or sub-
marines when they were attacked. I talked to him about how
he was like a transformer himself; he "transformed" from one
state to another. He liked being identified with transformers
because he saw these toys as powerful. I also told him how hard
it was for a transformer: how confusing it was to go from one
state to another and how disorganizing it was not to be able to
control the fast changes. Over many months I introduced the
idea that we could look at events that occurred just before he
"transformed" to understand why they happened, and that

understanding would make the process more in his control and less scary.

Although at first I had to guess about the precipitating event, Eric became quite adept at telling me what had angered or upset him. I, in turn, became better at understanding the nuances of his sensitivity. On some occasions, the precipitating event was that Eric had crossed paths with another patient. This was especially true if he saw me with girls, whom he assumed I preferred. At other times, I simply might have asked a question to which he did not know the answer, or used a word he did not understand. In each case, however, the common denominator seemed to be an event that stimulated his feelings of worthlessness. As we explored these feelings that made him transform, outbursts did not disappear, but Eric recovered from them more easily, and the alliance between us became less tenuous. The act of putting things into words was integrating, and helped Eric to delay action (see Katan, 1961).

One of the things I came to notice early in the analytic work was a lack of continuity and coherence within the sessions. Although this had not been true of our initial sessions, it became true once the analysis got under way. Eric was rarely able to maintain an alliance with me. Sudden changes of mood could disrupt our sense of being together. Eric might enter my office in a friendly mood, but then want to leave, without my having a clue as to what had happened. Continuity between sessions was also fleeting. Eric seemed volatile and sensitive to many things that took place outside the sessions. If we had a productive session one day, I could not count on a residue of good feeling or an atmosphere of safety lasting until the next session. Nor did Eric continue to use the same toys or to elaborate the same themes from session to session. Things felt fragmented. I wondered if the incoherence I experienced was a communication about Eric's inner state and/or a reevocation of the quality of some early object relationship, representing an early nonverbal transference. I tried to find ways to address this discontinuity with Eric that would elicit his curiosity. I told him that I did not know which Eric I was going to meet in the waiting room. I tried to describe the different "Erics" he could be.

Sense of Defect

Our early therapeutic relationship had a highly ambivalent quality to it. His relationship with me was one in which he provoked, teased, withheld, and kept "secrets." He derived pleasure from ordering me around, showing me up, proving me stupid, and manipulating games so he could win. During some sessions there was a more mutual interaction, a more genuine affection, and themes were more oedipal. However, this was the exception rather than the rule.

Eric elaborated in many different forms a fantasy that there was something wrong with him. It was often his brain. For instance, he played a doctor game in which there was something wrong with a boy's brain. Although it was never clear exactly what was wrong, various operations were performed to fix it, including brain transplants. Sometimes the boy was "crazy," sometimes the boy was "stupid" or "out of control," and sometimes the boy had "a learning problem."

Several times Eric expressed the fantasy that his brain got "stolen" and that revenge by "stealing back" might be a solution to the problem. He often demanded that I draw the same thing he was drawing. He then liberally "borrowed" my ideas and incorporated them into his own picture. We often played a game where we both built Lego houses. He saw himself as a good builder. Nevertheless, he needed to incorporate whole sections of my house to improve his, although there were plenty of unused Legos. He told me he was "mugging" (i.e., stealing from) me but he "needed to." I agreed and then suggested that it would be helpful to understand what he needed and why he believed his own was not good enough.

Eric's fantasy that there was something wrong with his brain functioned on many different levels. At the most surface and conscious level, Eric saw himself as "dumb" because he had been "left back" in school and had been told that he might have a learning disability. However, a defective brain also became the nidus around which other concerns coalesced. From an early age, Eric's chronic inability to regulate his affects, master his impulses, and control his behavior left him with a deep-seated sense of failure. These difficulties evoked many negative responses from his parents, leading Eric to believe that he was not the child his parents wanted. A defective brain became interlaced with this earlier image of inadequacy. Finally, there were more specific conflicts over his aggression, competition, and sexuality. These conflicts troubled him in their own right, and made him feel "bad" and deserving of punishment. A castrated self or defective brain could, therefore, also become the compromise solution to a conflicted set of neurotic wishes. The fantasy of a defective brain could be used to keep in check aggressive desires and threatening wishes for oedipal victory.

About eight months into the analysis, Eric made a book about a boy who was courting disaster by standing on the roof. His mother helplessly warned him to be careful, but she was too far away and he fell off. He hurt his brain and needed to go to the hospital for an operation. The doctor took out his brain, examined it, and pronounced that there was nothing wrong with it. Eric worked under great pressure to finish the book before the end of the session, because he wanted his mother to see it. When I commented on the pressure he seemed to be under, he yelled at me, "My mother wants it to be perfect!" He then rushed out of the office with the book.

What he really needed to show his mother was that there was nothing wrong with his brain—that it was "perfect." I noticed only after he returned the book to his box, that he had mistakenly written, "and the doctor said there was nothing," leaving out the last words: "wrong with his brain." In his haste, he had made an error that clearly had psychodynamic meaning. His fear was that there was "nothing" where a brain should be. For the first time, however, Eric had found a new solution: the doctor would cure the boy not by doing a brain transplant, but by declaring that the boy's own brain was okay. This was his curative fantasy of the analysis.

Since the learning disability was not truly diagnosed and in fact never materialized, I could not take it up in a straightforward, matter-of-fact way. However, I told Eric that he had a "wrong idea" about himself and that his troubles in kindergarten were not about being "dumb." In fact, I told him that I thought he was a "smart kid who didn't think he could do a lot of things he really could do." In our sessions he both underestimated his abilities and "played dumb."

In contrast to the learning disability, Eric's impulsivity was something very apparent in our interactions. I did not address this as a "brain issue," although perhaps it was. Instead I addressed the inner experience of being out of control. I told him that he had a hard time stopping and saying "no" to himself even when he really wanted to. I talked about it as a limitation that he needed to acknowledge and that we could better understand.

During the first year of analysis, Eric's behavior at home and school improved dramatically. Eric developed a good relationship with his new kindergarten teacher who genuinely liked him. Outbursts at school were a rare exception. He had friends at school for the first time, and he was apparently learning without difficulty. His behavior at home also improved considerably. He had transferred much of his negative behavior into the analysis, freeing himself for growth on the outside.

At the same time the parent work with my colleague, which continued for a year-and-a-half, succeeded in helping Eric's parents to cooperate in firm and appropriate limit-setting. It became clear to the parents' therapist that bitter, unresolved resentments toward each other underlay much of the parents' arguments about limit-setting. However, the parent work never effectively dealt with the deeper marital issues, which were left to fester.

In my work with the parents, the marital issues also went untouched. I saw the parents on a monthly basis. In the beginning, I was helpful in presenting them with a different view of Eric. I pointed out many of his strengths, including his obvious intelligence. The analyst's genuine, positive opinion of the child patient can significantly mitigate the sense of failure in both parent and child who are involved in a cycle of negative interaction. I also helped the parents understand Eric's behavior, which was difficult to comprehend and to manage without becoming provoked. As his parents understood more about his motivations, they found more effective ways to respond to his underlying needs. I saw my work with the parents as being an advocate for Eric and the analysis, while compassionately listening to the difficulties they faced, both in responding to his challenges and in making the analysis possible.

Defenses

Because Eric believed he was defective, his main concern was defending against his sense of vulnerability. His predominant defense was an identification with the aggressor. If we played school he was the teacher, bossing me, restricting my movements, and calling me "dumb." My homework received bad marks and scribbles all over the page. He did to me what he was afraid would be done to him. If I expressed upset in my role as the child, he could not be sympathetic to my plight. Likewise, he could only be the older sibling beating on a younger one. At this time in his life he was able to communicate, but unable to identify with the victim's point of view. His sense of smallness and helplessness was disavowed and split off from his awareness.

I told him that I could see how much better it felt when he was the hitter and not the doll being hit, or how much better it felt to call me dumb than to feel dumb himself, or how good it felt to win and how bad it felt to lose. Occasionally Eric confessed to me that when he lost he felt like "the worst kid in the world." Sometimes I played the role of the helpless one and verbalized what this experience was like.

Eric also used grandiosity to deal with his feelings of vulnerability. He exaggerated what he was capable of doing. He looked to the future when he would become a major league pitcher or superstar basketball player. Anything less than perfect was devalued. If his favorite pitcher lost a game, he "stunk." Eric could not get a realistic perspective on himself: he was either the best or he "stunk." I frequently pointed out to Eric how he felt someone became garbage and had to be thrown out the moment they made a mistake or had bad luck. I said that he treated himself in the same way, that he gave himself a hard time. I interpreted that it was difficult for Eric to not know something, even though it was a position necessary in order to learn. I said, "You would like it if you could know everything, because not knowing makes you feel little and dumb. But it's a funny thing, that the people who learn the most are the people who can say what they need to know."

Because of our work on these defenses, Eric tentatively began to articulate his feelings of vulnerability, mostly in displacement. Eric told me the following fantasy. When he was a baby the family had a puppy. This puppy was very wild and out of control. It would jump all over the place. One day a passerby shot the dog because he thought the dog was a "mad dog" and dangerous. In the story the puppy's behavior was misunderstood and feared, and so the puppy was eliminated. To Eric it was dangerous and confusing to be "wild." It meant he was "mad" in the sense of being both angry and crazy, and he worried that it would not be tolerated.

In another story Eric told me that originally he belonged to another family and that his current parents were in fact his adoptive parents. They had wanted to give him back early on, once they had found out what he was really like. However, the deal had been "no backsies" so they were stuck with him. Here again Eric expressed the painful feeling that he was unwanted and unlovable, and the unstated threat of abandonment was in the wings. This was an interesting version and inversion of the familiar family romance.[1]

Crazy Man: An Analytic Hour

The following material comes from a session that took place in the eighth month of the treatment. This hour was unusual for its coherence. It thus foreshadowed the cohesion of a deeper analytic process that was to come. It is a good example of the work during the first phase of the analysis when Eric's out-of-control behavior was a major focus of our interest. It illustrates

---

[1] In the traditional family romance, the child is adopted, but comes from a family of much more exalted status than his own. While the details of the family romance fantasy are unique for each individual, the motivation for such a fantasy is often similar. The fantasy expresses rivalry with the parents, resentment toward the parents for excluding the child, and a struggle to separate from the overidealized parental imagos of one's earlier years (Freud, 1909).

well Eric's preoccupation with the physical experience of hyper-activity and its psychic meaning to him, as well as the way in which he used this state defensively to ward off other threaten-ing feelings.

In this session Eric introduced a character he called "Crazy Man" by making a drawing in which the lines were wobbly, jerky, and out of control. The image he created was not coher-ent and was barely recognizable as a human figure. It was the way the lines jerked that seemed to convey the essence of "Crazy Man."

I asked, "What makes Crazy Man crazy?"

Eric demonstrated by making more jerky lines. "His body goes all over the place, like this. Out of control." Eric then drew Crazy Dog and showed me that his markers kept going off the page and onto my table as he drew. He then suggested that I make something crazy too. He made a boundary line that he wanted me to cross over. I drew and veered over the line impulsively to Eric's delight.

I asked, "What happens when Crazy Man goes crazy?"

Eric said, "He feels like he is going to explode. BOOM!"

"Like a bomb exploding?" I asked.

"Like a rocket going off into space," said Eric.

I inquired, "Does Crazy Man know when he is going to feel like a rocket that suddenly takes off?"

"No," said Eric.

"That must not feel too good," I said. "Suddenly this ex-ploding feeling just takes him over."

"Yep."

"It would probably feel a little better if he knew when it was coming. If he could get ready for it, he would feel more pre-pared."

"Yes, it would," said Eric.

Eric then began to draw a bird. "I'm drawing a bird. Isn't this a good bird?" he asked.

"Yes," I answered.

Eric added, "I didn't plan it. It just came out this way."

"Without planning?" I said.

"Yep." He continued, "Hey I'm doing this very fast. I'm winning by going the fastest. Faster than you. You go fast too."

"You want me to see what it feels like when things go so fast that there is no time to plan." I began to draw very fast, but my bird did not come out so well. I said, "Oops! My things come out a little better when they don't go too fast." As I slowed down and continued to draw, Eric looked at my picture and grabbed the pen out of my hand roughly.

"I am stealing your things," he said.

"You are mugging me again," I said.

"Yep."

In this sequence, Eric conveyed to me in a very vivid and creative way what it felt like to be unable to make his body do what he wanted it to do. I thought that Crazy Man represented his experience of what it felt like when he was hyperactive. The disintegrative and disorganizing aspects of this experience were communicated in the way that the jerky movements made it impossible to draw a coherent form. In Eric's mind, the out-of-control body experience was associated with transgressing and being bad, as in going out of bounds and drawing on the table, as well as being deranged, defective, and "crazy." These themes—out of control, crazy, and bad—were frequently inter-changeable in Eric's play and associations. When Eric mentioned his "rocket" feelings, I wondered to myself whether he was also making an unconscious reference to phallic sensations and erections, another body experience that may have felt out of control to him.

I believe that Eric's intent in this analytic hour was to get me to share his experience. He wanted me to be "Crazy Man" too. He wanted us to be together in the experience so that he could be understood, not isolated, and so that his feelings could be made more manageable. Complementing his desires, I too wanted to understand Eric's experience so that I could help him put it into words. I felt this would be integrative. I could offer him verbal symbols that could help organize his feelings and make them less overwhelming.

When I participated in his experience and verbalized it, it led to a deepening of the material. Eric then talked about another experience of being out of control, drawing fast without planning. This time he moved to talking directly about himself. Again he wanted me to experience what he was feeling. In this case, I probably did not stay with his experience long enough. Instead I tried to "educate" him about the consequences of going too fast, which he needed to ignore and deny. He experienced these remarks as threatening. He responded by aggressively stripping me of what I had, in a "mini" loss of control. When I tried to address this in the moment, he interrupted me with, "Shut up." However, the play was not disrupted for long.

Eric then went on to make a third drawing, "Crazy House." A father is in the house, a boy in front, and a mother in back yelling, "HELP!" Eric said, "Her boy is about to fall off. The way he is holding on isn't safe. Her boy is about to get hurt."

I said, "The mom is pretty far away from her boy. Will she be able to help him?"

He replied, "The boy doesn't want her help. He wants to control himself."

"He wants to be in control of himself, but at the same time he is making himself unsafe," I said.

Eric responded: "Oh well, another boring trip to the hospital."

In this material Eric elaborated a story/memory that was related, at least in part, to his childhood accidents. In his drawing Eric metaphorically portrayed what had gone wrong in the family. There was a boy making himself unsafe. The mother could not help the boy stop. The boy and his mother were too far apart. The father, who was in a position to be potentially of help to the boy and his mother, also did nothing.

Interestingly, this story followed Eric's aggressively and impulsively snatching my pen. At that moment I must have reminded him in the transference of his mother, too far away and unable to help. Eric expressed his aggression toward me by snatching the pen, but immediately retreated to a story/memory in which he put himself on the receiving end of something bad that was happening to him. He had now turned the aggression on himself. In this particular association the boy's courting dangerous out-of-control behavior seemed to have a defensive component to it, namely a way of keeping his own aggression at me under wraps and out of focus.

In the final play sequence of this session Eric picked up the play figure of a boy and gave me the mother figure. He said, "It is Christmas." He put a Christmas tree in the room. "The boy likes Christmas but he gets too excited." Eric made the boy into Crazy Boy, jumping around the room. Eric told me that the mother worried that the boy would do dangerous things and get hurt. Suddenly the boy took his bicycle and rode to the top of the roof. Using the mother doll, I was directed to yell for help. The mother tried to stop the boy, but the boy did not listen to her. The boy became increasingly aggressive to her and finally ran her over with his bike. When I asked Eric what was happening between the boy and his mother, he avoided any acknowledgment of the aggression in the play. He said that the boy was "overexcited" and the mother wanted him to "stop." "She has to call the police ten times a day because he is out of control ten times a day." At that moment, Eric dashed out of the room to check on his mother. When he returned, I said, "You needed to see your mother right in the middle of your story. Something in the story made you worry. It was just when the boy was giving his mom a hard time. You worried that a hard time could hurt your mom."

In the final play sequence, Eric allowed himself to be much freer in expressing his anger at the female figure as he rammed her with the bicycle. This figure probably represented some composite of mother, sisters, and analyst. The ramming may also have included a disguised sexual component. However, the expression of the aggression immediately became "too real." Eric had to interrupt his play, actually leave me, and check again to see that his mother was okay.

As one can see, the session started out with Eric communicating about the body experience of hyperactivity, which made him feel like Crazy Man—helpless, defective, and endangered. It ended with Crazy Boy jumping around and endangering himself to disguise and control his sexual and aggressive aims. Here we see how the symptom of hyperactivity was drawn into the child's fantasy life in a number of interrelated ways.

Middle Phase: Supplies and Demands

As the analysis continued, Eric began to acknowledge that he wanted things from me. He began to ask for food during his sessions, especially at times when he was frustrated or trying to avoid an uncomfortable feeling. At first I was interested in how his hungry feeling had happened to come up at that moment. I do not ordinarily have food in the office and I was not eager to make it part of our analytic exchange. However, Eric was persistent in needing something concrete from me. I eventually provided food, hoping that we would be able to analyze this demand in the future.

During this time, Eric became more able to show his affection. He would frequently station himself close to me and brush against me, establishing physical contact. He had much less need to be active in the office as a way of avoiding feeling. One of his frequent games during this period was to play at being a puppy who needed to be cared for by me. This "stray" puppy had no family, and I was supposed to take him warmly into my home and adopt him. In repayment, the puppy would defend me and my office against robbers. For one stretch of time we went into the restaurant business together and he was the dog/cook, sharing secret family recipes with me. He was a trick dog and together we became a performing team. He was obedient at first, but as the play developed he would suddenly be overtaken by different moods. He became excited and out of control, or he pretended to bite. We then had to renegotiate the relationship in the wake of these transgressions, but they never led to abandonment. I would try to reconstruct with Eric what had made the puppy lose control or bite. I interpreted the puppy's conflict over being wild or disobedient, the strength of his wishes, and his fear that this behavior would lead to his abandonment.

I felt that the puppy-Eric was trying to communicate the wish for an idealized early maternal experience in the transference. This included being fed, cared for, and made to feel powerful. Another important aspect of my role was to admire

puppy-Eric endlessly and to be gratified by having such a mar-
velous dog. This included my acknowledging all his feelings
and accepting them without judgment. In the play sequences
I freely interpreted the puppy's wishes, fears, and conflicts in
relationship to me. However, I left my remarks in the displacement of the play. I did not say that these feelings were Eric's
feelings, because such direct interpretations would have been
totally unacceptable to the 7-year-old Eric at this point in time.
They would have stimulated a defensive denial. I felt sure, however, that Eric implicitly understood that I was talking about
him as well as the puppy.

Our work and the progressive push of development
brought about a burgeoning of more appropriate latency defenses and interests. These developments became part of the
analysis. Eric had many collections of baseball and basketball
cards. He spent time organizing the superstars and painstak-
ingly keeping records of their statistics. For Eric there was a
tremendous sense of mastery in this. It also gave him a new
way of having control (obsessional control) in the analytic situation. He needed to resort to excessive activity and his old control battles much less frequently.

Despite these changes, whenever Eric felt threatened he
had a great deal of difficulty. His sense of vulnerability was
organized around tremendous castration anxiety. Eric did not
actually verbalize a fear of losing his penis, but the fear of
castration seemed to be represented symbolically in his play
and associations.

In the fifteenth month of analysis, six weeks after we resumed our work, I injured my back and needed to cancel our
sessions for four weeks. When Eric returned to treatment he
was very solicitous. He said I had "broken" my back and that
I was like him in that I, too, had "bad luck." Several times,
he worried that he had caused my back injury through my
association with him. When I was clearly recovered, he was able
to elaborate more of the negative transference.

This began with Eric's constant demands for food. At the
beginning of each session he wanted me to list the menu of
what was available to him. He elaborated the fantasy that this
food belonged to my children and that he was getting what did

not rightfully belong to him. He also felt that the "really good food" was secretly being kept from him. When he was beside himself, he yelled that even my own children could not stand my food. The food never tasted right if there was enough, and there was never enough if it tasted right. This "witch" transference became increasingly elaborated in the hours. Several times he drew me as a witch and showed me how he wanted to stomp on me and rip me into little pieces.

It was not always easy to talk about this with Eric, because in the middle of elaborating his feelings he could become totally out of control. On the other hand he worked very hard during this time and was always eager to come and see me. As our work continued, the witch became more specifically a mother who demeaned him and wanted to get rid of him. In one session he drew a witch pointing at a boy and saying: "You stink!" Eric was convinced that I had actually said this to him "once a long time ago." I suggested that he had perhaps felt that way when I had been unable to see him because my back was hurt. I do think that the back interruption influenced the timing and intensity of the emergence of this negative transference.

Eric also tested me time and time again by making a total mess of the food I gave him—spitting it out, mushing it around, and even getting it on me. He named this behavior his "disgusting-puker" self. For better or for worse, I had a tolerance for this. I told him that he needed to know that I accepted every part of him, even his "disgusting-puker" parts. Maybe as a little boy he had been worried that he would not be loved because of these parts of him.

Out of this work emerged an interesting elaboration of Eric's preoedipal conflicts and his struggle to resolve them. Eric was a true analytic partner, sustaining an analytic alliance for a much longer time. Together, we produced puppet shows. One of the main characters was a dragon puppet who wanted more and more food. The other main character was a mother bear who was unable to tolerate the insatiability of the dragon's demands. This led to her setting harsh limits, demeaning the dragon, and eventually throwing him out.

Eric switched his identification so that at times he was the hungry dragon and at times he was the strict mother trying to get things back under control. At times he tried to resolve the problem by magic. A witch put a spell on one or the other, transforming the dragon so he was never hungry again or changing the bear so she could deal with extraordinary demands. As soon as one was fixed, however, there were other puppets who became insatiable. There was also a father wolf with angry eyes who lost his temper in a scary way. Sometimes Eric gave me all the puppets with "problems" to take care of because he could not figure out what to do. On one memorable occasion the dragon became so insatiable that he ate up the bear and then, still unable to get enough, started eating himself alive in a most grisly way.

This material made clear Eric's internal conflict. He worried that his neediness and aggression would destroy the people he loved and needed. In my interventions I was appreciative of the difficulty of the problem. I commented that if there were such a thing as magic it could solve the problem. In real life, however, such problems need time and understanding to fix.

Eric's conflict about the strength of his needs and his anger when they were frustrated moved from the puppet play into the transference. This was illustrated by the following material which comes from a session in the eighteenth month of treatment.

Eric entered the office carrying the cover of a *New Yorker* magazine from my waiting room. Without looking at me he said, "Bring me all the food in the house." After a brief negotiation about what he actually wanted, I brought him a bowl of grapes. He ate one and fell to the floor in a death swoon.

I said, "What's the matter with the grapes?" He replied, "They are sweet. They killed me." I tasted one myself. "Ugh! They are sour," I said. I broke into a song, "She gave him sour grapes. . . . " Eric added the next line, singing, "She gave him bellyaches. . . . " He continued to sing, "She gave him poisoned grapes that gave him bellyaches. . . . " Eric then ate a grape, pretended to choke, and collapsed on the floor. He repeated this many times.

I asked, "Why did she give him poisoned grapes?"

He replied, "Because he asked for *all* of the food."

"You mean he wanted too much?"

"Yep," said Eric, "He was too hungry. He wanted everything in the *whole house.*" Eric continued to play being poisoned and falling to the floor. He then informed me, "There is no food in my house. Really. Nothing. Only one piece of candy and everyone is fighting over it. Everyone only gets so much." He squeezed his fingers together showing me that it was so little that it could not even be seen.

I said, "So when you come here, you have such a big hunger that you want everything in my house."

"Right," said Eric. "But then I'll eat everything and you'll have nothing left for you. Or even your children. So you poisoned me with those grapes. So that's the story."

I interpreted, "You worry that your hungry feelings will be too much for me and that then I'll want to kill you. I think it's not only hungry feelings that you are talking about."

Eric went into the playroom and discovered a necklace left by another child. "What's this?" he asked as he held it up. I commented, "That's another child's necklace. Girls' things are invading your space." He said, "Girls' things are yukky. Get rid of it." He sang, "She gave him poisoned grapes that gave him bellyaches. . . . "

I chimed in, "Because he asked for more. . . . "

Eric sang, "For everything in the store."

The session ended with an elaborate puppet show in which Dragon (Eric) could not get enough food from Bear (me) and became transformed into a vampire, eventually sucking all Bear's blood out.

During this session Eric seemed to have a fairly sophisticated understanding of the "as if" nature of the transference relationship. He talked about his fears and wishes from me at the same time that he was "just playing." I believed these mirrored the early conflicts that he experienced toward his mother and his wish to possess her totally. However, at other moments, Eric would ask me for concrete evidence of my affection, inviting me to come to his school play or birthday party. While I was clear about not complying with these wishes, at these moments Eric, like many other young children, did not understand the nature of the boundaries of our relationship. At these times he did not differentiate me from any other real person in his life to whom he was attached. I suspect it was the strength of his wishes for me to be more than an analyst that blurred things for him in these moments.

As we continued to explore Eric's greedy wishes and hungry feelings, he stopped asking me for food in his analytic hours. In this phase of the analysis Eric's sense of defect and badness was focused on his fear that he could destroy those he loved with his voracious oral–aggressive wishes. There was much less focus on his hyperactivity or his fears of having a defective brain as elements that caused him trouble. However, these elements continued to appear at least to some degree until the end of the analysis.

INTERRUPTION

In the middle of this work Eric became ill and was diagnosed with a chronic physical problem. This occurred in the thirty-third month of the analysis, at which point the analysis was interrupted for two-and-one-half months. My vacation occurred during that period and extended the time of the interruption. I was unable to meet with Eric regularly during his hospitalization, although I visited him several times. Eric felt contaminated by "bad luck" and told me that he regarded himself as a great burden to his parents and me. "What a bad present I gave my mother for Christmas," he said, referring to the fact that he was born on Christmas day. He drew a puppy with a skull and crossbones on his sides, indicating that people should stay away from him. Eric returned to treatment after his recovery.

This interruption had a major impact on what ensued. Not only did Eric experience the interruption as an abandonment, but in addition I could not help him sort out the hospital experience, which was scary and painful. Eric's illness was nonprogressive, but he was vulnerable to episodic recurrences. This enhanced an old feeling of defect.

TERMINATION

During the last month of the interruption, while I was on vacation, Eric's mother reported that he had reverted to his old behavior. He was very irritable and lost control easily. When I returned, Eric did not want to come back to analysis. However, once we started to meet again regularly, he settled down into his new second grade class.

The last eight months of the analysis were very different from what had come before. Although Eric continued to do well outside the analysis, he kept me at arms' length. He was not interested in revisiting any of the more regressive positions of the past. He resisted all my interpretations about the separation and about his obvious disappointment with me and everyone else who had "failed" him. His sense of vulnerability about his illness made him resistant to discussing it at all. It seemed to become the main locus of his sense of defect, but not one that could be directly addressed. Nevertheless, Eric continued to keep his friendships at school, played sports, and apparently had no trouble learning to read, write, and do math. In fact, he was quite proud of his academic skills, particularly his reading and his memory. He also was quite talented at drawing.

In the analysis Eric wanted to play competitive games with me. He invented many board games for us to play. There was a game of "Life" in which various mishaps befell the players. Eric called this "good luck" and "bad luck." In this game we came the closest to discussing the bad luck that had happened to him. There were also memory games and drawing contests between us. Eric created a baseball game that could be played in the office, in which paper bats were used to hit crumpled up paper balls and there was a complicated way of scoring hits. No running was involved.

Eric avoided all forms of imaginative play. Even the subjects of our drawing contests were realistic renditions of common objects, rarely leaving room for a more open-ended symbolic communication. Moreover, the games were often not very playful, because Eric was driven to win, and extremely agitated if he did not. Sometimes these games were fiercely competitive and seemed to recreate the rivalrous and sadistic aspects of the relationship that Eric had with his middle sister. Other games felt like space-fillers, ways of avoiding feelings or keeping them rigidly controlled.

For several brief periods during this time Eric used drawing to convey some of his inner life to me. For instance, he drew a series of grotesque monster faces, insisting that I draw equally grotesque ones. He then said that mine were "sicker" than his. I interpreted to Eric that he was very critical of the thoughts and feelings that were inside him and he worried that I would be turned off if he revealed himself. He then drew a series of war cartoons with a huge U.S. Army bullying a smaller country's soldiers and tanks. We talked about how vulnerable the weaklings felt and the kind of sadistic revenge they wanted.

We ultimately stopped the analysis because Eric became increasingly resistant to coming. Five months after the interruption, we set a date three months in advance and terminated at that time. The analysis had lasted two years and seven months. In anticipation of ending Eric expressed both relief and sadness. In the last weeks of the analysis we looked together at his large collection of drawings and other creations, a collection that spanned the course of his treatment. He was eager to bring everything home with him and, while organizing his things with great care, he commented on what he remembered about the times when he had made each item. He called termination his "graduation" and was very invested in treating his problems as a thing of the past.

FOLLOW-UP

I had mixed feelings about Eric's termination because I believed we had not finished our analytic work. In my view Eric's resistance to continuing was multidetermined. He seemed to be particularly intolerant of the regressive forces that he associated with the analytic work. The fear of regression was especially intense because Eric was trying to deal with a difficult reality, his physical illness and its aftermath, as well as trying to maintain his entry into a new developmental stage, latency.

In addition, the disappointment with me during the second interruption made his anger at me too difficult to overcome.

Eric fared well during seven years of follow-up. His conduct disorder did not return; his behavior remained improved at home and at school. Hyperactivity and impulsivity were no longer reported as symptoms. A learning disability never materialized and Eric never required tutoring. He got B's and occasional A's, but apparently never fully applied himself to his schoolwork. In his parents' view, he could have been an A student if he had fully committed himself. He participated in and excelled at sports, and had no further episodes of his physical problem during this time. He had a good social life. Although his parents had concerns about him at times, they felt his development was now on track.

SUMMARY

Eric's problems did not fall into a single diagnostic category. The diagnosis of ADD was equivocal not only at the beginning, but throughout the treatment. I believe that Eric's difficulties with impulse control had both constitutional and environmental underpinnings and these factors reinforced each other.

Eric came to analysis with the fantasy that there was something wrong with his brain. His difficulties with impulse control, his body experience of being out of control, his neurotic conflicts, and his sense of badness, all wove in and around this central motif of defect. This is illustrated in the section "Crazy Man." Analysis helped to modify his compromised self-image. However, when a real physical problem was diagnosed, it confirmed Eric's well-ensconced self-perception that something was concretely wrong with him. This made the fantasy of defect more resistant to analytic inquiry and more resistant to a more complete modification. Despite this, with the help of analysis, Eric made substantial changes in his behavior at home and at school, made friends, and became a well-functioning child.

Chapter 12

Discussion of Eric's Analysis

Dr. Yanof's vivid and evocative report of the analysis of Eric highlights several very interesting issues. One is the efficacy of Eric's treatment, despite the persisting uncertainty about his diagnosis. More specifically, the questions of whether there was neuropsychological involvement or an Attention Deficit/Hyperactivity Disorder were never clarified. As we stated in chapter 1, the diagnosis of ADHD is elusive insofar as it is based on a checklist of signs and symptoms. Psychological testing may support the diagnosis and reveal a learning disability, as well as suggest dynamic conflicts that interact with the neuropsychological condition.

Dr. Yanof permits us to grasp the multidimensional work she did with her patient in analyzing the complexities of his presenting problems in behavior, including his distractibility, impulsivity, and hyperactivity. She very sensitively explored his internal experience of these clinical states and the way they became incorporated in his unconscious fantasies. This perspective was coupled with the analysis of Eric's defenses against the discomfiting affects associated with these states; in addition, Dr. Yanof interpreted the ways in which these states were employed defensively to reduce the unpleasure associated with her patient's other conflicts.

Eric's diagnosis remained uncertain throughout his analysis. The psychologist who examined him when he was 6 years old labeled his condition Attention Deficit Disorder (ADD). She was obviously thinking that he was of the hyperactive type, but the diagnostic nomenclature of the time did not permit the clinician to specify this. Dr. Yanof was not convinced of this diagnosis as she grappled with the task of determining "whether psychological or neuropsychological factors dominated the clinical picture." At other junctures Dr. Yanof indicated her belief that "Eric's difficulties with impulse control had both constitutional and environmental underpinnings," a position with which we agree. Certainly the fact that Dr. Yanof did not personally see signs of ADHD during her consultation must have contributed to her skepticism. In this regard it is important to keep in mind that a patient's potential for distractibility and disorganization may be relatively obscured (at least for a period of time) in the one-to-one setting of a private office, when compared with the atmosphere of the classroom or home. After the analysis began Dr. Yanof did, of course, encounter Eric's impulsivity and difficulty in focusing cognitively.

Although Dr. Yanof reported many of the traits of ADHD, not enough of the DSM-IV criteria were met to make a definitive diagnosis (APA, 1994). Eric's second kindergarten teacher, who taught him after the analysis was in progress, did not see him as hyperactive. However, many of Eric's features are strongly suggestive of this diagnosis. His mother provided a history of his having been hyperactive since he could walk, always on the move and in danger. He was oblivious to his surroundings when immersed in his feeling states. At home, as well as in the classroom, Eric could not sit still long enough to complete tasks. During the testing, his squirming and poor impulse control, coupled with his extreme sensitivity and distractibility by outside sounds, seriously compromised his ability to perform. It is possible to argue that many of Eric's symptoms were manifestations of oppositional behavior (for instance, his kicking his teacher during a tantrum), or fearfulness; in this regard his activity could be viewed as an expression of and defense against anxiety and/or depressive affect. However, in our view, the long-standing nature of this picture strongly argues for a constitutional contribution.

There are a number of ways the psychologist who evaluated him prior to referral to Dr. Yanof could have supplemented hcr testing and perhaps clarified the diagnosis. Even though Eric was very young at the time of diagnostic testing evaluation, it would have been useful and optimal to further investigate a number of possibilities (e.g., visual sequential memory and visual discrimination). A follow-up evaluation by the middle of the first grade year to rule out subtle difficulties in the acquisition of basic academic skills also might have clarified the diagnosis. Had Dr. Yanof prescribed medication, this might have served as an additional diagnostic instrument. If there were an immediate ameliorative effect, the justification for a diagnosis of ADHD would have been fortified.

We lean toward a diagnosis of ADHD as well as the possibility of a circumscribed specific learning disability, based on the fact that Eric manifested directional confusion and difficulties with speech articulation and handwriting, which can reflect fine visual–motor coordination problems (or as the psychologist put it, "mild to moderate difficulty with all perceptual–motor tasks"). While in this particular case making the diagnosis of ADHD may not have resulted in a difference in the final outcome for Eric, arriving at such a diagnostic conclusion may be more important with other patients.

As it turned out, Dr. Yanof's approach was extremely fruitful. She was able to develop a therapeutic relationship with Eric without the complications the administration of medication might have produced, and the analytic work proceeded satisfactorily. Although administration of stimulant medication is not incompatible with the patient's participation in an analysis, prescribing it may in some cases contribute to a patient's reluctance to seek insight when medication appears to be the analyst's preferred method of treatment. However, there are instances when medication is strongly indicated (though this was not the case with Eric). As Dr. Yanof has stated, medication is indicated when the patient's hyperactivity, distractibility, or impulsivity too seriously compromise his ability to engage in an analytic process, to manage the demands of school, or to participate pleasurably and reasonably in family life. When this is the case, his resistant responses to medication will necessarily become a part of the analytic work.

Dr. Yanof's follow-up information bore out the effectiveness of this analysis, despite the fact that it was not complete and was terminated sooner than Dr. Yanof would have liked. She states: "Eric fared well during seven years of follow-up. His conduct disorder did not return; his behavior remained improved at home and at school. Hyperactivity and impulsivity were no longer reported as symptoms. A learning disorder never materialized and Eric never required tutoring." Eric achieved "B's and occasional A's [his parents thought him capable of A's, were he to have committed himself], but apparently never applied himself to schoolwork."

In our view, in the absence of diagnostic tests for a neuropsychologically based specific learning disability at a time further along in his academic sequence (e.g., in the second half of first grade and in third grade), we cannot be certain of Eric's cognitive state. It remains a possibility that he had a persisting subtle (and not clinically obvious) specific learning disability and/or ADHD which compromised his optimal level of functioning. It is also possible that Eric's parents expected more of him than was realistic and/or that remaining psychological issues interfered with his optimal performance. If a persistent subtle learning disability were to have been found, remediation may have been added to Eric's treatment plan.

Dr. Yanof has made a masterful contribution to the literature on psychoanalytically informed approaches to clinical work with ADHD patients, notwithstanding her uncertainty about the suitability of ADHD as Eric's diagnosis. She has provided an exemplary model of exploration in her efforts to analyze Eric's bodily sensations and the ideas and emotions connected with them. With great insightfulness and sensitivity she helped Eric become familiar with his inner experience of being impulsive, destructive, and changeable, experiential—behavioral phenomena that we assume to be, at least in part, neuropsychologically based. For example, she dealt with his rapidly changing state by saying he was like a transformer, the toy he loved and played with.

Together, Dr. Yanof and Eric came to appreciate many facets of these experiences: Eric's sense of confusion about transitioning from one state to another without a grasp of the "why's" of these changes, his sense of being out of control, his sense of helplessness and of being endangered without the assistance of others who could reliably protect him. Added to this were his experiences of being "defective" and "dumb," of being destructive, and too much for others who could be overwhelmed by his desires and his activity, which could even hurt them.

Dr. Yanof also appreciated that a complement to Eric's high level of activity and distractibility was his tendency to more fleeting and less organized perceptions and play, contributing to the lack of continuity within and between analytic hours. This is akin to Anthony's (1973) finding that hypoactive (as compared with hyperactive) children who were asked to take a walk around the same block and then report what they saw, conveyed a richer and more subtle texture of affective and interpersonal observations. Not only were the impressions of the hyperactive child characterized less by nuance, but they were also more disorganized and unpredictable and, therefore, less likely to be assimilated and internalized.

Eric was remarkably adept at portraying his experience of hyperactivity, impulsiveness, and lack of control. He drew a figure of a Crazy Man using wobbly and jerky lines. He got Dr. Yanof to draw crazy figures with lines that she seemingly could not control. He said that Crazy Man was going to explode, like a rocket going off into space suddenly and without warning. He, and things around him, moved rapidly. It was dangerous. Excited, aggressive, and out of control, he could fall and be hurt. His parents could not help him. In fact he could run over his mother and hurt her. Anxiety accentuated hyperactivity.

Although Dr. Yanof had to prohibit Eric's aggressive behavior at times, for the most part she maintained a stance of trying to "figure out" the meanings of things. She addressed his impulsiveness, his difficulty saying no to himself, his sense of being defective, dumb, crazy, or mad. She described his activity within the session to him, and tried to guess what had prompted his feelings; gradually Eric joined with her in ascertaining the precipitating events for his transmutations. By emphasizing precipitating events, "Eric became adept at telling . . . what had angered or upset him," and Dr. Yanof became increasingly aware of "the nuances of his sensitivity."

Dr. Yanof also explored with Eric the defenses he employed against his self-experience of being "dumb," "crazy," and the like. Several examples were Eric's tendencies to grandiosity in the face of his sense of inadequacy and to drawing the analyst into feeling inadequate; he frequently "turned the tables" on her and identified with the aggressor, treating her as defective, for example.

Dr. Yanof also helped Eric understand himself in another sense. She elaborated the meanings he had attributed to the bodily and affective experiences associated with hyperactivity, distractibility, and impulsivity, and the ways in which they had become woven into his unconscious fantasies, including his fantasies of cure.

Eric harbored a central fantasy that something was wrong with his brain. He imagined that his brain was defective, or that it had been stolen and he had to steal it back. He felt his parents wanted him to be perfect and have a perfect brain, but believed he had failed; he had no brain at all. While this had many facets and served many psychological purposes, in our view it had some truth to it. We believe there *was* a neuropsychological substrate to his hyperactivity and distractibility, and that Eric *may* have had a circumscribed learning disability. In addition, Eric's belief that his brain functioned poorly probably grew out of his sense of his parents' disappointment in him, as well as experiences of being told he might have a learning disability, of being left back in school, and of recognizing that he could not control himself.

Eric hoped he would be cured by Dr. Yanof's fixing his broken brain (thereby making him "smart" rather than "stupid" or "crazy") and telling him that his brain was perfectly fine. To a degree she did that. Since she believed there was no evidence that he had a learning disability, she told Eric with confidence that he had a distorted idea about himself; he was actually a smart boy who thought he could not do a lot of things that he actually could do. Dr. Yanof's reassurance put things in perspective. In fact, whether or not Eric had a learning disability, he did indeed have a distorted idea about himself.

It is important to note that Dr. Yanof never explained to Eric that his transformations might be neuropsychologically determined. Presumably she was not sufficiently certain that this was true. She may also have felt that, even if it were true, telling him this would not be helpful; the concept might be beyond Eric's comprehension and, further, it might derail the analysis by emphasizing a seemingly unalterable aspect of his difficulties rather than the part that could be modified. It might also discourage him from trying to understand the ways in which personal interactions affected him, as well as his effect on others.

During the first nine months of the analysis Eric concentrated on his brain as the defective part of his body. Although his brain *was* important, some of the concern about the brain was likely to have resulted from displacement. As Dr. Yanof herself noted, Eric's concerns about his brain became "the nidus around which other concerns coalesced." That is, these worries masked and expressed in displacement other worries.

A great deal of analytic work was also devoted to the analysis of Eric's use of his view of himself as defective, his hyperactivity, and his distractibility for defensive purposes. To illustrate, Dr. Yanof interpreted that Eric (unconsciously) attempted to keep anger and aggressive wishes under control and out of focus by such means as courting danger and via the lack of continuity within and between analytic hours. Eric's high level of activity was also a disguised expression of, as well as an effort to control, sexual and aggressive aims. In addition, Eric's self-endangering behavior and fantasies, and his sense of having a defective brain, satisfied superego demands for punishment for his imagined badness. In Eric's mind he had made the analyst sick, he was a "bad Christmas present" for his mother when he was born, and he asked too much and was generally overwhelming and dangerous to others. This was seen in his play in which a puppy feared abandonment as a punishment for being wild, disobedient, and prone to bite. More specifically, having a "castrated self or defective brain" served as a punishment for oedipal wishes and defended against the likelihood of achievement of such desires. Additionally, there were self-preservative aspects of these self-experiences and fantasies. Eric harbored the idea that his mother and father would want to abandon him because he was too overwhelming or dangerous to them.

Along with Eric's defensive view of himself as defective, he tried to deny the presence of a defect. Early in the analysis he wanted to prove that he was perfect. He wrote that a "doctor took out his brain, examined it, and pronounced that there was nothing wrong with it." In addition, in grandiose moods he sometimes exaggerated what he was capable of achieving.

When the analysis was terminated after a total of two years and seven months because Eric was so resistant to coming, he was a remarkably changed boy. His manifest concern about his brain was minimal. He was involved with worries over being left and being ill, which he more successfully mastered. He was less obviously invested in his representation of his head and more focused on his body which had come to the forefront as a danger to his well-being. He was no longer hyperactive, and achieved decent school marks (B's and occasional A's), but perhaps (as his parents believed) did not live up to his potential. Loss of control appeared in the analytic setting occasionally but not at home or in school. He remained reasonably well controlled in the analysis as he discussed his feelings about termination and, as he said, graduated from the analysis.

Chapter 13

Rebecca's Analysis

Karen Gilmore, M.D.

PRESENTING PROBLEMS

Rebecca R was 12 years old when she was referred to me for consultation. She had previously been evaluated and treated at 9 years, 2 months, when an acute symptom picture similar to the present one emerged. Then, as now, she approached the beginning of the school year with panicky anxiety, temper tantrums, generalized irritability, and demands for a school change. Her parents understood this as Rebecca's predictable response to transitions; the annual September reentry into school was especially troublesome. These reactions seemed to worsen over the years, and her parents felt increasingly unable to calm or console her.

These "crises," so named by the R's, were recognized as exacerbations of long-standing difficulties of a broader scope. Rebecca seemed unable to sustain friendships because of her hypersensitivity and readiness to feel insulted. The R's felt that she was too often the "victim" (her mother's word), becoming preoccupied with and stirred up by social conflicts at school. All too often, she was the target of hostility and ostracism among the girls.

Rebecca's prickliness affected her performance in other arenas as well. She wanted to be viewed as perfect, but was

313

often unwilling to work. As a consequence, she readily gave up on her pursuits. These difficulties, which recurred year after year at school, also spoiled her experience of summer camp, Hebrew school, and lessons in tennis, swimming, and guitar. The R's also touched on some other concerns, namely Rebecca's fears of birds and the dark, and her avoidance of sophisticated books with mature content.

PREVIOUS TREATMENT AND PSYCHOLOGICAL TESTING

Rebecca was initially brought for evaluation at 9 years, 2 months by her parents, when her school observed her distractibility, her overreliance on teacher support to tackle her assignments, and her poor handling of the usual social tensions within her peer group (i.e., she was overreactive to teasing, and avoidant). A child psychiatrist saw her in diagnostic interviews and, having obtained a history from the R's, asked that they fill out a Conner's Rating Scale (a self-administered questionnaire concerning behavioral observations pertinent to Attention Deficit/ Hyperactivity Disorders). This, along with neuropsychological testing, was recommended as part of the evaluation to determine whether she had learning or attentional problems.

The battery of tests included the WISC-R, Ravens Progressive Matrices, Wide Range Achievement Test (Reading, Spelling, and Arithmetic), Gilmore Oral Reading Test, Peabody Picture Vocabulary Test, Oldfield Test, Forer Sentence Completion, Paired Associates Learning Tasks (Word Pairs, Visual Braille, Morse Code), Neimark Memorization Strategies Test, Trail-making, Matching Familiar Figures Test, the sound blending portion of the Illinois Test of Psycholinguistic Abilities, the spelling portion of the Peabody Individual Achievement Test, Wepman Test, Beery-Buktenica Test, Purdue Pegboard, Izard Test, and a basic neuropsychological screening. Unfortunately projective tests were not included in the battery, presumably because the psychological component of Rebecca's difficulties was thought to be clear-cut. The tester noted, ''We could find nothing to explain her social difficulties; she is sensitive to people and has good insight. Possibly lacking the controls of other children her age, she is unable to interact with them at the appropriate level.''

Rebecca obtained a Full Scale IQ of 121 (with a Verbal IQ of 125 and a Performance IQ of 109), with the lowest scores in Digit Span, Arithmetic, and Coding, the classic triad for distractibility. Rebecca's next lowest score was on the Picture Completion subtest. Her highest scores were in verbal and nonverbal conceptualization, expressive vocabulary, and comprehension of social situations. Rebecca's achievement scores were adequate but not consistent with her potential. Spelling was her greatest weakness, compounded by the fact that the strategies she employed to cope with her deficit relied heavily on word blending skills, which was another weak area. Similarly, Rebecca's low arithmetic score reflected poor strategizing and her failure to check her work. In addition, she attempted to guess at problems well beyond her level of knowledge.

Closer examination of Rebecca's language abilities revealed a somewhat inconsistent picture. There was evidence of auditory processing difficulties reflected in requests for multiple repetitions of words and linguistic errors in responsive naming. She also showed relatively weak memorization skills and failed to use her conceptual skills to improve her performance. Interestingly, on tests requiring planning skills, she *did* seem to mount strategies and manifested little impulsivity. Tests requiring visual tracking of alternating sequences showed some breakdown of her attentional skills, which were otherwise average on direct assessment. Tests of motor and graphomotor skills showed some right–left confusion and marked overflow and dysrhythmia on repetitive alternating finger movements. Rebecca's hand–eye coordination was adequate, but her fine motor skills were consistently poor.

Thus in addition to a positive history for ADHD (distractibility, poor attention span, and low frustration tolerance), corroborated by the results of the Parents' Questionnaire of the Conner's Rating Scale, test findings were supportive of this diagnosis. At the conclusion of this consultation, the psychiatrist's recommendations were focused on medication, tutoring, the structuring of learning situations, and brief supportive psychotherapy, consisting of weekly sessions for about eight weeks,

with diminishing contact thereafter. The R's' understanding of
the therapy was that it was aimed at psychoeducation in regard
to Rebecca's diagnosis and adaptation to the medication. The
above-noted social deficiencies did not seem to be directly addressed by the recommendations, possibly because it was assumed that medication would ameliorate her social difficulties,
particularly those arising from poor frustration tolerance and
impulsivity.

Ritalin was instituted and the consultant followed Rebecca
for the next several months, monitoring her response to the
medication and providing reassurance. Rebecca herself remembered little of that treatment. Her school was advised of
some of the findings, which corroborated her teachers' concerns about her anxiety in the classroom. In response, her classroom placement for fourth grade was selected for greater
structure. Rebecca made a good adjustment to fourth grade,
progressing from a "defeated attitude" at the end of third
to a "wonderful and productive" fourth (as described in her
school report).

While her academic performance at her relatively demanding but ungraded progressive school had always been considered good by her parents and teachers, Rebecca's attitude
toward learning had been poor. At this time it was considered
to have improved. She was described as more self-motivated,
less demanding of teacher support, and more enthusiastic
about academic materials. Rigorous academic assessment was
not part of the curriculum at her grade level, but overall Rebecca's performance was viewed by her school as commensurate
with her potential at this time.

This improvement was evident despite the fact that not all
the recommendations were followed. Rebecca did not receive
formal tutoring, but was instead tutored by her physician father, who had an exemplary school history. Similarly, Dr. R
determined the amount and frequency of the Ritalin she took.
These choices were explained on the basis of convenience and
finances. However, they also reflected a subtle form of elitism
on Rebecca's parents' part, as if only *they* could know how best
to help her.

PAST HISTORY

Rebecca's early development was described as essentially unremarkable, with two exceptions. She was verbally precocious, which was a quality greatly admired by her intellectual and rather austere parents. She was also viewed as hypersensitive from early infancy, with a pronounced startle reaction and marked aversive tactile sensitivity that made her unable to tolerate many fabrics and articles of apparel.

Rebecca immediately responded to the birth of her brother, Scott, when she was 21 months old, with a pronounced maternal solicitousness. This sometimes bordered on bossiness but did not involve overt aggression. From age 4, when Rebecca began preschool, she was similarly unassertive, though "mesmerized" by others' aggression. She was routinely drawn to dominating girls to whom she would "accommodate" (mother's word) herself, only to feel resentment. Medical history included the onset of allergic asthma about one year previously, requiring daily Theo-Dur. Menses commenced at age 11.

In the years following Rebecca's initial treatment, her teacher's concerns about her school adjustment dropped off. Her school reports showed generally positive commentary about her self-motivation and capacity to stay on task. However, she continued to struggle with emotional upheavals in response to new situations, family arguments, and academic stresses, e.g., homework assignments that she seemed to experience as overwhelming. The R's reported that Rebecca was "hypersensitive" and "overreacted." She was easily frustrated by adversity in social or academic endeavors and lacked resources to manage, instead choosing retreat. She often responded to father's efforts to tutor her with indignation, argumentativeness, and door slamming. She seemed to experience competition from her peers as vicious attacks.

The R's described Rebecca's difficulties with a complex mixture of empathy and criticism, of psychologizing and then resorting to explanations involving purely biological causation and intervention. Recognizing the repetitive nature of her difficulties, the R's viewed Rebecca's despondency and urgent wish to change schools that had precipitated the referral as her typical reaction to newness and change. She had difficulty with the overall unfamiliarity of a new school year and the introduction of a new classmate, whom she experienced as a threat to her delicately maintained friendships. The R's felt Rebecca all too regularly fled in the face of frustration and anxiety. In addition, her father's increasing her Ritalin dosage at this time without any clear rationale underscored the R's implicit view of the medication as a nonspecific "crutch" (their word). Rebecca's parents gave little consideration to the possibility that she was responding, in part, to the specific cognitive challenges of each new academic year.

In fact, throughout Rebecca's history and continuing during her psychoanalysis, there seemed to be both too little *and* too much made of Rebecca's cognitive difficulties, their specificity and repercussions, and their exceedingly complex relationship to her psychological adaptation. Formal remediation, recommended by the tester and again by me, was never pursued by the R's. Indeed it was only much later, and even then only for a brief period of time during her analysis, that Rebecca was able to break away from daily tutoring sessions with her father by seeking tutoring from an older student; this was still a poor substitute for professional remediation.

Father's subsequent involvement in the administration of her Ritalin seemed to be a related phenomenon. Rebecca's father neither consulted me about decisions involving Ritalin nor informed me about how much he gave Rebecca and how much she took. I only heard through Rebecca about her acquiescence and refusal, which generally depended on the climate of her relationship with her parents. Certainly, a pattern of overinvolvement and overcontrol contaminated both interventions, so that Rebecca's remediation and use of medication was highly conflictual well before her treatment with me began. This was perhaps best exemplified many years after the analysis ended when, after briefly consulting with me about Rebecca's collapse in her freshman year in college, the R's elected not to pursue my recommendation for a repeat neuropsychological examination, but instead encouraged her to drop out of college.

CONSULTATION WITH THE ANALYST

In our initial meetings, Rebecca appeared at once childlike and adolescent. She was eager to solicit my support and to defend herself, pouring out her complaints about her classmates with her big blue eyes focused above my head, as if in prayer. She conveyed a feeling of internal pressure and prickly defensiveness characteristic of children with attentional problems, which contribute to anxiety, impulsivity, and unfocused attention. As is true of many of these children, Rebecca seemed to be struggling at a deeper level with a conviction that she was being blamed and was defective. However, she was also clearly oriented toward the interpersonal, seeking and making emotional contact despite her defensiveness. This quality was occasionally obscured by her tendency to retreat. Nevertheless, it consistently reappeared to sustain our relationship through difficult periods.

In our early meetings, Rebecca enviously described her arch enemy at school—the new girl—as "spoiled, pampered, and babied." These were terms she readily linked to her brother Scott whom she viewed as indulged and overprivileged. She complained that he was still getting his clothes laid out and playing with GI Joes. Rebecca guarded against her own desires for such caretaking by a self-pitying but virtuous abdication. She said she was not popular because she was not that pretty and because her good grades inspired envy.

This last mentioned idea exemplified the kind of misperception which both reflected wishful fantasies and contributed to her social difficulties. Rebecca was never a consistently superior student. In reality, it was mostly her virtuous and submissive behavior toward authority that provoked resentment in her classmates. Her holier-than-thou posture toward her peers, associated with her rigidity and reaction-formations, contributed to this "goody-goody" reputation.

Behind this thin veneer of virtue lay Rebecca's intense interest in, excitement at, and fear of violence and sexuality. Her vivid fantasy life and predisposition to phobic anxiety kept her exhilarated and anxious. At times Rebecca's impulsivity overwhelmed her concerns about authority. She described compelling desires to "punch out" (her words) an especially provoking newcomer at school and admitted that she and this girl had actually engaged in a pushing contest. This was especially remarkable in a school known for its pacifist philosophy.

Rebecca expressed several conscious fears. She alluded to a fear of birds, which I came to understand as one facet of her agoraphobia. She anxiously anticipated contact with the ubiquitous pigeon at every outing. Rebecca soon divulged an underlying preoccupation with kidnapping and molestation that emerged as the central determinant of her phobic avoidance of the street. Scott, with whom she stayed alone after school, served as her guardian. He escorted her to my office, a two-minute walk from school, for the first few months of treatment.

During the consultation, Rebecca reported a dream. She and Scott had to deliver something to a lady waiting in a car. As they approached her, she said, "Get in the back seat. There are big guys coming." Then she said, "Oh my gosh, look what they are doing." They were dragging Scott into the woods to molest him. Rebecca went on to describe some TV shows about "saying no" (the catch phrase used in advertising campaigns promoting children's resistance to pressure of all types) especially one where a male teacher molests a girl first, and the boy star thinks, "Uh oh, it will be me tomorrow." Rebecca readily acknowledged that she felt drawn to the idea of molestation, fascinated and terrified all at once.

I was immediately struck by the poorly modulated quality of Rebecca's impulses as they appeared in fantasy and impacted on her manifest behavior. Frightening sexual fantasies were not barred access to her awareness despite her agoraphobia. Similarly, despite her defensive efforts, aggressive impulses toward other children broke through and were barely restrained from action. I speculated that this faulty modulation was attributable to a number of developmental and biological factors. There was her developmental stage of heightened drive (adolescence) and her ADHD syndrome, including poor frustration tolerance, a low threshold for stimulation of intense reactions, and a predisposition to impulsivity.

In my experience, the combination of poor modulation of impulses, and their defensive projection in phobic symptoms which threaten reality sense, is common in the ADHD population. Children with this disorder are thus extremely vulnerable to disorganizing anxiety as well as to the eruption of impulses. The developmental histories of these children often reveal long-standing derangements in their biological patterning and self-soothing capacities. This contributes to complications in their adaptation to their environments and achievement of significant developmental tasks, both cognitive and interpersonal. On the other hand, and of course evolving in a dynamic relationship to these factors, there was ample evidence of conflict and recurring patterns of maladaptive defensive efforts in Rebecca's development. These included her use of aggression to ward off masochistic sexual excitement, her histrionic emotionality, her rigid reaction-formations, and her phobic and counterphobic tendencies.

The dream that Rebecca described during the consultation melded these trends in an amalgam of sadomasochistic excitement and revenge, thinly disguised by pity and concern. It introduced two major themes in the analytic work: Rebecca's resentment of Scott's birth and her competitive struggle with her mother. The latter previewed her typical resolution by taking a backseat to her and to other important women. I said that Rebecca worried so much about Scott, but got rid of him in the dream too; she must have a lot of different feelings about him. Oh yes, she concurred, she *does* worry about him much more than herself, but he also annoys her because he hits her and makes her wait on him.

Based on the information I gathered during the consultation, I recommended analysis to the R's. I cited the long-standing and recurrent nature of Rebecca's difficulties, her constriction and phobic anxiety, and the likely exacerbation of social problems as adolescence progressed. They agreed with some reluctance, epitomized by father's decision (which I learned about from Rebecca) to increase her dosage of Ritalin from 5 to 10 milligrams three times a day, thus expressing his preference for an organic solution. The lack of communication around the issue of medication remained a consistent, and certainly problematic, feature of treatment. My freedom to address this directly with her father was impeded by Rebecca's stated

wish to distinguish the analysis from the pharmacological intervention, as well as my sense that her relationship to the Ritalin
was already a complex psychological issue which required analytic exploration.

A clear picture of Rebecca's academic performance was
not available at that time. The absence of professional remediation and of a detailed assessment of her learning difficulties
left many things obscure. Her parents were not prepared to
have her retested, which I proposed in order to better tease
apart the psychological and cognitive issues. This was probably
due to a combination of finances and other factors unknown
to me (which led them to refuse testing much later as well).
However, I felt there was reason to believe that anxiety played
a significant role in Rebecca's avoidance of many cognitive
challenges and that analysis might help to clarify this and other
determinants of her academic difficulties.

COURSE OF THE ANALYSIS

First Year of the Analysis

In the opening phase of treatment, Rebecca attempted to demonstrate her victimization and impress me with her helplessness
and innocence. While she complained about the kids at school,
she quickly backed off from her determination to leave them
and reverted to another characteristic adaptation. She ignored
the snobby clique which disdained her, again misinterpreting
their teasing of her obsequious behavior as envy of her intelligence. She avoided the social scene, reading in the library during lunch period. She also exaggerated the importance of an
unstable relationship with an on-again, off-again girl friend
Judy who was, in part, a transference displacement.

At first, Rebecca dwelt on her family members, struggling
to maintain a balance between several feelings. One was her
deep resentment of her parents' (especially her mother's) perceived favoritism toward Scott. Another was Rebecca's painful
conviction that she disappointed her family by failing to live

up to their high and snobbish ideals. Because she fell below her family's standards, which later were understood to be set by the males, she felt "pushed around" (her words) and humiliated. Third, Rebecca wished to protect her parents from her rage, which made her particularly vigilant about possible criticism from an outsider, like myself.

I witnessed Rebecca's prolonged struggle with mother over swimming classes, which Rebecca felt mother insisted upon because she herself never learned to swim. Rebecca despised these weekly classes. She felt humiliated by her social ostracism (which she promoted by her aloofness) and her slow swimming. She ranted unsuccessfully at mother, who was unmoved. On swim class day she came in looking tormented. I pointed out to her that she was angry at her mother, but that she seemed to feel helpless and hopeless, resorting to tantrums or pathos to obtain leniency. She seemed unable to address mother directly and incapable of channeling her resentment to plead her case in a more grown-up way.

Rebecca made clear in this context that managing the emotional intensity of arguing with her parents was beyond her. She was unable to discuss disagreements or mount a campaign without feeling overwhelmed and bursting into tears, which were often rageful in tone. We gradually understood this to derive from a number of sources. One was Rebecca's potential for disorganization under the sway of strong affect. I began to connect this in my own thoughts to her neuropsychological endowment. In discussing it with her, I gradually linked it to her history of tantrums, her low frustration tolerance, and her aversive response to unexpected stimulation. Opportunities to address the very fundamental issue of her intolerance of excitement, and her difficulty maintaining linear thinking in moments of high affective arousal, frequently arose as Rebecca often arrived from school in upheaval over conflicts with teachers or peers. Very gradually, over the whole course of treatment, these aspects of herself were examined with Rebecca and became part of our dialogue as factors to take into account, just as she might come to recognize certain recurrent emotional responses.

In the current situation, I could observe to Rebecca how she recruited this historical constitutional vulnerability for current defensive purposes. I had the feeling that she wanted me to intervene for her, despite her adamant preference for my limited contact with her parents. In this way, she implicitly insisted that she was really unable to negotiate and to stand up to her mother; independence was fraught with danger. I suggested to Rebecca that she might also resent having four appointments per week. She might feel pushed around and humiliated, as if there were a consensus that she was a "real nutcase" (her own term which she dreaded applying to herself), yet she dared not complain directly to me. Moreover, the contribution of this conflict to some of Rebecca's struggles with her parents was gradually understood. We discovered that she was apprehensive that her parents would be only too willing to end what they experienced as her expensive dependency on me, which (from their perspective) threatened their importance to Rebecca. Furthermore, despite her potential to experience the analysis as yet another form of victimization at the hands of her parents, Rebecca openly valued her access to me.

No doubt complaints about feeling forced by her parents were expressed through the vehicle of her objections to swim class. They also ultimately surfaced around the question of her Ritalin, which she more openly viewed as containing the insulting message that she had what she disparagingly called "a mental problem." In this context, as in others, we had the opportunity to observe how Rebecca sought to reduce her awareness of painful insights and internal conflicts through action. She decided to refuse her Ritalin, which did not result in marked deterioration of her school performance, at least as far as was reported to me. However, Rebecca's association of Ritalin with failure and defect may have made it difficult for her to notice differences in her functioning on and off the medication. Moreover, because her father administered the drug himself, the question of the medication's efficacy was contaminated by feelings of submission to parental judgment.

It was subsequently possible to show Rebecca how she seemed to find herself in a similar quandary about the analysis, since complaints could backfire and deprive her of something that she valued. In fact, she very rarely articulated resentment about the number of sessions. However, she did fashion the treatment as a potent source of humiliation by unconsciously inviting Scott (who escorted her to her sessions for months) to tease her about her "shrink" and to view her as a "kook" (his words).

However, I gradually became aware of an equally important component of guilt, for which Rebecca unconsciously expiated via this same humiliation. It soon became clear to me that she was covertly "rubbing Scott's nose in" her special treatment, something *she* got and *he* did not. Her reaction-formation against her anger, her guilt, and her masochistic submission was certainly at work in her compliant attitude toward treatment. In retrospect this attitude also reflected the importance of a number of hidden gratifications. One was the willingness of her tight-fisted parents to spend money on her. Another was the feeding of her object hunger and her yearning for the nonjudgmental adult companionship that I offered.

Rebecca's guilt about the pleasure derived from treatment may have been incompletely addressed analytically, and may have figured decisively in her inability to fight successfully for further treatment when her parents agitated for termination. This pleasure, with its quota of guilt, was almost immediately detectable in the deep warmth of her relatedness to me and her craving for my interest and attention, which withstood all the inevitable chills to come. The intensity of Rebecca's pleasure contained painful implications about her parents' withholding and stinginess (emotional, as well as financial) and her feelings of deprivation. As might be expected, Rebecca tolerated such deeply disturbing feelings poorly.

Rebecca was often aware of feeling guilty, especially about any aggression focused on family members. She was less conscious of the way in which she indirectly punished herself for her anger and her desires. A dream early in the analysis, typical for its catastrophic representation of her impulse life, showed her struggle with her rage and her self-punitive solution:

I was going to a Bat Mitzvah and I heard someone say, "There's a bomb, an explosion," and I saw all these skeletons hanging from the ceiling. Everyone had been killed, except the family. Then I heard a TV voice saying they were going to kill me, or not me, but whoever's body I was in; I tried to hide but this man grabbed me and told me why he was going to kill me, like they do on TV, "because you did this and that." I woke up, but I wasn't scared.

The dream came back to Rebecca in the waiting room when the previous patient, a little girl, left saying emphatically, "I heard you!" Rebecca misheard this as "I hate you!" She thought of a TV show about the Dreyfus case and insisted that people "make such a big deal of these things," i.e., the persecution and murder of underdogs, like Martin Luther King, because of how guilty they are about their own suppressed bigotry.

After voicing other thoughts linking guilt to her violent fantasies, she repeated "I was in someone else's body" in a way that drew my attention to the phrase. It had been her way of describing the male experience of intercourse. This suggested the contribution to her thoughts of guilt about sexual fantasies. When I pointed this out, she said "yuck" and then told me how she had heard about a boy grabbing a girl "by the hair down there" and the girl slapped him. Rebecca added, "I told my mother right away so now I don't have to think about it anymore!" Thus one determinant of her need to remain a child was to secure mother's protection against the dangers of sexuality, from within and without.

Sex loomed as terrifying, in part, because of Rebecca's own denigration of her genitals in particular, and her femininity in general. Her conviction that her family devalued sex gradually emerged as well. Her father was apparently a child prodigy—a brilliant student, a Hebrew scholar, and a concert-level pianist. Rebecca felt she was continually compared to him, in the process of which she experienced defeat. Scott's arrival added insult to injury.

Over the years of the analysis I was repeatedly able to show her how she characteristically expressed her resentment by "cutting off her nose to spite her face." For example, she said she "preferred" to get under par grades (70's and 80's), decided against a Bat Mitzvah, and gave up the piano despite her talent and interest. Despite these efforts not to care, which also served as a defense against her guilt about her exhibitionistic wishes, Rebecca suffered deeply when she felt she disappointed her family. She was convinced that everyone viewed Scott as much more satisfactory.

Rebecca's stance of not caring was no doubt also an expression of her experience of some real cognitive weaknesses and deficits in higher executive functions. These were well camouflaged by neurotic defensive operations but contributed an important element to her masochism and abdication. While the component of anxiety was considerable, it was nonetheless apparent that she had tremendous difficulty in approaching complex material, in structuring her time and thoughts, and in developing realistic strategies. This became much clearer later, when Rebecca returned to consult with me as a senior in high school. It was evident, especially in retrospect, that she always feared she was incapable of doing well, particularly in tasks that required sustained attention and progressive efforts toward a distant goal.

To the extent that I understood the complex web of factors operating at the time that interfered with optimal functioning, I attempted to explore Rebecca's experience of her cognitive functioning, the reality of its limitations, and the layers of defensive operations that obscured these and possibly were promoted by them. Certainly, a measured and reasoned approach to what was really difficult for her was almost impossible to achieve in the early phase of treatment, and any attempts quickly became diverted to transference issues of narcissistic injury and humiliation. This problem underscores the usefulness of ongoing professional remediation simultaneous with analytic work, providing an arena where these cognitive weaknesses can be addressed and supported with diminished transference distortion.

Occasionally, Rebecca brought schoolwork to the hours and showed me her moderate disorganization and immature conceptualization of her assignments. It seemed that the strategies she employed failed to exploit her strengths, as adumbrated in her testing. For example, Rebecca approached a long-term assignment for a seventh grade research report by not making an outline or selecting key ideas. Instead she used a motley collection of references to produce a motley collection of facts. She also demonstrated her difficulties to me as she anxiously described her approach to studying for exams (given for the first time in seventh grade) and showed me her report card which contained her marks in black and white. Rebecca's tendency to take frequent breaks while studying seriously compromised the possibility of maintaining her focus. Her defensive posture toward her mediocre grades on these exams was typical of her: "This is good for the first time I have exams; I don't expect to do better."

This type of material created the opportunity for Rebecca and me to examine her struggle with her parents over her work, as it was reenacted with me. Rebecca's attempts to elicit interventions that she could experience as intrusive attacks by her parents, especially her father, were repeated in our relationship. She would bring in homework, for example a report assignment, and show me her elaborate plans for supplementary artwork, leaving no time for focus on the text. Descriptions of her preparation for tests did not include outlining or other study aids, but repeatedly focused on the timing of breaks. I pointed out her indirect request for guidance and her inevitable feeling of insult should I succumb. We could begin to see that Rebecca was deeply invested in these immature approaches which involved a sadomasochistic interaction with her parents and then with me.

Rebecca's lack of pointed focus needed to be gradually understood to derive from these and many other sources, anatomical as well as cognitive. So many of Rebecca's feelings of inferiority and conviction of second rate status were connected to her feelings about being a girl. Rebecca perceived a disparaging family view of the value of girls. Themes of gender inevitably became entwined with issues concerning her intellectual endowment.

Indeed in this opening phase of treatment, deep in the throes of her early adolescent sexual development, Rebecca was primarily concerned with the gender-linked aspect of her feelings of inferiority. We clarified her vague awareness that her mother was dissatisfied with herself as a woman, making half-hearted attempts to look attractive, by dieting and coloring her hair. However, Mrs. R was simultaneously contemptuous of such efforts and intolerant of "girlish" interests. "My mother is always trying to make me make up for where she failed," Rebecca observed. Through her critique of her mother, she could also retaliate for her mother's criticisms of her preferences. Both Rebecca's parents, but especially her mother, denigrated Rebecca's interests in doll play, cosmetics, clothes, romance novels, and her teenage crushes on popular TV and movie stars.

For much of the first year of analytic work, Rebecca maintained that she did not like being a girl. In her view girls were mostly "prisses" except for athletic types. The topic of sexual interest in boys was invariably greeted with "Yuck." Rebecca revealed a phobic attitude toward her own genitals. She was afraid to look, to feel, and to know. For example, she scornfully informed me of the meaning of "popping a virgin": "the translucent membrane over the fallopian tubes is torn," she explained, and then lapsed into confused silence.

I told Rebecca she felt outdone by the males in her family and that she viewed her mother as saying (in my paraphrase), "Us girls are all in the same lousy boat and need a lot of improvement." Scott's birth felt like a slap. Rebecca thought her parents wanted a better child, one with a penis. After expressions of disgust, Rebecca told me that she actually remembered the night he was born. She slept at the house of a family friend where there was a boy about her age. When she stood up in the crib, he copied her (i.e., stood up) and then he called his mother to tell on her because she was not supposed to do so. The boy's mother came in stark naked, combing her long hair over her breast. This recollection, probably a screen memory, emphasized visual excitement in the context of her brother's birth. It suggested both her exposure to primal scene and envy of what she unconsciously thought of as her mother's many penises (husband, baby boy, breast, and hidden phallus), as well as Rebecca's preoccupation with genital comparisons and inadequacy.

Elaboration of these ideas was accomplished over the entire analysis. Since Rebecca regarded me as a doctor and a female more openly and less conflictually invested in my own appearance than her mother, she experienced me as an enviable woman, the early mother, with both phallic and feminine qualities that made me intact and superior. At first this was manifested in her curiosity about me. She wondered whether I was married and had children, and where I lived. Mrs. R, who asked Rebecca these very questions, promoted her daughter's inquisitiveness. Although unwilling to share her fantasies, Rebecca displayed her admiration. I told her that she made me out to be one of the popular girls who, we had come to understand, she believed "had it all." I suggested to Rebecca that her curiosity about my private life had a history in her interest in her parents' private, i.e., sexual, life. This was met with the adamant denial, "My parents are old and boring! They had sex twice in their whole lives!"

Gradually, and perhaps hastened by the frustration of my not providing information in response to her questions, Rebecca identified with her mother whom she experienced as aggressive. She did to me what she felt her mother did to her. She began to pick me apart, especially in regard to my appearance. Rebecca dissected my color choices, my shoes, my makeup, my wrinkles, with disdain. She made every effort to embarrass me as she felt her mother embarrassed her. For example, her mother told her she was fat around the middle and grew impatient if Rebecca expressed a wish to window shop or buy *Seventeen* magazine. Complaints about mother's insensitivity would be followed, within the hour, by an all out assault on my person and office. I told Rebecca that she was giving me a taste of what she got and that it was hard for her to allow herself pleasure in girls' things because she felt that her mother enviously viewed them as second-rate and put her down for it. I added that she joined in with mother, rather than risk losing her altogether. But she was of two minds here too. Rebecca liked some of these very things that she scornfully saw me enjoying. However, she felt guilty and disloyal in doing so.

Toward the first summer break when Rebecca was 13, she became more directly competitive and wanted to play games. It was no accident that she settled in with jacks, at which I am very competent. Thus she was repeatedly compelled to acknowledge my supremacy. Rebecca guarded against feelings about the coming interruption with her typical scorn, "Miss you? You've got to be kidding!"

At this time she became more focused on her peers, at once a deflection of the transference and a developmental step away from her intense family preoccupation. Judy, whom she endowed with idealized feminine and phallic properties, was a better boy *and* a better girl than Rebecca. She was pretty, the daughter of a beauty editor of a women's magazine, an excellent athlete, and a mediocre student. Judy had a "big ego" (in Rebecca's words) and Rebecca looked up to her, envied her clothes and her dating single mother; she felt deeply possessive and competitive. Rebecca described a number of incidents involving Judy, characterized by her own guilty interest in intrigue and her proclivity for masochistic and highly exhibitionistic public humiliations. Rebecca hung out with some popular girls and joined them in bad-mouthing Judy for her "big ego" and her flirtatiousness. Then she called Judy to apologize and yielded to her demands that Rebecca identify the others.

On another occasion, she was again with the same group of girls engaged in critiquing Judy. When she saw Judy coming, Rebecca ran to her side and denounced the others in their presence. They retaliated by calling her names, e.g., "scum sucking dog," and ostracizing her. In talking this over, she acknowledged her anxiety that Judy was becoming more popular. In protecting Judy, focusing the hostility on herself rather than her friend, she also tried to seize the spotlight in her familiar "cutting off your nose to spite your face" manner. This was a characterization we had come to use as a shorthand for her familiar defensive management of her aggression.

Rebecca grew extremely irritable in the course of my efforts to address her pivotal role in these, and countless other, incidents. Even as she allowed me to show her how she recreated her humiliation with me, she cast me in the role of the sadistic witch who calls her foul names and shames her. The intensity of Rebecca's response derived, in part, from her difficulty tolerating strong affect (here, for example, her feelings of guilt and responsibility). We linked this to her history of externalizing painful affects in temper tantrums or righteous outbursts (both of which tended to relieve her internal tension and reduce her own sense of conflict). We also examined her outmoded idea that she could not tolerate thinking about her own contributions to difficult situations while feeling so bad. Rebecca began to be able to recognize her fear of her emotional life. I was also eventually able to show her her excitement in this victimized posture, painful as it was, since it touched on a prominent sadomasochistic theme. Rebecca indignantly recalled an incident when, innocently roughhousing with some classmates, they tied her to a desk, tickled her, and invited everyone to see. Reference to being "tied down and tickled," another term we came to use, was a useful shorthand in pointing out many similar incidents where she arranged her exciting, public humiliation.

Second Year of the Analysis

Over the second year of treatment, the peer focus persisted, as Rebecca visibly matured and tolerated the emergence of sexual interest in boys. Direct expression of her interest actually began while she was on vacation on a teen bike trip without analyst or parents around. At home, Rebecca was more driven to create distance from her parents, spending a lot of time locked in her room, even refusing dinner with them for weeks running. Thus she transformed her former avoidance of her peer group to avoidance of her family.

Rebecca also withdrew from me, propelled by the combination of her guilty loyalty conflict, her competitive transference position, the developmental imperative of establishing herself as a grown-up, and her need to gain distance from her homosexual transference feelings. All these themes occurred to me in turn as I reflected, sometimes silently and sometimes out loud, on how, during this phase, Rebecca successfully "turned me off" (as I phrased it to her) and made sessions an ordeal. She relentlessly teased me, calling me a rich fake and a rip-off artist, and complaining of boredom. She sat in my analytic chair, hummed and held her ears if I said anything she did not like. She regaled me with interminable stories, replete with intrigue, sex, and violence, from TV soap operas, which she secretly watched behind locked doors and against parental orders.

Rebecca's determination to distract our focus and to fragment themes of her own sexuality and interest in intrigue with a perseverative focus on TV ultimately provided useful grist for the mill in terms of analyzing Rebecca's fantasy life. However, I also viewed it as a window into her experience of her attentional problems. I guessed that the boredom, distractibility, and irritability she was both demonstrating and inducing in me were exacerbated when she felt anxious and threatened. I observed that while Rebecca was busy derailing my efforts to focus our work and seemed intent on boring us both to distraction, she was also getting to dwell on all the things that excited her without recognizing them as her own fantasies. She reduced this all to being naughty (according to her parents' values) by watching TV and "dissing" (disrespecting) me.

This assertion was supported by what Rebecca *did* tell me, since she continued to at least report events which lent themselves to further analytic work. Rebecca's brief relationship with a new boy in class was associated, in rapid succession, with a sense of her triumph over other girls, her discomfort with the specter of the dangerous and exciting possibilities of sex, her rapid disillusionment with the boy, and her relief upon escaping the relationship. Her impulsivity and her anxiety vied with each other as she accepted this boy's verbal overtures on a class trip. Rebecca seemed to be aroused and excited by the public victory of obtaining a boyfriend. However, a movie date alone a week later proved too much for her. She fled the scene and broke off the burgeoning romance.

Rebecca's friendship with Judy limped through the year, with eruptions precipitated by her envy of Judy's increasing involvement with the popular crowd. Despite Rebecca's resistance, we were able to develop an understanding of her chronic social struggles, amplified now by her growing sexual interest.

Many of her dreams reflected her oedipal guilt. Rebecca chronically struggled with her mixture of competitive, angry, yearning, and sacrificial feelings toward mother and other women and her compromise in a scary injurious image of sex. This expressed her castration fears and her masochistic penance for pleasure and exhibitionistic gratifications. For example, she dreamt of feeling sick at a school assembly, standing up and yelling, "Daddy, help me." Exploration of this dream led to Rebecca's memories of early problems with asthma where she clung to mother, not father, despite his being the doctor. This dream was initially understood as a disavowal of her yearning for maternal protection. Subsequent discussion of the dream allowed us to link it to Rebecca's sense of inadequacy as a female and her surrender to a view of herself as sick to merit her father's attention. Finally, we came to understand it as a manifestation of her sadomasochistic compromise solution to oedipal longings.

Rebecca dreamt of dancing with a desirable older (i.e., inaccessible) boy, feeling his erection even though he was much taller (indeed "as tall as [her] father"), and then being tied up at a table by villains who touched her, "changed" her (as she put it), and then changed her back again. Here her associations led to a soap opera involving a girl's plot to kill the mother of a lover and steal her money.

Rebecca and I were further able to discuss her guilty feelings about competitive struggles with her mother and her desires for mother's privileges, as well as her own fears that she would suffer bodily for them. She then dreamt of sending a note to the same older boy asking to get to know him. He responds positively, but then Judy finds out and tells the whole class, after which he says, "Forget it." I was able to observe Rebecca's histrionic, loud attempts to attract the attention of the yearned-for older boys as she recreated this in sessions. I recognized the familiar signature of her unconscious guilt, in her efforts to make herself seem like a self-conscious little sister.

Analytic work on these issues allowed Rebecca to begin to examine her body, especially the dreaded genital area (in the context of struggling with tampons), and to recognize her hostile competitive strivings toward her girl friends, against which she defended with guilty defeat. Rebecca became less phobic, freer to come and go on her own, and less self-defeating in her attitude about schoolwork, which stabilized at an above average level.

Rebecca's standoffish posture with me was impacted significantly by her parents' contemplation of interrupting the analysis at the close of the second year (she was then 14). The R's thought of ending treatment because Rebecca's social situation had improved and her defensiveness had diminished. They also feared that she "used treatment as a crutch" (their words) and felt she should stand on her own.

As Rebecca and I discussed this, she began to adopt a more mature posture toward the analytic work, recognizing her ongoing struggles, her continued resentment of Scott, her feelings of humiliation and inferiority, and her fear of sex. While she refused to participate in a meeting between her parents and myself to discuss the issue of continuation of the analysis, Rebecca did discuss the matter at home in a distinctly different way. Rather than engaging in childish tantrums at the possibility of being deprived, behavior which served to get her parents off the hook, she participated in a number of conversations with them. She was especially able to communicate with her father, who was warmer and less moralistic about Rebecca's needs. In the end, I think it was her father who facilitated acceptance of my recommendation of a minimum of one more year of treatment.

Third Year of the Analysis

By the time the second summer interruption approached, Rebecca was less hostile and relentlessly critical of me and more able to consider that she would miss me, as she looked forward to a finite relationship. No doubt, the prospect of the interruption relieved her homosexual anxiety, as well as her chronic loyalty conflicts and her ambivalence about dependency on me. I also wondered if a perceived weakness in me, my failure to intervene successfully, brought me into a more manageable perspective.

Again while vacationing on a teen trip, away from parents and analyst, Rebecca had some real sexual experiences. She French kissed and allowed boys to touch her breasts. It was of note that she had developed abundantly, and took pride in her large, attention-getting breasts. However, her forays into sexual activity proved to be at once forced and impulsive, exhibitionistic, and ultimately painful. She went from one boy to the next "like a butterfly" and developed a "reputation" that followed her (briefly) back to school. These designations, her own, also highlighted her moralizing tendency.

The third and final year of treatment allowed Rebecca and me to consolidate insights about her conflicts around sexuality, competition, and guilt. Also salient was the emergence of a far softer and yet more grown-up Rebecca as she negotiated the experience of loss in the termination phase. Early in the year, she dreamt:

> I was with a new boy in my class, Jim. [He was more accessible and thus represented a step forward as a crush.] We were some place with my mother and Scott. My parents were divorced. Jim and I decide to leave, not because I wanted to go to my father, but just because I didn't want to be stuck there. My mother was trying to stop us, setting up road blocks. Jim and I escaped and kissed.

Rebecca told me how furious she was with her father for not defending her when she misbehaved with his mother, her grandmother. Consequently she was refusing father's help with homework and now had failed a French quiz. I told her that she was keeping her distance from her father, especially after having successfully used her influence with him to get something mother did not want her to have, i.e., further analysis. Despite her need to punish herself for being a young woman with growing sexual power in life, she allowed herself both an independent course and a thrilling kiss in the dream. We later came to understand her failing the test as an indirect and self-defeating demonstration of her neediness—a testimonial that acknowledged the importance of her parents, even while it also reinforced the importance of continued treatment.

Over the year Rebecca repeatedly described examples of her parents' deprivation, infantilization, and withholding, as if attempting to master traumata. To illustrate, they refused to let her go to France on a short exchange program, citing money as the reason. They argued against her interest in resuming clarinet lessons, saying first that she would only drop it again and then simply that mother did not like the idea of lessons with a young man. Her parents resisted her determination to get a part-time job at a popular clothing store, which she managed to override. Ultimately she rented the clarinet with the money she earned there.

Increasing focus on her experience of loss in regard to the analysis was painful for many reasons. Recognizing her parents' limitations was certainly a contribution, leading Rebecca to disclaim sadly, "I'm not a deprived child!" At the same time she fantasized about coming back to me when she was self-supporting. Thus she would be on her own *and* my equal.

Rebecca's tendency to express her anger in a panoply of self-destructive ways was repeatedly worked through. These ranged from her spiteful TV watching to her renunciation of her reasonable desires, such as for a professional haircut instead of the inept job mother did. Rebecca's tolerance of her femininity and her willingness to experience pleasure through her body increased considerably. She examined her genitals with a mirror, conquered the dreaded tampon, and was able to discuss well differentiated sensations arising from her clitoris and vagina in the course of shy descriptions of masturbation fantasies associated with teenage TV stars.

We also explored her conviction that she could never call or see me again. I linked her assumption that when treatment was over, it was absolutely over, to her experience of her parents' rigidity. No doubt her awareness of her mother's history of grudges, leading to decade-long family rifts, informed this fantasy. During the last weeks of her analysis, Rebecca played Solitaire while we talked, which I suggested was her metaphor for her future on her own. She surprised herself by not crying when she said good-bye, but was warm and genuine.

FOLLOW-UP CONTACTS

I have since heard from Rebecca several times. Once she requested a single visit because she wished to share a characteristic struggle with a girl friend, the familiarity of which she recognized when I pointed it out to her. I told Rebecca that she was sacrificing her own ability in order to let me know she cared for and missed me. Almost ten months later, she left me a message saying she had had a great year and a successful Sweet Sixteen party "and you know how hard it's been for me to enjoy my birthday!"

Almost two years later, as a senior in high school, Rebecca resumed treatment on a once per week basis. Her academic performance had deteriorated markedly and she described suicidal thoughts to her mother. We were able to understand her disorganization as, at least in part, a response to her enormous separation anxiety in anticipation of college. She had resumed her Ritalin use, but with little apparent benefit. This was perhaps because her difficulties derived more significantly from her psychodynamic conflicts and her learning disabilities than from her distractibility and impulsivity.

This greatly attenuated treatment was sufficient to help Rebecca to structure her time and planning and to recognize the irrational, counterphobic quality of her plans (for colleges which were too demanding and too remote). However, it could not help her resist her parents' pressure to apply for early admission to a local college which would keep her too close to home. Ongoing treatment was not supported by the R's. When Rebecca was unable to work and organize herself in college, her parents refused my strong recommendation for neuropsychological testing. Instead they attributed her difficulties to immaturity.

SUMMARY

In summary, Rebecca was in analysis from ages 12 to 15, presenting as a hysterical personality with phobias, inhibitions, and many prominent obsessional traits, in the context of a history of Attention Deficit/Hyperactivity Disorder. Certainly evidence of Rebecca's Attentional Disorder was prominent in her personality organization, as I would suggest is common in these children. In her case, as in others, treatment was able to modify some of this impact and to help her better understand herself, including psychological aspects of herself related to this disorder. Rebecca came to see how she recruited her school difficulties, such as problems in managing her time and learning how to master a body of material, to her neurotic conflicts around her femininity and her masochism.

Rebecca's impulsivity, her difficulty tolerating waiting and its associated anxieties, and her readiness to be overwhelmed by strong affect all seemed to be sequelae of her neurophysiological endowment. These posed special challenges for her in her life in general, and for us in the analysis in particular. Some of these characteristics became better modulated, although there was inadequate time to work through many of Rebecca's gains in the area of impulse modulation, cognitive disintegration in the context of anxiety, and distractibility. Even with the forced termination, she was able to use the allotted time to confront her feelings of loss and deprivation, to develop tolerance for the frightening experience of independence, and to consolidate earlier insights, especially those concerning oedipal conflicts.

However, my subsequent contact with Rebecca some years later suggested that problems remained with regard to her capacity to monitor her impulsivity and her tolerance for the sustained demands of academic settings in the context of emotional upheaval. In part this may have been attributable to her great difficulty seeking academic help in college from someone other than her father. Such support might have served a number of purposes, in addition to the cognitive, especially if her parents were able to support it. Most critically, it might have allowed her to disengage from the desperate clinging to her parents, through the availability of another concerned adult, to bridge the transition to more autonomous functioning. Unfortunately, with her parents' encouragement, she withdrew from college after less than a year of "trying to get herself together'' (her words) without any form of treatment. However, many years later I was informed that Rebecca had eventually returned to college, graduated, and was attending a specialized graduate school.

Chapter 14

Discussion of Rebecca's Analysis

Dr. Gilmore's portrayal of the analysis of Rebecca, an adolescent girl with an Attention Deficit/Hyperactivity Disorder and cognitive difficulties, offers an opportunity to consider several issues. Dr. Gilmore has conveyed her exquisite grasp of the convergence of her patient's struggles with her adolescent development, her ADHD, her learning disabilities with a neuropsychological contribution, and the conflicts particular to her early developmental experience in her family. Dr. Gilmore's conceptualization of the case and her interventions were strongly influenced by her understanding of the complex relationship between Rebecca's cognitive problems and her psychological adaptation, organized from the perspective of compromise-formation theory. For example, she demonstrated an appreciation of how Rebecca's actual cognitive difficulties were used for defensive purposes.

This case also underscores the way in which even seemingly detailed diagnostic testing evaluations can fail to take full advantage of the available data. When an accurate and compelling diagnosis is made (in this instance, ADHD), it is no less necessary to continue to investigate other accompanying possibilities: in Rebecca's case, the existence of a specific learning disability and/or psychic conflicts to which the ADHD is contributory and with which it is interwoven.

INTERRELATIONSHIPS BETWEEN THE
NEUROPSYCHOLOGICAL AND PSYCHIC
CONFLICT

The DSM-IV diagnostic criteria for an Attention Deficit/Hyper-activity Disorder include a specific number of manifestations of "inattention" and "hyperactivity-impulsivity" (these were detailed in chapter 1). When looked at from a psychoanalytic perspective, we are faced with the problem that any of these behaviors may also be expressions of psychic conflict involving anxiety and/or depressive affect. Conflicts over aggressive and sexual wishes may present in the form of self-defeating behaviors and inhibitions which are manifested in the above-delineated forms. Therefore, a careful assessment of the many possible sources of this manifest clinical picture is necessary.

Dr. Gilmore (we believe correctly) accepted the diagnosis of Attention Deficit Disorder (the diagnostic term at the time) made by the psychiatric consultant who saw Rebecca three years before, after a sufficiently in-depth diagnostic testing assessment. However, she went on to consider that there were many additional factors (intrapsychic, developmental, and familial) which contributed to Rebecca's presenting difficulties. Having done so, rather than dismiss the significance of ADHD since there were "alternative" explanations, she carefully attended to the way in which having ADHD, and prior to that a proclivity for hypersensitivity and hyperreactivity, had contributed to Rebecca's experience of herself and her world. (This was also an important aspect of the analytic work done by Drs. Miller and Yanof in chapters 4 and 7.)

One could also think about how Rebecca's characteristics might have shaped her parents' experience of her and of themselves as parents. Rebecca had an early history of hypersensitivity, including a pronounced startle reaction and marked aversion to tactile stimuli, including many fabrics. Thus in all likelihood she had not found the earliest physical contact with her parents pleasurable either. She had also suffered from allergic asthma beginning at age 3. Parents with such children may be overprotective in recognition of their vulnerability. They may also feel insulted by the child's apparent rejection of normal parental wishes to soothe, particularly via physical contact.

Dr. Gilmore presents a rich conceptualization of the multiple derivatives of Rebecca's experience of inattention and impulsivity. Among them were Rebecca's predisposition to anxiety, her sense of internal pressure, her prickly defensiveness, her poor frustration tolerance and generalized irritability, her trouble with self-soothing, and her poor modulation of impulses. The latter was evident in many forms. Rebecca's tendency to temper tantrums, her fear of and excitement in relation to violence, her intolerance of excitement in general, her potential for disorganized thinking under the sway of strong affects, the ease with which disturbing and exciting fantasies were stimulated, and her too ready access to such fantasies. One specific example was the ease with which Rebecca would feel overwhelmed, burst into rageful tears, and feel unable to manage the emotional intensity of arguing.

Dr. Gilmore also emphasized her clinical experience that such patients have a greater than ordinary tendency to defensive projection of their impulses in phobic fantasies. In Rebecca's case, this took the form of fears of birds, of the dark, and of sophisticated books with mature content, which she avoided. We can add to this the likely contribution of Rebecca's ADHD to her proclivity for other defenses. One example is the way in which inattentiveness to aspects of the environment and information may serve as a substrate for failure to consider significant features of a social or intellectual experience, and thus promote denial. Rebecca's denial of her own contribution to her difficulties with her peers (she imagined that she was not popular because she was not that pretty and because others envied her good grades) serves as an illustration.

Dr. Gilmore was fundamentally in agreement with the view of the original consulting psychiatrist and psychologist that characteristics associated with ADD were central to Rebecca's social and academic difficulties. Rebecca's ability to sustain friendships was compromised by her hypersensitivity and readiness to feel insulted, and thus to experience herself as a "victim." She became overly stirred up by and preoccupied with social conflicts at school and consequently handled social tensions poorly. In the school setting per se, negotiating transitions could have been affected by the experience of drivenness and distractibility common in ADHD. As schoolwork becomes more demanding, additional difficulties may develop, such as problems in interpreting complex material, structuring time, organizing vast amounts of material, and mounting realistic problem-solving strategies.

It is also necessary to add to this that, prior to the analysis, Rebecca evidenced a typical preadolescent difficulty in coping with and identifying the intensification and confusing admixture of drive pressures to which they are subject. This (not uncommonly) provokes a regression which may manifest itself in schoolwork of a poorer quality and immature interpersonal relationships. Preadolescents may provoke their friends and become increasingly attached to their mothers. In Rebecca's case, this expectable developmental trend combined with her ADHD and learning disability, along with her parents' special traits, to complicate her preadolescent experience. As an early adolescent at the onset of the analysis, these preadolescent traits continued to manifest themselves in interaction with the effects of her ADHD and learning disability.

Dr. Gilmore recognized that, in addition to ADHD, there were likely to have been specific cognitive requirements with which Rebecca had difficulty. These, along with anxiety deriving from other sources, figured into her repetitive dread of each new school year. However, deprived of a carefully defined picture of the nature of Rebecca's cognitive functioning, Dr. Gilmore could not analytically explore these specific features with her patient. Since Rebecca and her father (in different ways) isolated the use of medication and tutoring from the analysis, the opportunity to integrate the meanings and effectiveness of these interventions within the analytic process was also greatly diminished. Rebecca reported conflicts with her parents over her academic work, tutoring, and medication. At times she used the analytic hours to plan her strategies for academic work. At the same time, she repeated with Dr. Gilmore the sadomasochistic struggles she reported with her parents. Asking for help, she refused to avail herself of it.

The fact that dosages of Ritalin were changed without any clear rationale and without mention to the analyst, and that Rebecca's parents repeatedly refused the idea of diagnostic evaluation and professional remediation, make it clear that powerful meanings were embedded in these practices. Several possibilities were suggested by the scanty data available. Both Rebecca's father and mother appeared to have had great difficulty tolerating the experience of their daughter having significant relationships outside their orbit (the analyst, female friends, a boyfriend, her departure for college and the like). Rebecca's custom of preserving as clandestine the experience of being treated by her father (along with some of Rebecca's associations to her dreams) was suggestive of the unconscious sexual meaning of this treatment. Refusing her Ritalin was an expression of a panoply of Rebecca's sexual and aggressive wishes and of her unconscious need to be punished for them. There was a highly charged sadomasochistic sexual aspect of her relationship with her father (refusing to take in his substances, to allow him to penetrate her), and unconscious wishes to potentiate her childlike and explosive qualities. Furthermore, declining any form of amelioration of her academic performance may have been an expression of her unconscious need to punish herself for her burgeoning sexual attractiveness and desires.

Dr. Gilmore also convincingly described her discovery of the ways in which Rebecca recruited her vulnerabilities and limitations for defensive purposes. She detailed Rebecca's reliance upon an array of defenses against her experience of failure to perform academically at a level of excellence. Rebecca assumed a stance of "not caring." She used a projective mode, in which she imagined that her peers rejected her due to envy of her intellect; implicit in this fantasy was the idea that excelling would bring her into conflict with significant others. We believe that Rebecca's tendency to half-hearted effort and to apparent complacency with little can also be viewed as an identification with her parents' belittlement of her abilities, and their unconscious pleasure in her mediocre level of achievement. This was seen, for example, in her statement, "It's [i.e., mediocre grades] good for the first time I have exams; I don't

expect to do better." This was related to her parents' denigration of females, and their need to control their daughter's active engagement with all aspects of her life. Rebecca seemed
to feel she *could* not do, *dare* not do, and did not *deserve* to do
any better than just above average.

We wondered, did she feel she owed it to her parents to
sacrifice her success as a testament to their superiority and their
crucial contribution to her progress in life? This was suggested
by Dr. Gilmore's comment that, once Rebecca became more
able to directly compete with her in games in the analytic
hours, she gravitated to playing jacks. This was an activity at
which Dr. Gilmore excelled; thus Rebecca had to acknowledge
her analyst's "supremacy." It was Dr. Gilmore's view, based on
what she saw of her patient's academic work, that Rebecca did
not make use of her conceptual strengths. The analyst also
considered Rebecca's "preference" for "under par" grades as
a defense against her exhibitionistic wishes. Unfortunately, in
the absence of a well-delineated assessment of Rebecca's cognitive picture, it is impossible to assess whether she was performing at (or considerably below) the level of her potential,
once the more pronounced psychological conflicts over performance were successfully analyzed.

Dr. Gilmore observed that Rebecca used her "moderate
disorganization" and "immature conceptualization" of her assignments for defensive and aggressive ends. She induced in
the analyst the "boredom, distractibility, and irritability" which
were aspects of her own experience of her ADHD and possible
specific areas of neuropsychological difficulty. Not making
good use of the analysis, and/or threatening to alienate the
analyst, could also be viewed as expressions of Rebecca's guilt
for having this special experience (one which her brother did
not have), and which she felt her mother (and probably also
her father) begrudged her. In thinking back upon this analysis,
Dr. Gilmore felt she saw in bolder relief how Rebecca invited
her brother's humiliating remarks about her being in analysis
as a form of punishment for having been given this special gift.

The account of this analysis richly portrays the ways in
which Rebecca's ADHD and her clear (although not well-defined) specific neuropsychologically based cognitive problems

contributed to, and became intertwined with, many other issues of central psychological significance. Most salient was Rebecca's sense of being defective as a girl in a family in which the male gender was regarded as superior. Rebecca also interpreted her "defects," and her need for treatment of them (medication, psychoanalysis, tutoring), as evidence that she was "a nut case." Rebecca felt "blamed" for being unable to live up to her parents' high standards.

Remaining a child, and performing at a level "under par" or "just above average," also protected against the imagined dangers of sexuality. Rebecca's proclivity for expressing feelings and fantasies in action helped to reduce her awareness of painful insights and internalized conflicts. As the analysis proceeded, Dr. Gilmore explored with Rebecca her "outmoded" idea that she remained unable to think successfully when she felt intense unpleasure. While this may well have been the case at an earlier point in her life (prior to the introduction of Ritalin and the preceding analytic work), her current view of herself now served defensive purposes. Rebecca's unconscious excitement in her resulting experience of being victimized was also interpreted.

DIAGNOSTIC TESTING EVALUATION

This is a case in which it would have been very helpful to have another diagnostic evaluation at the outset of the analysis. Dr. Gilmore recommended this both during her initial consultation and at a later time, but Rebecca's parents refused this recommendation. Reevaluation was indicated for two reasons. The initial evaluation done some three years before was problematic in a number of respects. Furthermore, even when previous evaluations are optimal, three years is a substantial enough period to warrant a reassessment; the clinical picture may have changed and some new cognitive demands are posed with changing academic requirements.

The report on the diagnostic assessment done when Rebecca was 9 years, 2 months old strongly (and for good reason) emphasized the significance of her Attention Deficit Disorder. The battery included the standard intelligence test for Rebecca's age, along with many tests permitting the examination of academic skills and specific neuropsychological functions which are the building blocks for these skills. Projective tests were omitted.

The psychologist concluded that Rebecca had difficulties sustaining her attention and concentration on the basis of the patterning of her test scores (the classic triad of relatively poor performance on the Arithmetic, Coding and Digit Span subtests of the Wechsler test), combined with her impulsivity, her failure to check her work, her poor strategizing, and her need for repetition of orally presented material. These findings were also corroborated by the results of the behavioral checklists diagnostic of ADD (Conners' Questionnaires) which were given to Rebecca's parents and teachers.

Once this diagnosis was made, Rebecca's conflicts about school and peer relations—including her tendency to be a victim, her inability to sustain friendships, her hypersensitivity, and readiness to feel insulted—were explained on this basis alone. Consequently, the resulting recommendations reflected this singular clinical impression. Rebecca was thought to require stimulant medication, brief supportive psychotherapy to help her adjust to the use of medication, more structuring of her school setting, and tutoring. The focus of tutorial efforts was not specified. The imbalance of this evaluation dovetailed with Rebecca's parents' preference for both *overestimating* the significance of her cognitive difficulties (including the role of ADD to the exclusion of matters of psychic conflict) and *underestimating* their importance (not having a clear picture of the landscape of her cognitive variations and, possibly, specific neuropsychological disabilities).

A close examination of the findings of this evaluation led us to several impressions. While it seemed to be a reasonable diagnostic conclusion that Rebecca had an Attention Deficit Disorder, there were also many suggestions of the possibility of a concurrent specific learning disability, along with the many elements of psychic conflict which converged with these difficulties. These aspects of the clinical picture were not adequately considered. When there is a prominent attentional disorder, it is often difficult (if not impossible) to accurately evaluate this possibility prior to a systematic trial on stimulant medication. If such a trial is effective, then partial reassessment, in order to parcel out disability from the effects of attentional fluctuations, is the most useful way to proceed.

Furthermore, many types of questions should have been asked of the test data reported. What accounted for the substantial ten-point discrepancy between Rebecca's Verbal and Performance IQ's? An array of possibilities exist. One is that she did not receive time bonuses due to her trouble sustaining attention and concentration. A second is that she had specific problems in visuospatial reasoning, sequencing, or visual discrimination, all of which were ingredients of some of the subtests on which she attained lower scores. Another question is, why were Rebecca's achievement test scores below the level expected for someone of her overall intelligence? Rebecca's spelling was reported to be particularly low, at least in part because (as was noted) her sound blending (i.e., the ability to blend discrete sounds together to form words, as in "c-a-t" is "cat") was weak. There was no mention of the reasons for Rebecca's lower than expected score in reading, even though reading seemed to have been examined in considerable depth via the multiple reading tests administered.

There were references to many other specific findings, the significance of which was not integrated into the diagnostic conclusions. "Auditory processing difficulties" (implying a problem in interpreting and/or discriminating stimuli of an auditory nature) were mentioned on the basis of Rebecca's requests for multiple repetitions of orally delivered material. It is worth noting that this same presentation could be equally characteristic of someone with an immediate auditory memory disorder or with an Attention Deficit/Hyperactivity Disorder. The psychologist did not indicate how the conclusion that requests for repetition were attributed to "auditory processing difficulties" was reached. This can (and should) be done, since these are distinctions of considerable import, in that the resulting recommendations would be quite different. There were also references to "linguistic errors in responsive naming" (presumably word finding problems), right–left confusion, and marked problems in fine motor coordination. Thus the many suggestions of specific areas of neuropsychological difficulty could have been followed up, and more detailed recommendations made for the focus of tutorial work.

Apparently Rebecca did respond well in many respects to the recommendations made for medication and increased structure. She was better able to stay on task, more self-reliant and enthusiastic about her work, and required less input from teachers. However, there was no diminution of her "emotional upheavals" in the context of new situations, the academic stress of difficult homework assignments, or social problems and family arguments. She retreated, or fantasized doing so, in the face of her easy frustration in social or academic matters. Consequently, these were the same problems for which she was brought to Dr. Gilmore three years later.

Chapter 15

Ms. Ames' Analysis

Roberta Green, M.D.

PRESENTING PROBLEMS

Ms. Ames came for evaluation at 36 complaining that she was depressed and unable to move forward in her life. She had been in supportive psychotherapy for 10 years without much effect. During the latter part of the therapy a psychopharmacologist prescribed antidepressants, antianxiety medication, and sleeping pills. Ms. Ames said that no medication had more than partially resolved her depression.

Six months before the consultation with me, Ms. Ames found a psychoanalyst whose analytically oriented psychotherapy was very helpful. To Ms. Ames' dismay she soon learned that this therapist had acquired a serious illness which disrupted the treatment. She therefore sought another analyst with whom to engage in similar treatment.

Ms. Ames' psychoanalyst, who preferred to remain anonymous and whom we have given the pseudonym of Dr. Green, decided to use a different approach from that of the other contributors. Rather than describe the analysis of her patient sequentially and fully, she chose to report aspects of the analytic work which clarified the dynamics and development of certain of the patient's symptoms. These symptoms appeared at first to be obsessive, but later were understood to involve primary cognitive disabilities as well. In her contribution Dr. Green first supplies background material, including an outline of the patient's complaints and history, as well as the analytic process. She then proceeds to emphasize the work involving her patient's learning disability.

CONSULTATION

After a prolonged consultation of six months, I decided the patient was analyzable, despite the serious nature of her depression which recurred when medication was stopped. Ms. Ames agreed to a five times a week analysis. During the evaluation a psychopharmacologist, in consultation with me, regulated the medication. Another half-year passed before we could convert the therapy to analysis.

Ms. Ames' history revealed that her symptoms were determined, to a significant extent, by the fact that her mother had suffered from breast cancer. The malignancy was discovered soon after Ms. Ames' parents returned from a vacation when she was 5 years old. Surgery deformed the patient's mother and chemotherapy caused her pain and misery until she died when Ms. Ames was 12.

COURSE OF THE ANALYSIS

Early in the treatment, the analysis of a nightmare on the anniversary of the patient's mother's death demonstrated the important contribution of these events to her symptoms and character traits. Ms. Ames became depressed and anxious at times of separation, including vacation times. She panicked at the thought that I might get sick and die. Since her family had hidden her mother's sickness from her, Ms. Ames was suspicious and hypervigilant as she suspected that her analyst might try to keep a secret of illness. Fearing disease and defect in herself and others, Ms. Ames sought perfection and feared any flaw. She defended against rage which was prominent but forbidden. As a child she had been furious at her mother for leaving her, neglecting her, and embarrassing her when mother displayed symptoms of her malignancy or the effects of her treatment. Ms. Ames recalled wishing her mother would die, but also loved her mother and wanted to keep her alive.

Ms. Ames' defenses included isolation and reaction-formation, giving an obsessive coloring to her character, in addition to her depressed demeanor. She even displayed obsessive–compulsive symptoms as a child. For example, as she prepared breakfast she felt she could keep her mother alive if she completed preparation of all parts of the meal at the same time. When she failed to get her mother's food prepared on schedule, she felt she was causing her mother to remain ill. After her mother died she kept her own clothes in the same place in the closet, even after she had outgrown them, with the fantasy that if her mother returned to life she would find something familiar in the house.

Magical thinking added to the obsessive cast. So too did her need for perfection in herself, which made her very slow in her schoolwork and inordinately slow in work as an adult. She also demanded perfection of others and became furious when people parked illegally, littered, or made errors when they made out bills. She became so upset when a cashier was slow or incorrect that she chose supermarkets according to the nature of the checkout person. She became so angry at violators of laws, including drug dealers, that she confronted them, thus putting herself in danger.

Evidence emerged that traits of Ms. Ames' family facilitated her need to seek perfection and her obsessive character. This allowed further analysis of the genesis of the defenses she favored, her character, and her symptoms. Ms. Ames' family was extraordinarily orderly, neat, and clean. Her house was immaculate and elegant with ornate woodwork. The patient's mother, Ms. Ames said, had beautiful, well-kept walk-in closets with special shelves for hats and shoes. Ms. Ames believed that her mother deserved the best because she was the victim of cancer.

When the patient was a small child her parents took her on magnificent trips in which they stayed at the best hotels and ate at expensive restaurants. She was expected to achieve high standards of etiquette and grown-up manners. Family meals were a torture. Even when the extended family ate together on holidays, they had to wash the dishes between courses. They could not tolerate having dirty dishes sit in the sink or on the counter.

Ms. Ames too was very neat. A needy person, she brought food to her analytic sessions to fortify and comfort herself. She was able to eat or drink while lying on the couch without spilling anything. Once while vociferously condemning both the children of parents in television situation comedies and children of her misguided friends who allowed their kids to be messy, Ms. Ames reacted to my interpretation of her envy of these children with a rare accident. She spilled the sugar she was putting into her coffee, but miraculously did not spill the coffee itself. She was astonished and relieved when she looked up and saw me smiling benignly rather than being furious at the mess.

Ms. Ames' psychodynamics appeared to explain her obsessional slowness as she, trying to live up to her parents' ideals which she had incorporated, sought perfection. Her superego was severe and firm. Analysis of these dynamics and the compromise formations involved brought some relief and a great deal of insight. But over time material emerged in the analysis which made me think that more was involved, that Ms. Ames suffered from cognitive disabilities.

I had known from the history Ms. Ames provided in her early sessions with me that she had had a school phobia which started when she was in nursery school. Her worry about her mother's getting ill, entering a hospital, or dying while she was at school had made her more fearful.

In addition, her mother demanded that she get excellent marks. As an adult, Ms. Ames searched for evidence of what her life was like as a child. She came across her report cards and learned more about her mother's high standards. When Ms. Ames was a child in second grade her teacher wrote on her report card that she was pleased with how well she did. Her mother wrote a scathing note on the card which Ms. Ames returned to her teacher: "Thank you for your lovely comments. However, we are disappointed that Betty is not doing better in reading. Books in our home are like bread and butter. It is really hard to understand why she would not be in the top reading group." Although at that time Ms. Ames could not read her mother's script, she seemed to discern what her mother's feelings were.

Ms. Ames and I now considered that, in addition to fearing her mother's demise, she also feared her mother's criticism for her failure to be perfect enough at school. Her parents expected her to receive only A's. Mr. Ames had a bad temper and resorted to physical violence. Betty was afraid of the rage she could set off if she made a mistake. Thus school and academic performance was a highly charged aspect of Ms. Ames' life. Again, psychodynamic perspectives alone could have been compelling. However, features of Ms. Ames' description of her experience at work, combined with some of her behavior in the analytic hours, led me to consider additional contributions. Indications that cognitive difficulties interfered with her skills at work appeared. She had held many clerical and secretarial positions over the years, but quit or was discharged repeatedly. Letters of recommendation from her employers emphasized her overall intelligence and skills in certain areas. Still she was very slow at work, seemed to try too hard, and aim too high. She took too long to do relatively simple jobs.

Examination of Ms. Ames' behavior at work filled analytic hours. She had trouble finding her way around the office. Each time she got a new job, she had to draw a map of the office to which she would refer to avoid getting lost. When she tried to file folders, she could not recall the alphabetical order. If someone asked her where a particular item was, she would take him to the object because she could not give directions for how to locate it.

Similar behavior occurred in the analysis. If I told Ms. Ames I would be away during a particular period, she could not readily grasp when that was. She had to write down the specific dates and occasionally even asked me to do so. At times I did so and learned that I had to be very exact in my explanations for her to be able to understand and recall. For example, if I said I would be away from September 2nd to 10th, she would remain uncertain as to whether I would return on the 10th or the 11th. When the psychiatrist Ms. Ames saw changed the dose or frequency of her medication she would often become confused and unable to follow his orders. Again, he had to be precise and unambiguous. Obsessiveness alone did not explain these characteristics of slowness and the need for precision.

As we talked about the possibility that she had a learning disability, Ms. Ames recalled her school history in more detail. She had worked very hard to get decent marks in elementary and high school. Her difficulties included mathematics. Despite mediocre boards she got into a very good college in California. At college she studied less and did less well, yet managed to squeak by and graduate. Ms. Ames, who was not in treatment during her college years, often felt depressed and overwhelmed. She tried to deal with this by self-medicating with "recreational drugs" like marijuana and Qualudes. She was also able to distract herself with an active social life. She had made many friends at college and was still close to them, over a decade later.

Diagnostic Evaluation of the Learning Disability

Ms. Ames agreed that a learning disability would explain more about many of her characteristics and considered taking psychological and educational tests, the nature of which I explained. Among other things, I told her that the tester would ask her questions about general information, vocabulary, and simple arithmetic. She would also have puzzles for her to solve and inkblot cards for her to examine and describe. Ms. Ames decided to pursue this evaluation to ascertain whether she had a learning disability.

To her surprise, the tests were more disturbing than she had anticipated. Ms. Ames became furious that the psychologist was late and, therefore in her mind, imperfect. She felt as though she were a captive whom the psychologist forced to do things. Only later did Ms. Ames calm herself by recognizing that she was *employing* the tester rather than being her slave. She felt as if she were in a school or job situation in which she was being judged. She also felt as if she were being tricked, particularly on the Rorschach Test. Ms. Ames could not trust the examiner, even when she told the patient that she did not have to finish parts of the tests if she truly could not do them. Determined, she persisted in trying to complete everything.

When I gave Ms. Ames a copy of the report of the test findings, she was appalled that it contained so many typographical errors. She deprecated the tester, proclaiming that she herself would never send out such defective work. Again, anger boiled within her. As we went over the findings, Ms. Ames felt upset that she was defective, but then was reassured that she really had a disability; her father had been wrong in accusing her of being lazy. With time we could come to understand how her learning disability affected her personality development and psychopathology.

The diagnostic battery included the Wechsler intelligence test, the Wide Range Achievement Test, tests of graphomotor functioning, and of an array of visual and auditory memory functions, as well as projective tests. The overall diagnostic impression was of an extremely bright woman with a marked ability to conceptualize. The psychologist who did the tests found that Ms. Ames displayed specific neuropsychological problems in visual–motor functioning, including cross-modal integration and visual memory. She thought that these had contributed to the patient's performance difficulties at work, and specifically to retrieval of visually encoded memories. The psychologist also emphasized the added contribution of Ms. Ames' inhibitions about knowing and seeing to difficulties in the visual area. Her concentration was compromised by anxiety, she added, but there was no evidence of an Attention Deficit/Hyperactivity Disorder.

Ms. Ames attained a Full Scale IQ of 107 (in the Average range as measured by the WAIS-R). Her Verbal IQ was 120 (in the Superior range) contrasted with her performance IQ of only 92 (also in the Average range). Examination of the subtests of the Wechsler disclosed that Ms. Ames possessed outstanding verbal abilities. She had an excellent vocabulary. Her grasp of abstract concepts, general factual information, and of societal conventions and principles was outstanding as well.

The only verbal subtest at which Ms. Ames did not excel (indeed her score was at a markedly lower level) consisted of solving arithmetic word problems. This task encompassed visuospatial reasoning, which was an area of neuropsychological disorder for Ms. Ames. If this score were omitted, she would have attained a Verbal IQ in the Very Superior Range.

The psychologist also commented on manifestations of anxiety and depressive affect on the Wechsler. Anxiety adversely affected Ms. Ames' functioning on the Arithmetic subtest. And at times the patient's depressive concerns were evident in the content of her replies on other verbal subtests, although these concerns did not compromise her accuracy for the most part.

Specific problems appeared in Ms. Ames' processing of visuospatial material, visual memory, and cross-modal integration. In addition, her efficiency, and sometimes her accuracy, on timed perceptual–motor tasks was reduced by the motor slowness which resulted from her depression and the compromising effects of anxiety upon her concentration. Constructional tasks (such as replicating block designs and assembling puzzles) and graphomotor tasks (such as copying geometric figures) were particularly affected. Tests which required visual discrimination without motor and/or spatial reasoning were performed well. However, the patient had difficulty when an appreciation of perspective and/or the interweaving of parts was necessary.

Ms. Ames demonstrated strength on portions of the achievement test she took. She did well in reading and spelling, but her performance on a written mathematics test was well below expectations based on her overall intelligence and education. This was essentially due to the limited number of items she completed within the time limit, rather than to computational or conceptual errors.

Projective tests revealed that Ms. Ames was a highly ideational woman with a good potential for delaying her impulses and reflecting on her emotional responses. At the same time, her marked attempts to ward off anxiety and depressive affect were sometimes poorly integrated and often unsuccessful.

Characteristic defenses were denial of hostile wishes in particular and the emotional significance of a situation in general. Looking and seeing, concretely and symbolically, were heavily conflicted. This was related to Ms. Ames' unconscious thoughts and fantasies about her mother's illness. To illustrate, her Rorschach record was replete with images of deformity.

Ms. Ames evidenced highly ambivalent feelings toward women. Longing for maternal nurturance, wishes to identify with the maternal object, only to fear having a deformed body, were prominent. The psychologist remarked that the "affective heart" of Ms. Ames' experience could be traced back to the period before her mother's death. The tester felt confident of Ms. Ames' capacity to make use of interpretations and to ultimately understand and master the traumas of her life.

Psychoanalytic Work with the Diagnostic Findings

Ms. Ames was both troubled and relieved by the report. She had begun analysis hoping that at termination she would no longer need antidepressants and also that her cognitive difficulties (which she was aware of but had not labeled as such) would be gone. The testing left her with a feeling that she had areas of defect for which she might be able to compensate, but which would remain a part of who she was. Before the testing Ms. Ames thought she was imperfect; now she thought she was imperfectable. By analogy, she believed that in addition to a biological component to her depression that might persist after the analysis and continue to require medication, there was also a biological basis for her cognitive difficulties which might remain. She had indeed dug up evidence of an inherited foundation for her depression. In exploring some of the many family secrets, she had learned that her maternal grandfather had suffered from severe depression requiring hospitalization; she was concerned that heredity was at work.

Ms. Ames also struggled with the question of how much of her past psychological and family conflict would haunt her in the future. She was distressed about the limits of analysis, just as she was concerned about her own limits. Ms. Ames became angry at the therapist she had seen throughout her twenties for his failure to talk with her about her mother or to discuss and analyze her rage. She was particularly angry about the wasted years because she felt that by this time she might have been able to be in a successful romantic relationship and to have had children. Hidden behind the anger at others was her fury with me for having brought her limitations to light.

On the positive side, Ms. Ames felt vindicated that she had not been lazy at school or on the job, but instead had actual difficulties with specific kinds of tasks. In her next few jobs she was able to use this information constructively. Her career remained a problem because the jobs for which she was eligible by training required the skills with which she had the greatest difficulty. She finally decided to take a less stressful, but also less lucrative, sales position.

The knowledge that Ms. Ames' cognitive difficulties involved trouble dealing with numbers led me to further thoughts about her dealings with money. Ms. Ames' father, who earned a modest amount of money when Ms. Ames was very small, became a rather wealthy man by dint of great effort and great intellectual capacity. The Ameses ultimately moved to a wealthy part of town, occupied a beautiful house, and lived a lavish life. They traveled widely, taking their daughter with them on expensive trips. Mr. Ames was sure that he would leave his daughter a large inheritance and thus promised her a fortune. When he died he left a considerable amount, but not the vast holdings he had vowed he would. Ms. Ames believed she had been left a great deal and so did I. Therefore, she paid a full fee.

However, following the diagnostic testing evaluation, my attention was drawn to evidence that things were not as rosy as Ms. Ames thought. In part because she had difficulty adding and subtracting, she avoided evaluating her worth and income and other financial facts. She spent large amounts of money without regard to whether she could afford to do so. For example, she did not add up her mounting credit card debt and had no budget; nor did she know about taxes. Although she had an accountant and financial advisor, she did not know the details of what he advised or what she paid in taxes. I began to wonder whether Ms. Ames possessed as much money as she thought. By paying careful attention to what she said about money and her incomplete references to what her financial aide told her, I was able to piece things together.

I realized that although her father had been very wealthy, the property he owned could not be liquidated at that time, and its value had fallen considerably before he died. Nevertheless he clung to his statements that his daughter would inherit a fortune from him. Ms. Ames did not try to ascertain how true his statements were, even when the will and surrogate proceedings *could* be evaluated.

Important dynamic aspects of Ms. Ames' blind spot supplemented the role of her deficient powers of observation due to her learning disability. She loved her father and wanted to believe that he loved her and had given her large amounts of money as an expression of that love. She had to deny that he had failed her, and thus keep from recognizing her rage at him for not leaving a truly huge inheritance. Eventually Ms. Ames realized that her accountant had been warning her that she was rapidly using up her money. She suddenly noticed that she did not have the money she imagined she had. Then she became angry at her father who, she felt, did not protect and love her. She felt guilty about her rage at him. Perhaps punishing herself for her anger, she reversed her course. Instead of spending excessively, she became penurious and spent even less than was prudent.

Denial was a prominent defense for Ms. Ames and her family. When her mother was ill and finally died, they avoided talking about it. The patient attempted to defend against anxiety and sadness by imagining her mother would return. We could now see that there was an amalgamation of her denial through identification with the defensive style of family members, with denial related to her neuropsychologically based difficulties in perceiving accurately.

Faced with her actual financial status, Ms. Ames and I had to deal with her analytic fee realistically. While the fee was obviously too high, lowering it would create complications. It was possible for Ms. Ames to maintain her high fee but come less frequently; this would mean that psychotherapy would replace analysis.

Or she could be seen in analysis four times a week at a lower fee. Ms. Ames was reluctant to follow either course. Analysis had been very helpful and she wanted to continue it; psychotherapy would be a poor substitute. On the other hand she felt that lowering the fee would be unfair to me. She would feel guilty. Further, she wondered if she would be able to express her hostility to me if she felt grateful and obligated. Would she be able to call me at night, as she sometimes had, if she paid a low fee? Would she be able to indulge herself, for instance, by taking a taxi at times, if she paid me less? In effect she would feel I was paying for her extravagance.

Ms. Ames also had to consult her financial advisor to get his approval; he had to determine whether paying for the analysis was financially sound. She reported that, although he was skeptical about the expenditure, he recognized that the treatment helped Ms. Ames. In the area of economics, he thought I was able to accomplish what he had failed to do. I had been able to convince Ms. Ames to examine her finances and deal with her money realistically. He therefore favored continuation.

After much discussion and analysis of her conflicting feelings, I agreed to lowering the fee and seeing her four times a week. Suspicious, she wondered what my motives were. Eventually she decided that I was a conscientious doctor who wanted to help her with the best treatment: analysis. The analysis continued. Ms. Ames felt she had to settle down and be an adult.

She examined her relationship to her parents in that regard. She felt that her parents discouraged her from being an adult. For example, by telling her she was a genius but lazy her father was treating her as if she could not grow up and achieve things in a realistic manner. She was an exception who did not have to follow the usual adult rules. She was exempt because she was both "defective" *and* "superior," a member of an elite family. Her parents considered themselves above others. Not only were they clean and orderly, aiming for perfection; they were intellectual. They did not watch television, which they considered lowbrow. They listened to only "the best" radio station, which played classical music. There was the expectation that in being "superior," Ms. Ames could indulge herself; however, she was simultaneously chastised for it.

The analysis helped Ms. Ames to mature and face preoedipal and oedipal desires with less anxiety. I will touch on a few themes that we dealt with in the subsequent years and then discuss the way the tests helped me in my analytic work.

Along with using denial, and thus failing to perceive important aspects of her environment, Ms. Ames was often hypervigilant. As we got to understand her denial, she became more able to investigate in an adaptive manner to further the analysis. For instance, she supplemented her knowledge about her childhood experiences by asking relatives and finding documents, such as her report cards and letters that her parents had written. Ms. Ames had the feeling that her mother had had a miscarriage when she was 4 years old. She came to realize that her mother's crying, which she had attributed only to the pain her malignancy and chemotherapy produced, was also a result of the loss of her baby. This enabled Ms. Ames to reconstruct her childhood wish to destroy potential siblings and the guilt these desires entailed. She imagined she was responsible for the miscarriage and, therefore, should not have children herself. These conflicts appeared in the transference; she hoped to keep me from becoming pregnant.

Especially in the first year of analysis, Ms. Ames would explore the office carefully and stealthily. She noticed where books were located and was alert to any change in their placement. On the one hand this was understood as a compensation for her cognitive defects. On the other hand she was searching for clues and secrets, as she had wanted to do as a child, to find out about her mother's illness and evaluate her chances of losing her mother. Thinking there was a destructive aspect to her looking, she warned me not to leave any written information in the open, lest she find out about my patients.

Ms. Ames also tried to find out about my personal life. She heard the doorman to my office building say that I was a nice person, and then saw a newspaper that had my home address on it. She subsequently hung around the apartment house in which I lived, but was unable to get further information there.

She looked at the building, but did not like it. It was too modern, not like her charming childhood home. She noticed a black marble slab that decorated the lobby, and said it looked like a tombstone. My home was associated with death, her mother's death, and the family she wanted to be part of, my family. Early in the treatment, Ms. Ames enacted such wishes by actually eating her breakfast in my office; later (as noted earlier) she ate food and drank coffee while lying on the couch. Early in the analysis Ms. Ames dreamed that she looked into my refrigerator and saw quarts of homemade chicken soup there.

She wanted to be my child, to be fed by me and to enter me. Although she had wanted to be taken care of by her mother, she was dissatisfied with her, felt her mother and her mother's sisters were cold. In many ways she preferred her father who was warmer and more maternal.

Ms. Ames' separation anxiety was accentuated in the context of groping with her feelings about a friend, Dorothy, who suddenly died of meningitis. Ms. Ames herself had developed a sore throat with severe laryngitis which prevented her from speaking for a considerable period. During the time she could not talk to Dorothy, she did not know her friend had been very ill and uncared for. Ms. Ames subsequently learned that Dorothy eventually went to an Emergency Room, where the doctors kept her waiting; it was there that she died. Ms. Ames' reactions were complex. She felt very sad, blamed herself, and criticized her friend for neglecting herself and the doctors for letting her die. The episode reminded Ms. Ames of other losses: two cats she owned some years ago who had been abused (like herself, she thought), and of course, the deaths of her mother and father. As the end of the analysis was approaching, Ms. Ames also worried about losing me.

As the analysis came close to the termination phase Ms. Ames dealt with cognitive concerns which intertwined with conflictual oedipal issues. This was exemplified by her work with a dream she reported in the sixth year of the analysis in which she was at a party in my apartment:

You [the analyst] were in the kitchen with your mother and several other women. I was in the dining room with your husband who was telling me something amusing. I laughed and caught your eye. I felt you not only could tolerate this social interchange between me and your husband, but you were proud of my lack of anxiety. I came into the kitchen and listened to you explain to the other women what was wrong with the stove. I was very surprised that I was able to follow your complicated verbal description without getting confused. I then went to the living room where I saw my aunt Ruth [her favorite aunt who was usually anxious and depressed] on the balcony with a drink in her hand clearly enjoying herself.

Associating to the dream, Ms. Ames said that she now knew that her cognitive difficulties were exacerbated by her anxiety. In the dream I (Dr. Green) could tolerate her flirting with my husband and be happy for her without denigrating her, as her mother had done in such situations. When I could allow her that pleasure, Ms. Ames was able to be less anxious and to understand what I was saying. Her aunt's uncharacteristically enjoying the party meant to Ms. Ames that she did not have to feel guilty about enjoying herself, because she was not surpassing her aunt. In describing the dream she was also aware of her wish to be close to me and part of my family. Referring to the manifest dream, she said that in the dream my mother was much like the mother of one of her friends, a critical but loving immigrant. She added that I (Dr. Green) was being put on the defensive by my mother. Ms. Ames was thus implying that my mother, being like the critical immigrant, was attacking me, a mother substitute.

Oedipal wishes were quite clear as we analyzed the dream. Rather than being put on the defensive by her mother as she usually pictured she was, I, a mother surrogate, was the victim of maternal attack. Ms. Ames felt buoyed by the dream. She was more able to allow herself to show off to me and to playfully spar with me. In her bantering she could often best me. She experienced the dream as our granting her permission to be my rival without feeling guilty or risking the loss of our relationship. She subsequently became more interested in dating and made concrete efforts to find a man of her own.

The manifest dream contained a reference to Ms. Ames' cognitive disability: she was able to follow my "complicated verbal description without getting confused." In her first association she asserted that she knew anxiety had had an adverse effect on her cognition. She implied that, as she tolerated oedipal wishes to triumph over her mother without excessive anxiety, she could overcome her learning disability and possibly equal her mother in intellectual competition. In a salute to analytic thinking, she said that when she was anxious it was important for her to understand; when she was calm, she was capable of doing so.

Although Ms. Ames did not carry this line of thought further in the session described, these thoughts became more prominent as the analysis proceeded. Ms. Ames saw more and more clearly that her cognitive difficulties reflected an interweaving of cognitive disability and defense. The implicit and explicit demand that Ms. Ames not see how ill her mother was fostered a cognitive style that interfered with Ms. Ames' seeing other things around her, both literally and metaphorically. This interfered with her ability to compensate for her learning disability. In addition, a high level of anxiety further compromised her cognition. Insofar as she feared competing with her mother intellectually, she had further specific motivation to inhibit her thinking and perceiving. During the analysis she became less anxious and more able to tolerate awareness of distressing events and feelings.

This allowed her to better compensate for her areas of cognitive impairment, which, having a biological base, would never go away altogether. Ms. Ames remained disappointed by her difficulties in following instructions, alphabetizing, and working with numbers. While they interfered with her getting good jobs, she could better take this in her stride. She was able to find employment in which she could exploit her adaptive traits, such as her social skills, her affection for people, and her desire to be of help. Because her guilt and masochistic leanings diminished markedly, she berated herself for her shortcomings much less than previously.

DISCUSSION

I will conclude by commenting on the effect that my recognition of Ms. Ames' learning disability (through clinical observation supplemented by psychological and educational test findings) had on me as her analyst. I was pleased that I was able to broaden my view and not limit my understanding of her to the usual psychoanalytic perspective. I could understand her better as an individual coping with dynamic preoedipal and oedipal conflicts. Knowing the cognitive difficulties she had, I could understand more about her daily experience, the tension she had to deal with as she tried to cope with the world about her and her inner feelings.

I could thus make interpretations that took into account her actual experiences. Rather than jump to the conclusion that her tension resulted only from her difficulties with authorities who reminded her of her parents, I would recognize how her cognitive difficulties made her day difficult, as she tried to clarify her perceptions and organize her activities. In my interventions I could balance drive and ego aspects, with sufficient emphasis on cognitive factors. I had to be careful not to exaggerate the role of her obsessional character structure, but rather take her learning disability into account when assessing and interpreting her slowness.

Further, I became aware that I had to be especially careful to be specific in my statements. Ambiguity bred misunderstanding and confusion to a greater extent in Ms. Ames than in other patients. If I told her I would be away "through January 1," for instance, she would not understand me (i.e., it would be unclear to her whether I would be back on January 1st or 2nd) and a remarkable degree of confusion would arise in our relationship. As I developed a feel for the effects of Ms. Ames' cognitive difficulties and her resulting ways of thinking, I was able to help a difficult analysis run more smoothly.

Chapter 16

Discussion of Ms. Ames' Analysis

This case is exemplary in portraying an open-minded collaboration of analyst and patient as they search for an increasingly complex, broad, and in-depth understanding of the patient's experience. The process of discovery of the patient's learning disability, its evaluation, and the clinical value of this evaluation within the analysis are all beautifully described. Finally, the diagnostic testing evaluation performed was sufficiently comprehensive to permit an appreciation of the specifics of the patient's cognitive difficulties, and the interweavings of neuropsychological dysfunction and psychic conflict. The report of this case was written with the intention of giving greater emphasis to work surrounding the patient's learning disability (when compared with other aspects of the analysis and with other cases in this volume, except that of Mr. Young).

It would have been eminently possible to overlook the existence of a learning disability in this case. Much careful analytic work had been accomplished in the one-and-one-half years before Dr. Green and her patient considered that they should investigate the possibility of previously undiagnosed problems of a neuropsychological nature.

THE ANALYTIC WORK PRIOR TO TESTING

There were compelling, and by no means simplistic or reductionistic, intrapsychic explanations of Ms. Ames' symptomatology and character problems. At the age of 35, Ms. Ames had

369

not accomplished important life goals. She was not intimately involved with a partner, was unsuccessful at work, quite depressed, and manifested significant obsessional concerns. However, she had long-standing friendships and was a caring person.

Her history was remarkable. At the height of her oedipal phase, and following her parents leaving her to go on a vacation by themselves (about which Ms. Ames felt enraged, jealous, and abandoned), Ms. Ames experienced the horror of her mother becoming ill with cancer. For a period of six years, ending just as Ms. Ames went into puberty, her mother endured extremely stressful and disfiguring treatments. Unconscious fantasies of having made her mother ill and of killing her were an understandable outgrowth of this developmental experience. Ms. Ames' associated self-punitive trends to assuage guilt for her sense of herself as a murderer who had wished her mother dead, and gotten father all to herself, were prominent in Ms. Ames' clinical picture. So were obsessional traits, as seen in her marked slowness and meticulousness at work, which was so pronounced that she was sometimes fired. This further tempered Ms. Ames' sense of guilt, but also contributed to her depression and experience of herself as defective.

Ms. Ames' depression and sense of being defective had many additional psychodynamic sources. One was her identification with a damaged (severely ill, disfigured, and then dead) mother. Another was her inability to live up to the unrealizable standards set by her parents; she was to be a perfect student and a perfectly behaved child who could never be messy or childlike in any respect. Her parents felt themselves to belong to an elite group to which Ms. Ames was privy only via her connection with them. Thus she was especially privileged but at the same time did not truly share in the exceptional qualities of those with whom she lived. Her mother and aunts (who figured importantly in her childhood) were not warm. No doubt Ms. Ames' mother was also extremely self-involved due to her illness, which exacerbated her characterological sense of specialness and entitlement to be and have the best. Ms. Ames' father, who was more demonstrative, had a fierce temper, which Ms. Ames lived in fear of igniting. Ms. Ames too had a sense of righteousness and intolerance of the imperfections of others. This was also put to self-punitive ends, as, for example, when she put herself in danger by confronting law violators.

Ms. Ames desperately feared the loss of her parents. She felt rage toward her mother for being ill, for embarrassing her, for neglecting her, and ultimately for leaving her by dying. Childhood symptoms expressed and defended against these (and many other) wishes and fears. Ms. Ames had a school phobia, related to her chronic fear of returning to find her mother missing. She also evidenced prominent obsessive–compulsive traits. Ms. Ames anxiously prepared food on a particular schedule, with the fantasy that, if she failed in this endeavor, mother would remain ill. For years following her mother's death, Ms. Ames preserved the location in her closet of her own clothes, long outgrown, with the fantasy that this familiar remnant of the past would be reassuring to mother if she were to return.

Ms. Ames' description of her family's idiosyncrasies helped Dr. Green understand how her patient developed obsessive–compulsive characteristics. Ms. Ames' parents and other family members with whom she identified appeared to "teach" her to use these types of defenses. They were extraordinarily orderly, clean, and perfectionistic. These family traits also facilitated the use of denial. Again Ms. Ames identified with them in absorbing this attribute.

Ms. Ames was also not supposed to see or know the nature of the many problems at home, most especially the humiliating disfigurement of her mother, or even the fact of her illness. An air of secretiveness and denial permeated Ms. Ames' environment. Nor did this change following her mother's death. Ms. Ames functioned as if she knew nothing, but was nevertheless suspicious and hypervigilant, lest anything evade her notice.

Another analyst might have felt satisfied with this very rich and convincing conceptualization of Ms. Ames' psychic life. However, several observations of her behavior in the analytic hours and descriptions of the specific difficulties in her work life did not escape Dr. Green's notice and raised questions in her mind. For example, she noted Ms. Ames' confusion surrounding announcements of dates when she (Dr. Green) would be absent. While this could have been understood solely as an expression of Ms. Ames' need to deny the fact of separation, and the rage and anxiety associated with such experiences, Dr. Green felt there was more to it.

Dr. Green began to note Ms. Ames' descriptions of her need to draw maps in order to prevent herself from getting lost at work. She also reported having difficulty giving directions which involved spatial concepts; she preferred to accompany a person to a destination, unable to provide directions on how to locate it. She was overly deliberate in secretarial types of tasks, especially when it came to the sequential aspects of alphabetical filing, a task which would seem to be so elementary in nature. Ms. Ames' tendency to spend far more than the requisite hours at work, no doubt related to her family history of perfectionism, was necessary for her just to accomplish her basic responsibilities. Ms. Ames functioned very slowly, despite the fact that in other respects she was highly appreciated by her bosses, such as for her intelligence. In fact they had noted that she tried *too* hard.

These impressions resonated with reports Dr. Green had received from the psychopharmacologist about Ms. Ames' slowness, confusion, and deliberateness in precisely recording directions for the medication he prescribed. As a result, he often felt he had to do the writing for Ms. Ames. Again, this could have been construed as a repetition of the childlike position of incompetence and reliance upon her parents which had been encouraged, and/or an identification with her mother's increasing helplessness. It could also have been accounted for in terms of Ms. Ames' self-punitive trends; she experienced conflict over permitting herself to have the medication which, unlike her mother's uncurable illness, could make her better.

These data, combined with the school reports Ms. Ames found and her memories of having worked remarkably hard to achieve adequate grades in elementary and high school, seemed to Dr. Green to require additional explanations. She felt it was necessary to at least investigate whether neuropsychological factors were at play.

THE TEST EVALUATION

The diagnostic testing evaluation performed was excellent in most respects: its comprehensiveness and degree of integration of neuropsychological and psychodynamic considerations. The psychologist who carried it out sensitively portrayed Ms. Ames' sense of sadness, anxiety, and of "abnormality" in the context of taking tests which incorporated areas of specific cognitive difficulty: visual memory, visual–motor functioning and visuospatial reasoning in (two or three dimensional) constructional and drawing tasks. The psychologist also emphasized the convergence of Ms. Ames' neuropsychological dysfunction in seeing visuospatial relationships, her intense anxiety over what she might see, and her vigilance and experience of being tricked and deprived of essential "clues." Fundamentally, the testing situation was experienced by Ms. Ames as threatening to expose her "defects." The psychologist also appreciated the amalgam of intense psychic conflict and visual memory weakness in Ms. Ames' tendency to have difficulty in retrieving visually registered memories.

There were only a few ways in which this very fine evaluation fell short of ideal. It would have been instructive to evaluate whether there were problems with Ms. Ames' ability to deal with sequential information in the absence of a demand for memory. In addition, a more detailed examination of the nature of Ms. Ames' difficulties with math could have been carried out. According to the examiner, it was the spatial, and not the computational, aspects which were problematic; this could have been further explained and documented. Had this been done, more light may have been cast on the nature of Ms. Ames' difficulty in managing her finances, which also had important psychodynamic significance (as we will discuss below). Finally, the psychologist did not seem to consider that Ms. Ames' responses to the Rorschach would find contribution from her problems in visuospatial organization; imposing organization on the amorphous Rorschach inkblots is, among other things, a visuospatial task. It would have been optimal to look at the anxiety Ms. Ames experienced in carrying it out, and the content of her responses (for example, the preponderance of "deformity" responses), from this perspective as well.

Working with the Findings: Impact on the Patient and the Analyst

Significant analytic work centered around Ms. Ames' reactions to the findings of the diagnostic evaluation. Furthermore, the delineation of specific areas of neuropsychological dysfunction brought to Dr. Green's attention several areas previously unexplored in the analysis.

Ms. Ames was able to analyze her distress surrounding the process of being tested. She and Dr. Green came to see that it recalled for her the intensely discomfiting experience of working in school. She felt as if she were being judged and forced to do things (she experienced herself as a "captive," a "slave"), and persisted even when it was clear that she could not succeed. The power of her wish to please her parents with their unattainable standards, *and* to express her fury about this, was appreciated. This potentiated the analysis of Ms. Ames' perfectionism and overwork in the present, followed by her rage and frustration. She also felt "tricked" as if there were "clues" being withheld from her by the psychologist; this resonated with and repeated her childhood experience of not being told many things, including the nature of her mother's illness and death.

Ms. Ames' initial response to the test findings was to feel she was defective. She also expressed a "boiling" rage about the tester's imperfections (her typographical errors in her report, her lateness). Ultimately Ms. Ames felt reassured that her father's view of her as lazy was erroneous. He had been wrong; something really *had* been the matter with her which was not a function of her degree of effort. As she confronted her rage toward her father and her mother, who had expected too much of her and been unsympathetic to her difficulty, Ms. Ames became aware of other objects of her rage. The therapist who had worked with her in a supportive psychotherapy throughout her twenties had wasted crucial years, and in this sense contributed to Ms. Ames' childless and unmarried status. She also raged at Dr. Green for having "revealed" her limitations.

In the context of receiving the findings of the diagnostic testing evaluation, and the analysis of her reactions to these findings, Ms. Ames had a dream which she reported in detail and associated to amply. This dream was about being with her analyst and her analyst's mother and husband. Among other things, this dream incorporated Ms. Ames' awareness and integration of her cognitive disabilities (in that she was able to understand the analyst's complicated verbal explanation of what was wrong with a stove) and aspects of central conflictual issues. Ms. Ames was also able to pleasurably and safely spar and compete with her analyst. In this dream Ms. Ames felt Dr. Green could enjoy her flirtations with Dr. Green's husband, and her (Ms. Ames') ability to grasp the meaning of Dr. Green's explanation of what was wrong with the stove. Although the nature of the explanation was not detailed by Dr. Green, presumably this would involve some grasp of visuospatial relationships, one of Ms. Ames' most compromised areas of functioning.

One could speculate about many other meanings of the stove image: a bodily metaphor for something broken that can presumably be fixed, an enclosure in which things are cooked in the heat (possibly a metaphor for the uterus), a representation of Ms. Ames' efforts to contain her boiling rageful and sexual feelings, and the like. In these respects Ms. Ames, now at the age of 40, could have been expressing wishful fantasies of repair of her neuropsychological difficulties and childlessness.

This dream, and the analytic work surrounding it, seemed to represent advances for Ms. Ames. How did they come about? Could it be that putting her learning disability into perspective better enabled Ms. Ames to make developmental progress? Furthermore, did the analysis of Ms. Ames' antagonism toward her mother in relation to the learning disability help her to better tolerate her antagonistic rivalry toward mother without a comparable degree of associated anxiety about being a murderer?

From the standpoint of the analyst, Dr. Green found that the test findings clarified several areas in her work with Ms.

Ames. A detailed knowledge of Ms. Ames' cognitive functioning assisted Dr. Green in listening to her patient's thoughts
about future work planning. The finding that Ms. Ames had
major difficulty in dealing with numbers also brought to Dr.
Green's attention that she and Ms. Ames had overlooked another important aspect of Ms. Ames' life, her neurotic dealings
with money. Up until then Ms. Ames' handling of numbers
had been unrealistic, self-destructive, and informed by wishful
fantasies about her father, who had proclaimed himself capable
of taking care of her financially forever. As Dr. Green began
to listen to incomplete allusions to money, she and her patient
discovered that Ms. Ames had denied her increasingly precarious financial status. While she was by no means poor, she would
inevitably run out of funds well before the end of her life,
unless she made significant changes.

One question we have, in light of the diagnostic testing
findings, is the degree to which Ms. Ames continued to work
at a level considerably below her potential due to the persistence of dynamic conflict. Dr. Green felt that the jobs for which
Ms. Ames was eligible required just the skills with which she
had greatest difficulty. From this perspective Ms. Ames was left
with the option of taking a minimally stressful sales position in
which she could avoid her areas of deficiency, but earn little
money. It was true that, according to the diagnostic findings,
Ms. Ames could not manage work significantly dependent upon
a grasp of visual memory, visuospatial relationships, or mathematical reasoning. However, the test results also suggest that
Ms. Ames' pronounced strengths in verbal expression and processing and in verbal conceptualization should have permitted
her to find many other avenues of interest and proficiency.
That is, her neuropsychological picture does not document
that she needed to be confined to working on a relatively me-
nial level.

Thus the question remains whether the presence of pronounced areas of disability was used for defensive purposes.
Many related questions arise. Did Ms. Ames unconsciously retreat from competing with a disabled mother? Was earning
a significant amount of money experienced as damaging or

denigrating father? Father acted as though he wishfully believed he would take care of his daughter forever and, as a corollary, that she would be unable to take care of herself. It appears that Ms. Ames, who denied the declining value of her investments until Dr. Green enabled her to begin to analyze her avoidance, was sustaining a pathological tie to her parents based on the fantasy that she could not be a competent adult. Instead, it seems, she felt like an "exception," both because she was "defective" and because she derived superiority from her attachment to her elite family.

Dr. Green asserts that Ms. Ames wanted to think her father left her a vast fortune because his doing so would signify that he loved her. She could thus avoid rage at him for in fact failing to be truthful to her and to provide for her as he had promised. We suspect that Ms. Ames harbored the unconscious fantasy that, through possessing her father's money, she could preserve her mother and father intact and never lose them. Interweaving with these dynamic explanations of Ms. Ames' fantasies about her economic state lay her difficulties with math as shown on diagnostic testing.

It became clear to Dr. Green that Ms. Ames' use of several other defenses was overdetermined. She had previously appreciated how Ms. Ames' family's perfectionism and cleanliness facilitated her obsessive–compulsive behavior. Ms. Ames' identification with her parents, who tried to hide and overlook painful reality which appeared in abundance in their lives, fostered denial. Now Dr. Green could see that Ms. Ames' learning disability, which involved distorted perceptions and created scotomata, also facilitated her ignoring of actual reality (i.e., denial).

During the analysis it became apparent that Ms. Ames' learning disability contributed to the particular types of attachments she formed to others. For instance, unable to follow directions adequately, she induced her analyst to write instructions for her. At work she could not give people directions, but instead personally took them to places they asked about. It is not unreasonable to assume that Ms. Ames similarly needed to be close to her parents as beacons guiding her in a cognitive (and especially spatial) haze, although this was not reconstructed in the analysis. However, it *was* clear that she wanted her mother to take care of her and became panicky when she (her mother) separated from her. This panic was accentuated by Ms. Ames' fear that her mother's illness, as well as the imagined dangerous impact of her hostility toward her mother, would take her mother away.

When Ms. Ames felt her mother or a substitute did not take care of her, she became enraged. Her learning disability punctuated this rage, as it interfered with her achievement of many of her goals. "Anger boiled within her," Dr. Green wrote when, following the psychological testing, Ms. Ames realized that she *did* have cognitive difficulties. Projecting, she accused the psychologist of being defective, just as she (Ms. Ames) had previously attacked people for their errors and misdeeds. Later in analysis the oedipal contribution to her hostility emerged as well.

Ms. Ames' learning disability also augmented the harshness of her self-judgments. When she failed to live up to her parents' academic standards, she chastised herself severely. Her parents in turn exceeded the school's demands, producing in Ms. Ames, who identified with them and their ideals, even more stringent standards for herself. When her second grade teacher found Ms. Ames' reading satisfactory, her mother was nevertheless disappointed because she thought her daughter should be in the top reading group.

At the same time, Ms. Ames' learning disability sometimes enabled her to defend against her self-judgments. Unable to add and subtract well and, therefore, unable to understand her financial status, she could indulge herself by spending excessively. Later, when she realized her financial predicament, she deprived herself excessively because she exaggerated her poverty, and thus punished herself.

Ms. Ames in this sense felt she was an exception. "She was exempt [from adult rules] because she was both 'defective' and 'superior.' " Her learning disability both caused and was evidence of her sense of defectiveness. Since she belonged to a superior, clean, orderly, intellectual, perfect family, she was (as her parents pronounced) a member of an elite group.

Thus Ms. Ames' learning disability played an important role in influencing the development of her drives and super-ego. As we have seen in our discussion of other aspects of her personality and psychopathology, other developmental and dynamic factors played an interweaving role as well.

Chapter 17

Mr. Young's Analysis

Roberta Green, M.D.

PRESENTING PROBLEMS

Mr. Young was a 28-year-old, single paralegal referred for consultation by a psychopharmacologist while he was undergoing a trial of medication for a severe depression. When, at the same time that he was having a prolonged evaluation by me, he did not respond sufficiently to medication, I recommended psychoanalysis to which he agreed.

PAST HISTORY

Mr. Young was the only child of parents who separated when he was 3. Mr. Young believed his parents divorced because his

---

Dr. Green, who also analyzed Ms. Ames, wanted anonymity, and hence has been given a pseudonym. As in her other case, the author did not present a fully chronological account of the analysis. Rather, Dr. Green started with a brief history and then described the events that led to psychological testing and the patient's reactions to the tests, as well as some of what analyst and analysand learned of the effects of Mr. Young's learning disability on his personality and psychopathology. Finally, abandoning the chronological approach, Dr. Green concentrated on major themes in the analysis.

mother was very sensitive, and his father was unusually emotionally distant. After the separation Mr. Young's father remained active in his son's life. However, Mr. Young
experienced his father as dutiful rather than truly interested
in him. He was not demonstrative or giving of himself, although
he was quite generous with money.

Mr. Young's mother was an independent woman who was
able to support herself by working as a teacher. She was quite
anxious and polyphobic, encouraging her son's fearfulness by
expressing her exaggerated fantasies of danger. Mr. Young's
mother complained that the men in her life, his father included, abused and disappointed her, and warned against his
becoming like these brutish men. Rather Mr. Young should be
emotionally sensitive and kind to women. In contrast she
"sugar coated" realistic problems in order to be falsely reassuring. For example, she refused to acknowledge that Mr. Young
was having trouble with girls during adolescence and denied
that he was relatively short. Her repeated reassurance that his
problems were "a phase" and would spontaneously disappear
seemed Pollyanna-ish to her son.

It was unclear when Mr. Young's depression had started.
However, he reported a number of difficulties as a child. Mr.
Young had a persistent sense of having greater than usual difficulty following instructions and learning new tasks. His parents
and teachers always reassured him that he was intelligent but
needed to be more diligent. He complained that many activities, such as Hebrew School and karate, were too hard for him.
While his parents encouraged him to continue these activities,
they allowed him to stop them when things got too tough and
when failure appeared to be inevitable.

Mr. Young was an average student at public elementary
school, where he was more interested in sports than academics.
He transferred to a "progressive" private school which allowed
students to pursue their own areas of interest (such as video
and film) and to ignore major formal academic subjects such
as math, English, or foreign languages; these were areas of
weakness for Mr. Young.

Mr. Young felt his father and mother never investigated
the nature of his difficulties. When he was a child he thought

his parents were permissive. In retrospect he decided they were neglectful. This notwithstanding, they had him tested when he was quite young; the psychological tests were reputedly perfectly normal, although a report of findings was unavailable. In addition, Mr. Young briefly saw a psychologist during latency because his mother thought he was unable to adapt to new situations.

Until Mr. Young was 8 years old his father was only moderately successful. Then he joined an extremely successful law firm and became very wealthy. His own daring enterprises contributed strongly to the firm's affluence. Mrs. Young worried that her son would be spoiled by the availability of his father's money. She encouraged him to live solely on what he earned, fortifying his own conflicts about using his father's money. She herself had made a point of refusing alimony, and accepted only child support.

After his divorce and spectacular financial success, Mr. Young's father began to lead an increasingly active social life. This coincided with his son's adolescence. At a time that Mr. Young could not get a date, his father was dating women his son's age. This sparked angry, rivalrous, and hopeless feelings in Mr. Young who was often attracted to these women. This was the more galling to him because he saw himself as nicer to these women than was his father. Indeed Mr. Young often became a confidant to his father's girl friends, as he had earlier been with his mother and with female classmates in high school. Each of his father's girl friends ultimately left Mr. Young's father, complaining that he refused to become emotionally intimate with them.

When retired, the elder Mr. Young continued to lead an adventurous life, traveling and spending money on women he dated. Mr. Young felt his father encouraged him to act without considering the consequences. Mr. Young's father was as daring and adventurous as his mother was inhibited and phobic.

Mr. Young had had several additional treatments in late adolescence and early adulthood. He began group therapy in college in an attempt to understand his difficulties with women. After graduation he saw a woman therapist for six months; it was unclear why he started and why he ended this treatment.

From ages 24 to 27 he was in individual and group therapy with a psychologist, Dr. R, who was a friend of his father. This was primarily a supportive and directive treatment in which Dr. R frequently revealed details of his own social life, including the fact that he was divorced. He also attended social gatherings at which the patient and his father were present, both during the treatment and after it was concluded. While the therapy was in progress Dr. R remarried. Mr. Young said that prior to that Dr. R had a "roving eye."

Shortly after his therapist remarried and while he was away on vacation, Mr. Young sought psychopharmacological help from Dr. S. It is possible that this was an act of revenge against his therapist. When a number of trials with different antidepressants failed to produce relief, Dr. S recommended psychoanalytically oriented psychotherapy with me rather than a return to Dr. R. It appeared that Dr. R was not dealing adequately with an intense paternal transference with positive and negative oedipal resonances; certainly he was not interpreting it.

THE EXTENDED CONSULTATION AND BEGINNING OF THE ANALYSIS

I was initially rather cautious in my approach to Mr. Young. We engaged in a prolonged consultation which lasted about six months before I recommended analysis. This consultation involved my offering interpretations intended to assess his analyzability; it was therapeutic as well as evaluative.

Despite a vagueness of speech which made many sessions hardly comprehensible, and made me worry that Mr. Young had a thought disorder, I was sufficiently able to follow his meandering line of thought. He was also able to fill me in on a reasonable amount of his history, and to meaningfully elaborate several central concerns and conflicts. Mr. Young was attracted to women whom he considered deficient in some way, either due to their minority status or actual physical defects. Sometimes he risked being accused of unethical behavior by dating clients. (In fact, he lost one job as a result of this activity.) At other times he courted danger by going out with women who appeared physically ill.

Mr. Young also considered himself defective, inferior, and average at best. He felt he was a disappointment to his parents whom he regarded as intellectual powers. In his view everyone else was better than he, better endowed, better motivated. He complained that he suffered from a biologically based depression and, worse, antidepressants failed to help him; he regarded this as further evidence of his defectiveness.

Mr. Young complained that I had trouble paying attention to him. Indeed when he rambled I *did* sometimes fail, despite concerted effort, to understand what he was saying. Mr. Young needed a great deal of praise. He wanted me, his parents, and others to admire him for even the mundane aspects of life. For example, he wanted me to commend him for getting up and coming to the analytic sessions, buttoning his shirt, and for working. He wanted his friends to give him recognition for kindly acts, which they did.

After a while I offered a reconstruction. I suggested that when he was a toddler his mother had been depressed and thus could not pay enough attention to him. In her sadness, I proposed, she found it difficult to be optimistic and to praise or encourage him for things such as walking and talking, as a mother usually does. To Mr. Young's satisfaction, his mother confirmed the reconstruction. She had been depressed when he was 3 to 5 years old and possibly even earlier. Mr. Young was so pleased with my insight that his alliance with me strengthened markedly. He even stopped dating disabled women and went out instead with a woman who was not handicapped. He found this information about his mother so helpful that he asked both his parents to provide him with answers to questions he had about his childhood. His mother responded in detail, but his father ignored the request.

Mr. Young's complaints about himself continued. He had intellectual failings, and could not immediately understand things as others could. He regaled me with everything he could not grasp. In fact, from his perspective, there was nothing he *could* get. He also felt I was demanding too much of him, as his parents and teachers had. Analysis was the wrong treatment, he believed, one much beyond his capacity. He needed to be fixed, repaired.

I noted that there were inconsistencies here. He *had* held jobs. He even published some articles explaining practical legal matters in respectable popular magazines. Other people liked what he did and appreciated what he did for them. (He was a perpetual do-gooder.)

Mr. Young tried to refute my statements. He maintained that he just *seemed* to do things; he pretended. Others were well disposed to him so they let the fact that he did not do things slide. While there was *some* truth to his rejoinders, matters were more complex. For example, after getting an A on a school paper, he did not return the paper which prevented the teacher from registering the mark. Or Mr. Young did not submit the next paper when it was due. We agreed that there was a question as to whether he actually had a defect.

Mr. Young began to experiment with activities he had previously given up on to ascertain whether he could accomplish what he thought he could not. He simultaneously took driving lessons and instruction in ballroom dancing. However, he did so in a self-defeating manner. Explaining that he felt he should not use his father's money, Mr. Young sought the most inexpensive teachers possible. For example, he took automobile lessons with Spanish speaking instructors; since he knew only rudimentary Spanish and the teachers barely spoke English, he had inordinate difficulty learning to drive. It thus became almost impossible to ascertain whether Mr. Young could not learn because he was innately a poor learner, or whether he chose circumstances that made the task insurmountable.

To add to the confusion, his instructors would become furious at him for his ineptitude. They could not understand him and he could not comprehend what they wanted. At the same time that this was happening, Mr. Young confused me. I would become drowsy as he spoke less clearly. Only later, after the analysis was well under way, did Mr. Young tell me that this was a conscious strategy. He had similarly lulled his father or other paternal figures to sleep with his circumstantial speech. In this way those he regarded as potentially attacking could be rendered impotent. By putting them into a trance he could defend himself from their aggression while attacking them at the same time.

Chaos reigned in much of the analysis. Mr. Young tried to mislead me by talking about things he said he could not do, even though we both knew he *could* do them. For instance, he declared he could not write clearly despite the fact that he had definite skills in that area. He also withheld information in a way that prevented me from ascertaining what he was avoiding.

I was about to interpret this behavior to Mr. Young when he revealed something new. As he was trying to perform dance steps, he found it necessary to verbally repeat his instructor's verbal directions, which he had memorized. He was entirely unable to use a kinesthetic visuospatial approach; the verbal approach failed too. The same was true of driving. Mr. Young would repeat the teacher's words, which he understood poorly, as he tried to drive one step at a time. Such procedures did not become kinesthetically automatic.

At this point I felt confused. My dynamic formulations explained many things. I thought that the patient was protecting himself from fantasies of being attacked by aggressive, critical parents; he also anticipated this from me in the transference. Mr. Young had internalized harsh demands; just as no one was ever satisfied in his family, so he repeatedly criticized himself. Further, his identification with his mother's belief that no one deserved pleasure was very prominent. All the men she dated, including her second husband, had to be marred; my patient sought defective women and experienced himself as marred as well. In addition, his defective demeanor had aggressive and provocative elements. His behavior drove those who came into contact with him crazy and enraged them.

Mr. Young and I also noted that in feeling defective, he experienced himself as like his mother, a formerly depressed and (he thought) impaired person. In addition, Mr. Young's feeling that he was defective defended against an identification with a sadistic father. When he felt more powerful than his sexual partners, he treated them meanly, like the "brutish" person his mother warned him not to be. Further, he fantasized that being flawed, he could attract and attain his father.

As we discussed these analytic issues, Mr. Young kept insisting that it really *was* more difficult for him to do things than it was for others. I thought to myself, how could I be sure that this was not true? In an attempt to settle this issue so that we could get on with the analysis of it, I recommended psychological testing. I was convinced that the tests would at the most reveal some minor disability, in the context of basically sound cognitive capacities. After all, the psychological tests Mr. Young had taken as a child were reportedly normal. (Attempts to get these tests failed. Mr. Young's parents could not recall the name of the psychologist and they had not kept the report.) In addition, I hoped that testing would cast light on whether Mr. Young had a thought disorder, which was a persisting concern of mine.

In contrast, Mr. Young anticipated finding that he really *did* have problems. If this were so, he felt he would deserve not only remediation, but also reparations comparable to those a concentration camp survivor receives. It was only fair, he said, that he get a free ride. He was outraged that the Lighthouse for the Blind pressured the blind to work rather than simply taking care of them.

Psychological Testing

The test results surprised me and shocked Mr. Young. Mr. Young was administered a diagnostic testing battery which included the Wechsler Adult Intelligence Scale-Revised, special tests of an array of visual and auditory memory functions, motor (including graphomotor) coordination, and projective tests. Results indicated a major discrepancy between Mr. Young's generally above average functioning on verbal tests and his specific cognitive deficiencies in a number of nonverbal areas. These included visuospatial reasoning, visual memory, and graphomotor skills, again revealing problems with spatial planning and organization. The psychologist reported that this was consistent with "a visual integrative learning disability of childhood."

In light of the reportedly normal diagnostic test findings from childhood, this marked weakness in visuospatial reasoning in adulthood greatly concerned the psychologist who tested

Mr. Young. She felt it was necessary to refer him for a neurological examination to rule out grave pathology such as a brain tumor. Luckily, the neurological examination was normal.

The testing revealed an enormous contrast between Mr. Young's Verbal IQ of 113 and his Performance IQ of 79, giving him a Full Scale IQ of 97. The psychologist believed that he had a potentially higher Verbal IQ, in that his performance was compromised by his intense anxiety. Mr. Young was described as especially anxious and self-critical in the face of perceived inadequacies in his performance, most notably on structured tests. Nevertheless, he remained highly motivated to succeed.

The tester also concluded that Mr. Young's specific disabilities had contributed to his sense of inadequacy to deal with the ambitious strivings of his successful father. She felt that his avocational interests were more consonant with his abilities than were his vocational activities.

More specifically, Mr. Young demonstrated an above average fund of general factual information and vocabulary. His ability to form verbal concepts and to reason arithmetically were similarly above average. His demonstrated grasp of social norms and practices was compromised by a tendency to be impulsive and/or overly literal; this was seen in several of his responses which resulted in an average level score. Also at an average level was Mr. Young's performance on a task which involved repeating number series.

With one exception, Mr. Young's scores on tests of nonverbal abilities were well below average. He functioned in the average range when presented with a rote learning task, which required sustaining motivation and attention to reproduce the correct symbols corresponding to numbers as presented in a key. In contrast, he had major difficulty with other nonverbal tests which demanded abstract spatial reasoning and visuospatial abilities. When required to replicate block designs, Mr. Young manifested difficulty visualizing rotations on a plane, as well as in analyzing and organizing part–whole relationships. Confronted with unassembled puzzle pieces, he had trouble mentally envisioning the gestalt to be constructed. Tests of

graphomotor skills revealed uneven and poorly formed productions (in handwriting and copying Bender-Gestalt designs) as
well as poor planning and organizational abilities. When required to draw geometric figures which had been shown to him
for ten seconds, Mr. Young scored significantly below average
for his age, suggestive of a weakness in immediate visual memory. This was in contrast with his adequate recall of verbal stimuli on several tests.

Projective testing revealed no problems with reality testing
or thinking. At the same time, Mr. Young's perceptions were
frequently vague, and relatively unintegrated and unimaginative for someone of his intellectual abilities and educational
background. The tester also commented that Mr. Young evidenced a pronounced constriction of affect. Conflicts over aggressive impulses and competitive feelings in the context of
performance and interpersonal relationships were central. Mr.
Young was thought to express and defend against these wishes
in a number of ways. Intellectualization, rationalization, and
obsessive and phobic features were observed.

The psychologist also reported that Mr. Young evidenced
narcissistic self-preoccupation and an immaturity which contributed to feelings of dependency upon, and helplessness in
relation to, significant others. Furthermore, he was noted to
have unrealistic standards for himself and to feel subject to a
harsh and punitive superego. This contributed to his sense of
the world as a dangerous and critical place. There was also
evidence of significant depressive trends, including feelings of
hopelessness and chronic dysphoria.

The diagnostic impression was of a Mixed Personality Disorder with Depressive, Anxious, and Avoidant Features. The
psychologist felt that Mr. Young's combination of "socioemotional immaturity and primary cognitive deficits" had contributed to his sense of "global deficiency" which seriously
compromised his functioning in performance situations.

Immediate Responses to the Diagnostic Testing Evaluation

It was apparent that I had to modify my conceptualization of
Mr. Young's psychodynamics in light of these findings. While

the dynamics I had postulated were probably accurate, they were incomplete. I had not taken into account the contribution of Mr. Young's marked cognitive disability. This evaluation also confirmed my impression that, contrary to my patient's belief, he was not a complete failure. He had significant areas of competence.

At first Mr. Young was pleased that he *did* have cognitive problems which required fixing; he felt he could understand many of his difficulties in these terms. For example, he could see why he had trouble dancing and driving. Subsequently, he became grief-stricken at the likelihood that he could not be repaired; the idea that he might have to work in the analysis to deal with his learning disabilities was extremely distressing and precipitated a new type of depression. He was shocked that he had a type of defect that made people sit up and take notice. Something really *was* wrong with him!

Mr. Young never told his parents or anyone else about the test results. He was ashamed to expose his defects to those who knew him. Paradoxically, when he talked with me about the results, he emphasized his disabilities and did not want to look at areas of competence. He had difficulty tolerating the idea that in certain spheres he *was* capable.

The psychological tests broadened our analytic work. I was able to show Mr. Young that he defensively needed to undermine himself and to feel needy; this buttressed his wish to require others to do things for him. While Mr. Young's cognitive failings compromised some aspects of his functioning, he made matters even worse to further justify his desire to be looked after. He was willing to wait for others to take care of him and was conflicted about being independent.

CENTRAL ISSUES AS THE ANALYSIS PROGRESSED

Desire to be Dependent

Analytic exploration of Mr. Young's conflicts about his desire to be dependent revealed a number of ways in which his parents had contributed to this. The family philosophy had demanded that everyone act as part of a unit. Everyone and everything should be taken care of by others. Mr. Young should not have feelings different from those his mother experienced. If she were happy he should be so. If she were sad he should be melancholy too.

Mr. Young's need to be one with his mother involved intense separation anxiety. Early in the analysis—and later too—when I went on vacation, he missed sessions after I had returned. Thus Mr. Young turned passive desertion by me into an active rejection of me. At other times he turned on me with fury.

As the analysis continued, it became apparent that Mr. Young used his learning disability to fortify his need to be a dependent babylike person. Of course the fact that he had a learning disability made it wise for him to get additional help in some areas. However, Mr. Young also made use of this reality for defensive purposes. He firmly believed that he was an extraordinarily needy person who had to cling to his parents or substitutes. He was, he thought, biologically more anxious and impoverished than most people, and had been since infancy.

As we tried to understand this fantasy, which the existence of his severe learning disability contributed to and partially justified, Mr. Young's mother told him that both his parents had had demanding parents who had made decisions for them. Mr. Young's parents determined that their son would not have such a fate. They, therefore, attempted to avoid imposing their ideas on him; he would decide for himself what to do. Unfortunately they tried to make him independent before he was actually capable of autonomous decisions.

Reflecting these childhood experiences, Mr. Young as an adult misjudged children's capacities to be self-reliant. He was able to observe parent–child interactions in friends' families because in several instances he was treated like an intimate uncle who spent a lot of time with them. In his dealings with these children he always thought they behaved much younger than their actual age. This was largely based on his assessment that they were much more needy and demanding than children that age should be. For instance, he became angry when a child, whose parents had taken him to the zoo, refused to leave following a satisfying and pleasurable stay. The idea that the children did not get filled up and satisfied, but wanted to get pleasure from something else as well, irked and astonished Mr. Young.

At first he thought that the children he observed were deprived. However, when he noticed that the children of his half-siblings displayed the same childish traits, his convictions were shaken. The material he learned in a child development course further shocked him into reevaluating his concept of what normal children were like. He realized that it was not deviant for children to be demanding. Movies of children reinforced the instructor's assertions that these were normal children. Dejected and identified with his parents, he felt he could never be a parent; he could not tolerate his children's demandingness.

It was also very difficult for Mr. Young to believe that the demands he placed on his parents as a child were normal rather than deviant. He tried not to get angry at his parents who, he was beginning to believe, failed to satisfy some of his basic needs. By thinking normal children were not demanding and that his demands were abnormal, he avoided rage at his parents.

Mr. Young and I further concluded that his feeling of deprivation stemmed in part from his learning disability, in combination with his experiences of having been encouraged to be prematurely independent. His excessive desire to be cared for grew out of these experiences as well.

Mr. Young's parents provided additional information that enabled us to reconstruct the genetic (historical) background for his psychodynamic constellation. His parents divorced several years after his mother's pregnancy with him, a pregnancy his father did not want. Dutiful and conscientious, Mr. Young's father tolerated the pregnancy and birth of his son, and stayed with his wife and child for a few years after the birth. He continued to see his son regularly out of a sense of responsibility. Mr. Young craved and feared a powerful father. This was evident in the transference. Imagining I was such a person, he was at times reluctant to lie on the couch lest I subjugate him.

Mrs. Young, who had not expected to be and was unprepared as a single mother, did not understand the nature of children or how to raise them. She had little or no practical support from Mr. Young or her own family. However, there was one area of child rearing about which Mr. Young's parents *did* agree: that children should not be told what to do.

Mr. Young's belief that his parents had raised him normally, even when they treated him as if he were more mature than his age warranted, appeared in the analysis shortly after his psychological testing evaluation and recurred cyclically throughout the analysis. Even after he seemingly believed otherwise, he repeatedly surprised us by insisting that his parents had done well by him. Over and over again he forgot and then recalled what normal children were like.

On one occasion late in the treatment, Mr. Young visited a nursery school where he saw a grandmother and grandchild interact. When the little girl, who was finger painting, messed her clothing, the grandmother did not appear distressed and did not chastise her. At the end of the day, the girl insisted on staying at the nursery. Even though she cried hysterically, the grandmother was unruffled. She quietly assured the child that they would return in a few days, and that she could paint at home. Mr. Young was astonished that the grandmother did not strike the child, but considered her granddaughter's behavior normal. Although he did not think his parents ever hit him, he imagined they would have considered the child's behavior deviant, as had Mr. Young before our discussions of children's development.

On another occasion, Mr. Young, who was eager to do good works to such a degree that he considered it a hobby, took two children to visit their father in prison. When he saw how close the children were to their father, he became envious. He knew that his own father had always been distant to his (Mr. Young's) mother and failed to be intimate with his girl friends.

The Structure of the Analysis

As previously noted, a pattern became recognizable in the analysis. A theme would appear and be discussed in some detail.

Then it would be forgotten and dropped, often because the patient became depressed or anxious as he discussed the motif. Later the theme would appear again, be worked on for some time, and then dropped once more. Subsequent working through would gradually amplify the theme and often clarify its genesis.

Impulsivity and Closure

Early in the analysis, a tendency to impulsiveness appeared. Mr. Young's father, who was adventuresome, encouraged this by at times urging the patient to take premature action. For example, once he pushed Mr. Young to buy a time share on an island where he (the father) owned property. The patient immediately bought it even though he could not afford it.

A need for rapid closure, as seen in this action, was also connected with Mr. Young's learning disability. Finding it difficult to decipher a sentence, he tended to guess what was written. He would reach a conclusion quickly and prematurely, and often incorrectly.

The Role of the Telephone

During the third year of the analysis Mr. Young frequently wanted to have telephone sessions, a reflection of his desire to be cared for. Since he sometimes could not bring himself to the session and since he paid for missed sessions, he felt it was only fair for me to talk to him on the phone. At times I agreed to do so. We discovered that his sense of being unable to come to the sessions at these times had a complex of meanings. It was an expression of his feeling that he had to avoid being angry at me. Furthermore, talking on the phone soothed and satisfied him. Mr. Young revealed that as he talked he would lie coiled up in bed while he rubbed his cat. There was clearly a masturbatory aspect to this, as seen in concurrent fantasies which involved prostitution. In my giving in to him, satisfying him, and keeping him from losing money, he experienced me as a prostitute. Mr. Young also felt he was frustrating me by not attending sessions.

This was a specific expression of Mr. Young's more fundamental feeling that he was frustrating to everybody, including his parents. Even though frustrating people *was* aggressive, he simultaneously defended his parents from his rage by such acts. His thinking was: How could his parents not deprive him or get angry at him? Indeed he, being a biologically "defective" person, would even try the patience of a saint. He thus proved over and over again that nobody could take care of him, nobody could raise him well; if his parents had half a normal child they might have raised him properly. In the transference he tried my patience with his demands, and repeatedly attempted to get me to throw him out of analysis.

Rage and Ambivalence

Mr. Young and I talked a great deal about his rage. Not only was he furious at his parents, a fact he had to deny, but he was also angry at people he thought were deficient. Everybody had to be unflawed or they would be thrown out. He was upset by my interpretations which made him feel sad, and thus unloved. Hating me, he became frightened that I would end the analysis, and get rid of him.

Then something occurred that Mr. Young found incomprehensible and horrible, indeed beyond description. In the fourth year of analysis he started to feel love and hate simultaneously. He commented that it was the weirdest thing he had ever experienced. He wanted to quit analysis; it was impure and impossible. When he spoke to his parents about this, they indicated their belief that loving and hostile feelings could not coexist. They even warned Mr. Young that he would get into big trouble with such feelings. Mr. Young found it puzzling that I was not surprised by the new development. Indeed he later came to feel "that is what analysis is all about." He was going to have to tolerate these conflicting feelings and see the world in another way that was at odds with his family's view.

Mr. Young dealt with this conundrum by leaving long phone messages for me to listen to. In these messages he often criticized me for making interpretations about which he felt rage. Frequently he would react to his rage by returning home instead of going to work. He experienced this as *my* fault in that I was not more careful to avoid enraging him. Instead, like his parents, I overwhelmed him with interpretations he believed he could not handle.

Following these phone communications, Mr. Young felt he was getting something for nothing, since I did not charge him for the time I took to listen to them. He found it necessary to justify this as follows. He deserved to talk to me without paying. He had paid me a full fee for years and had not called me. Others, he thought, had done so all along. I interpreted to Mr. Young that in taking free time he was both trying to avoid knowing that he was angry at me and simultaneously expressing his anger.

Mr. Young worried that I would not pay full attention to him, that I would be only half with him. It turned out that he was testing me to see whether I would get angry at him. If I did he thought I was rejecting him. If I did not, I did not care. At that time it was inconceivable to Mr. Young that I was trying to help him understand himself, which involved caring.

Mr. Young expressed his anger on the tape not only by taking my time, but also by attacking me verbally on the phone. When he did not bring up in his sessions the thoughts he had said on the tape, I did so. I then learned that he could not recall what he had said, much of which involved anger. It was not until the fifth year of the analysis that Mr. Young was able to become angry during the sessions. At that time he did not pay his bill for several months, which was an extraordinary act of hostility for him. He said he wanted to hurt me, keep me from getting my money. Mr. Young withheld payment for as long as he could and then, fearful that I would retaliate, paid me. He had expected me to withdraw and become vindictive, as his parents did. While relieved, he was also disappointed that I did not do so; now he had to look at his parents in an unfavorable light.

Sadomasochism

Throughout the discussion, I have referred to Mr. Young's sadomasochism. He was provocative through much of the treatment. His practice of missing analytic hours and demanding telephone sessions instead was, in part, intended to irritate and test me. He frequently expected me to get angry at him. Once he arranged for a consultation with a senior analyst he believed to be my superior in order to protect himself from my errors and to retaliate for my leaving him; he also wished to intimidate me and irritate me.

On other occasions Mr. Young refused to use the couch for fear I would subjugate him; sitting up he felt powerful, as though he could intimidate me. As a child, he recalled, he had provoked his father by taking an extremely long time to tie his shoe laces. This was an example of using his learning disability to find masochistic and sadistic satisfaction. Although his masochism served to alleviate guilt and his sadism could discharge aggression, he found libidinal gratification in his masochism and sadism as well.

Sexual Fantasies and Avoidance of Competition

Another related theme concerned masturbation. The reader will recall that in the third year of the treatment Mr. Young talked to me on the telephone while he stroked his cat; in his sessions he associated this to prostitution. Later in the analysis, as he talked of his inability to accomplish things, he thought of sexual fantasies. For a while Mr. Young, finding satisfaction being with me, stopped dating. Then he became friendly with a married couple. Although he did not engage in overt sexual activity with either member of the pair, he in effect shared a sexual object just as he had done with his father and his father's girl friends. As stated above, Mr. Young's father had dated young women his son's age, much to Mr. Young's consternation. He became jealous as his father flaunted his relationships with his girlfriends at a time that my patient had difficulty dating. But soon they would draw away from his father, complaining that he avoided intimacy, and turn toward the son in whom they confided; however, they did not engage in sexual activity with Mr. Young.

Then Mr. Young remembered frustrating events of childhood. He had tried over and over again to accomplish things—schoolwork, puzzles, sports—but never succeeded. No matter how hard he worked, he failed. He developed a compensatory sexual fantasy that he would be loved for himself. Somebody would do it all for him. He would sit, surrounded by a half-dozen harem girls who peeled grapes for him. They would also feed him, perform fellatio on him, and more generally care for him in such a way that he did not have to lift a finger. In this fantasy Mr. Young was totally passive and did not have to deal with competitive feelings toward his father.

As a child he decided that competition was wrong for him, although he did compete at times. Indeed, as a child he was an excellent bowler, the best one on his team. He recalled being unmercifully contemptuous and insulting to other boys on the team who did not do as well as he. Nevertheless, even though he attacked and frustrated them, people liked him and stuck with him. As an adult he still retained many friends from childhood with whom he could discuss his past as the analysis proceeded. This made me believe there must have been a charming aspect to Mr. Young's personality, which was not evident during analytic sessions.

When he did become more independent and assertive his father would often try to restrain him. Similarly, at times when the analysis was effective, Mr. Young's father would try to disrupt it by demanding that he himself meet with me, threatening to withdraw financial support or insisting that he himself receive the bills.

CURRENT STATUS

The analysis is still in progress. As Mr. Young has found life more gratifying and has allowed himself accomplishments; he has talked about termination. The possibility of separation and independence has frightened him and led him to miss sessions, especially after I have taken a vacation. He continues to struggle with his disappointment over the revised and more realistic images of both parents which have emerged in the analysis. In particular, he now sees his father's thrill-seeking assertiveness as an effort to mask his significant anxiety and emotional isolation. Mr. Young has come to recognize his own ability to outdo his father in interpersonal situations.

In many ways he much preferred the earlier idealized images of his parents whom he alternatively adored and raged at. Now he sees them as flawed and more human. In fact, he can see many ways—good and bad—in which he resembles each of them. Associated with this is Mr. Young's growing awareness of my shortcomings and my tolerance of my own fallibility; with this recognition he is gradually developing a greater tolerance for his own imperfections.

Chapter 18

Discussion of Mr. Young's Analysis

As was true in her report of the case of Ms. Ames, Dr. Green's portrayal of the analysis of Mr. Young provides a rich opportunity to follow the complex process of discovery of the multiple meanings of her patient's sense of defectiveness. Dr. Green also presents unusually detailed data about the place of the diagnostic evaluation in the course of the analysis: both the reasons for its emergence and the nature of subsequent analytic work with its findings.

The climate in which the evaluation arose is distinct in some important respects from that of the other cases in this volume. Dr. Green had found ample psychodynamic factors to account for Mr. Young's conviction that he was disabled. The diagnostic work that demonstrated the presence of a learning disability as an additional significant factor was done after the analysis was well under way. Rather than truly expecting the evaluation to delineate the nature of her patient's learning disability, Dr. Green referred Mr. Young for testing to show him that he was *not* truly defective, i.e., that he did not have a cognitive disorder.

It is extremely unusual for an analyst working from Dr. Green's perspective—that there were ample psychological determinants of Mr. Young's view of himself—to suggest the possibility of a diagnostic evaluation. Instead analysts working in such climates usually continue to analyze the combinations of satisfaction and defense embodied by the compromise formations involved. In the two years of analysis which preceded the diagnostic testing evaluation, Dr. Green and her patient had explored many compelling determinants and meanings of his sense of "defectiveness": his intense conflict over sexual, competitive, assertive, and aggressive strivings. Had this conventional approach occurred in Mr. Young's case, the additional insight he and Dr. Green gained would not have come about.

A central theme in Mr. Young's analysis was not only his *feeling*, but his firm *belief* that he was defective. This conviction was analyzed repeatedly from many points of view. However, the role of his learning disability in the formation of this fantasy was not apparent until Dr. Green decided that psychological tests could clarify whether the cognitive difficulty Mr. Young claimed to have was actual or whether (as she thought) his beliefs were defensive. The evaluation revealed that Mr. Young suffered from major difficulties in visuospatial reasoning and visual memory, which affected selected aspects of learning.

Once testing affirmed Mr. Young's intellectual failings, the analysis deepened and broadened. One could then integrate the cognitive and conflictual determinants of his personality. Another important feature of the analysis at this point was the careful analysis of Mr. Young's reactions to the findings. Dr. Green was particularly skillful in her observations of Mr. Young's responses to being tested and learning of the results.

The nature of the analytic process in the early portion of the analysis of Mr. Young's feelings of defectiveness was not unusual. He agreed with the psychopharmacologist who referred him to Dr. Green for psychotherapy; they both believed his depression, while biologically based, had a substantial psychogenic component. When his depression did not respond to medication, Mr. Young's sense of himself as inferior became even more pronounced, to a degree greater than is characteristic of many depressed patients. This feeling was combined with his experience of the seriousness of his deficiency, based on a history of academic difficulties as he was growing up. The fact that his parents were dissatisfied with his failures etched the feeling of deficiency even more deeply.

On a deeper level, the analysis revealed that Mr. Young had an unconscious need to be inferior in order to attain his mother's and father's love. He had grown up in a family in which marital strife, which started early in his life, led to divorce. Both parents had irreconcilable values and were self-preoccupied. Neither parent was able to help Mr. Young adequately. His father was emotionally uninvolved, although committed to "doing the right thing" as a father, and his mother minimized Mr. Young's difficulties.

Mr. Young's mother, who was attracted to maimed men, communicated to the patient that he should be a weak person rather than a cruel person like his father; sadism and assertiveness were, she indicated, masculine traits which were to be avoided. In addition, Mr. Young unconsciously felt that through being defective and weak, and thus feminine in general and like his depressed mother of early childhood in particular, he could attract his father whom he loved. Mr. Young also identified with the maimed women he himself dated and loved.

There were defensive aspects to Mr. Young's sense of defect as well. He was extremely competitive with his father and feared being successful in this regard. When his father dated young women after his divorce from the patient's mother, Mr. Young became their confidante, as he had been his mother's. Thus he fantasized he could win them away from his father. But, fearing the consequences of such victories, he retreated from this position and became the deficient, powerless person who could not defeat his father.

Mr. Young's view of himself as a weak and injured person also served as a defense against his rage at his parents whom he unconsciously experienced as negligent. As a disabled person he posed no threat to them. Mr. Young's sadomasochistic conflicts played a significant role too. Trying to avoid sadism, of which his mother disapproved, he found a masochistic solution instead. He would provoke his father and thus attain his love (father being sadistic himself), and be punished for forbidden wishes. Mr. Young's masochism was also evident in his tendency to put himself in threatening situations, dating clients, for instance. In that way he not only risked contracting AIDS, but also being fired for grossly inappropriate behavior.

That was more or less where things stood when Dr. Green, hoping to demonstrate to Mr. Young that his sense of deficiency was a defensive stance, suggested psychological testing. Dr.

Green had reason to believe that Mr. Young, if he had a learning disability at all, had a rather minor one.

Mr. Young's psychological testing as a child revealed no disability, according to his family. Since we do not have a report of the childhood findings, it is impossible to know whether the parents' statements about them were accurate. Nor can we know the basis for such conclusions, if the psychologist had indeed reached them. Years ago (and even today) it was not at all uncommon for testing to be quite brief and not inclusive of an assessment of academic skills or specific and subtle tests of neuropsychological functioning. Therefore, a false negative finding of "normality" could easily emerge. Mr. Young's "average" performance in elementary school seems to have been attributed to his greater "interest" in sports than academic matters. However, it is conceivable that his undiagnosed neuropsychologically based difficulties with some aspects of academic requirements contributed to his apparent lack of interest. Mr. Young's attendance at a progressive school which permitted him to navigate around areas of disability may have further obscured these undiagnosed problems. This would, of course, combine with the above delineated psychodynamic constellation to fuel conflict over performance.

The diagnostic testing evaluation performed during the analysis revealed that Mr. Young was of average intelligence. However, there was some reason to believe that his IQ was actually higher. Anxiety, the tester reported, interfered with Mr. Young's achievement. His Performance IQ was lower than his Verbal IQ. He had pronounced difficulty with most nonverbal tasks, especially those involving visuospatial capacities (encompassing visuospatial organization and the execution of visuospatial tasks such as copying geometric figures) and immediate visual memory.

The evaluation performed was reasonably comprehensive, consisting of an intelligence test, tests of specific memory functions, and projective testing. Optimally several additional features of Mr. Young's functioning could have been examined. A detailed assessment of academic skills would have permitted a more specific determination of the extent to which his visuospatial and visual memory weaknesses had compromised selected aspects of academic achievement. We can certainly assume that academic subjects which rely heavily on visuospatial concepts (e.g., geometry, geography, and physics) were exceedingly difficult for Mr. Young. However, the testing did not fully define the impact (or lack thereof) of specific disabilities or other aspects of learning. For example, we cannot know if Mr. Young's visual memory weaknesses impacted on his ability to retain in immediate memory material he had just read. Nor did the assessment elucidate whether, and if so how, visuospatial reasoning deficits affected the spatial demands of math.

In addition, in some respects the optimum integration of cognitive and emotional findings was not achieved in this evaluation. For example, it is important to bear in mind when interpreting the Rorschach record of a patient such as Mr. Young that his visuospatial weaknesses will contribute to his difficulty organizing the amorphous visuospatial configurations of the inkblots. When the tester reported that "several of his (Mr. Young's) percepts were vague and impressionistic, lacking the kind of articulation and flexibility characteristic of mature insight and psychological mindedness," and that "his productions were limited by a marked restriction of affect, resulting in rather trite, concrete, and unimaginative percepts," we need to consider these observations from the combined perspective of neuropsychological and psychological functioning. Similarly, the production of figure drawings by a man with visuospatial reasoning and graphomotor weaknesses will inevitably be affected by these cognitive disabilities. This component was not acknowledged in the psychologist's statement that Mr. Young's "human figure drawings reveal a primitive, poorly differentiated perception of self and others." Furthermore, in the psychological sphere disabilities in visuospatial reasoning and visual memory are likely to have shaped Mr. Young's experiences of object constancy, and his sense of security in his surround and in navigating in unfamiliar places. At the same time, the psychologist *did* elaborate the interrelations between some of Mr. Young's cognitive disabilities and his sense of being deviant, "damaged," depressed, and, in turn, his heightened sensitivity to real or anticipated criticism and his tendency to elicit sadistic responses to his masochistic orientation.

At any rate, the starkly stated results of the diagnostic evaluation tests Dr. Green arranged "surprised" Dr. Green and
"shocked" Mr. Young. The findings were so pathological (especially in light of the fact that the childhood assessment was
reportedly normal) that the psychologist referred Mr. Young
to a neurologist to rule out a brain tumor. The normal results
of the neurological examination reassured all concerned, but
the powerful impact of the psychologist's report persisted.

The diagnostic test findings relieved Mr. Young at first.
He was pleased to have a handy explanation for many of his
problems, such as his childhood difficulty in tying his shoelaces
and his current trouble learning to drive and dance. But it was
simultaneously apparent that he accentuated his failings, in the
past as well as the present, for psychological gain. In childhood
he had used his difficulties in dressing to provoke his father
and, as an adult, hired instructors with whom he did not have
a common language, thus impeding his mastery of driving to
an even greater degree. In these ways, Mr. Young also turned
passive into active, apparently *choosing* to be disabled (when he
actually experienced great difficulty in selected skills).

At the same time, Mr. Young, who found satisfaction in
the *fantasy* that he was defective, gradually became aware of
being quite upset that it had, in his view, been confirmed. Why
should this have been so, given his lifelong claims of difficulty?
One answer lies in the discovery he and Dr. Green made that
he became disorganized when he experienced or understood
matters in a way different from his parents. In their view, there
was really nothing wrong with him.

Another answer is that confirmation of Mr. Young's sense
of disability also potentiated his rage at his parents, rage which
he was highly invested in denying. He unconsciously felt they
both neglected him and used him to fulfill their own needs to
keep him close in some respects. Neither Mr. Young's mother
nor his father could comfortably tolerate his separateness from
them, emotionally or functionally. Among the many other ways
in which Mr. Young felt his parents had failed him, they had
not helped him find out about his cognitive disabilities, and
had not intervened on his behalf to offer him assistance with

these disabilities. Mr. Young felt anger at people whom he perceived as "defective," which was in all likelihood both an identification with his parents' stance and a displacement of his feelings toward his parents. In this way he expressed and defended against his experience of his parents as flawed caretakers who were unable to tolerate his disabilities, or the limits of his normal developmental capacities as a child. In addition, Mr. Young could not tolerate the imperfections of others, with whom he identified. This was analyzed in the transference in Mr. Young's tendency to become angry at his analyst whenever he noticed any type of failing.

The depth of Mr. Young's fury at his parents was conveyed in his associations to concentration camp victims who required reparations. Mr. Young felt he deserved payment for damages. This emerged in the transference in his view that his analyst could not and would not help him, that she required of him more than he could do. A view of Dr. Green as caring and helpful in catalyzing his ability to help himself contrasted with, and reflected negatively on, his parents. Mr. Young's recognition of this contrast disrupted his denial of his rage toward his parents who he felt to be poor caretakers.

Another aspect of the disturbing effect of the test findings was that Mr. Young had not imagined himself to be as defective as the tests revealed him to be. He had hoped to be defective, but correctable. The test results disrupted the balance between his self representation as potentially capable and adult on the one hand, and babyish and needy on the other hand. Mr. Young was concerned that he could not be repaired, and disappointed that he would have to work actively to improve rather than be passively fixed by his analyst.

New determinants of Mr. Young's feeling of deficiency emerged following the diagnostic evaluation. His parents, who had wanted very much to raise him as an independent person, misgauged the degree to which parents had to help their children. Trying to let him accomplish things on his own, they demanded more than he could accomplish and neglected him as well. In fact, in view of his belatedly diagnosed learning disability, he must have required more, not less, help. Instead his mother minimized the degree and significance of his disability.

In this sense the existence of Mr. Young's learning disability accentuated his feelings of deficiency, and hence his rage. Because he unconsciously blamed his parents, and further was angry at them because he was unable to please them and to rely on them sufficiently, his anger became excessive. Conflicts between his aggressive wishes, his love for his parents, and his superego were magnified, requiring intensified defensive activity.

Mr. Young's defenses against his anger at his parents for their neglect were complex. He, too, overestimated children's capabilities and underestimated the degree of help they needed. He buttressed his denial of rage by imagining that his parents had not misunderstood his capacities at different developmental levels. He preferred to believe that *he* had been defective, through not living up to their expectations. Indeed, Mr. Young regarded his adult immaturity as proof that his parents were correct in their assessment of children; he had been defective and to blame all along in not being able to achieve, despite their sound child rearing practices. Thus he exonerated his parents.

This defense involved denial and the distorting of his perceptions. As his parents had failed to perceive other children's achievements correctly, and thus expected too much of Mr. Young, so he as an adult misevaluated children's developmental achievements. For example, when he saw a woman calm her crying grandchild by reassuringly telling her that she would return to the nursery school in a few days, Mr. Young was surprised that the grandmother was so patient and tolerant of the child's age appropriate immaturity.

We believe that Mr. Young's use of denial was based on his identification with his parents, as well as his tendency to confused and distorted perceptions which was one feature of his specific neuropsychological disabilities (his pronounced difficulties with visuospatial organization and visual memory). In the analysis Mr. Young gradually became capable of making more realistic observations about normal child development and rearing.

Dr. Green and her patient discovered another remarkable defense, also expressive of Mr. Young's anger, after she noted that she repeatedly became drowsy during analytic sessions. Mr. Young was lulling his analyst to sleep, thus simultaneously weakening her so she could not attack him and attacking her as a transference object. His rambling style, which Dr. Green once regarded as a manifestation of a thought disorder, served to sedate and confuse her. This was analyzed as Mr. Young recalled that he had consciously attempted to weaken his father in similar maneuvers in the past.

There were several additional interferences with Mr. Young's learning which combined developmental and neuro-psychological determinants. One was his defensive need to be dependent, which compromised his autonomy and activity. These are important components of learning. Mr. Young's neuropsychologically based learning difficulty, which affected his grasp of spatial relationships and his memory of what he saw, contributed to his dependence on the adults around him. Mr. Young's impulsiveness also compromised his learning. Although a biological tendency to excessive impulsiveness and a related need for rapid completion of tasks (what Dr. Green calls closure), may have been present, we can find no evidence of that. Mr. Young was not a hyperactive, distractible, or impulsive child who could not concentrate. Rather we observe that his father was an active adventuresome man who encouraged his son's impulsiveness, as in the purchase of property he could not afford. Dr. Green also observed that her patient tried to cope with his failure to comprehend the material he read by guessing what it said, often so rapidly that he reached incorrect conclusions.

Thus in complex ways Mr. Young's neuropsychologically based cognitive disorder interlaced with his childhood environment to produce marked inner conflicts and maladaptive defenses.

Chapter 19

Mr. G's Analysis

Antoinette Ambrosino Wyszynski, M.D.

PRESENTING PROBLEMS AND HISTORY

Mr. G, a 27-year-old white male, complained of difficulties in relationships with women and "irrational fears" (all words within quotes are those of the patient, unless otherwise indicated) which began six months prior to his consultation with me. Soon after a short plane trip with his parents, he became phobic about flying; he worried that he would be trapped for several hours, "hyperventilating," and creating a "public spectacle" in which he would "go crazy." Mr. G's fears then became more pervasive. He experienced anxiety about eating in restaurants where he anticipated "difficulty swallowing, especially meat getting stuck in my throat." Mr. G gave up his tickets to stadium-based sports events that he had traditionally attended with friends for fear of "going crazy" in a public place. More generally something about leaving his apartment made him anxious. He was barely able to use his car to travel to business meetings because he feared tunnels and had to suspend all trips (business and leisure) that required flying. He also had

Acknowledgment. The author is grateful to Shelley Orgel, M.D., for his helpful suggestions.

difficulty traveling in elevators to his skyscraper office and apartment. At that time Mr. G abruptly stopped using his regular "escort service," both because he worried about contracting AIDS and felt it was "morally wrong and abnormal" to be involved with prostitutes.

Dr. A, the psychiatrist who referred Mr. G to me after a several session consultation, had seen him briefly in psychotherapy at the age of 14. Mr. G returned to him as an adult because of his current difficulties. Dr. A sent me the results of recent psychological testing which he had suggested Mr. G undergo. The report stated that there was "evidence of mild organicity consistent with the residual effects of minimal brain dysfunction, probably present since childhood." Dr. A regretted not having made this diagnosis during his brief contact with the patient as an adolescent. Although he had suspected a specific learning disability and/or an Attention Deficit Disorder at the time (based on the school record of difficulties in math), Mr. G had dropped out of treatment before the workup could be undertaken. According to Mr. G, Dr. A summarized the results of testing by saying "everything was normal," except that there was evidence of a "mild learning disability" from childhood.

In the consultation with me, Mr. G described always having had "worries," although he denied childhood phobic symptoms. He was known as "waterworks" as a boy, because he frequently burst into tears when anxious or frustrated. He recalled wishing he could have "acted like a man," but was instead "more sensitive" than other people, a trait that has been "a mixed blessing."

Mr. G grew up in an affluent family. His father, a successful businessman, was rarely home. His mother dominated the family scene and used the family fortune to "make things easy" for him and his sister who was three years his junior. Mr. G had many failures and learning difficulties, especially in math. His mother, a former college administrator, took a "bite the bullet" approach to his academic problems, which she assumed to be the result of a lack of effort and perseverance. Mr. G commented, "She would put me in a room to do my homework until she saw beads of sweat on my brow." She would not help Mr. G with any schoolwork, "probably because she didn't want me to be a Momma's boy, though I probably was anyway." Mr. G commented that this approach taught him to be "stoical." He described his mother as "overly involved in her children's lives," but nevertheless maintained that she was "like any normal mother."

Because Mr. G's parents could not understand why he was not more academically successful, they transferred him to a challenging private grammar school when he was 14. He felt he was no match for his public school friends who were all "superachievers and superbright." There followed a particularly difficult period for Mr. G. Although he did not recall the specific problems, "it had something to do with low self-esteem." Mr. G saw Dr. A for four months at this time because he "wasn't coping well. The anxiety surfaced then . . . I felt as if I were leaving boyhood friends behind." Mr. G remembered crying often in the principal's office so that his mother would have to come to get him. At sleep-away camp that year he was "miserable" because he wanted to come home. His parents insisted that he "tough it out."

Mr. G gradually adjusted to private school and precipitously dropped out of treatment with Dr. A. In high school Mr. G became a sports trivia expert and joined the debate team, at which he was quite successful. An "above-average" athlete, he had many friends and was considered "funny," popular, "tall and nice-looking." Nevertheless he could not approach girls to date them. Instead he "hid behind sports and being funny." "Impatience" and distractibility, his nemeses, limited him scholastically and socially.

Mr. G completed four years of college as a history major. He wanted to go to graduate school but his Graduate Record Exam score in math precluded this. He entered law school for a year but suffered crippling test-taking anxiety, causing him to flunk out. Mr. G then decided to work in his father's company, where he remained at the time of consultation with me. Although moderately successful, he continued to be plagued by his father's public outbursts toward him and had little confidence in his own abilities. Mr. G was unhappy being a salesman and wanted to pursue another line of work helping people. However, he was "terrified" of the idea of leaving the family business and felt there were few realistic alternatives.

The history was not suggestive of hyperactivity, or of early extended or unusual separations from either parent. Mr. G was color blind and left-handed. He had no significant medical history as an infant, child, or adult. There was no history of drug or alcohol abuse. He had never received tutoring until college.

All of Mr. G's adult sexual relationships with women had been with call girls or "one night stands." He maintained that he had no idea what it meant to be "in love." Yet he described one college relationship where he experienced both sexual and loving feelings toward a woman by whom he was rebuffed. Mr. G's first intercourse occurred after college with a call girl. He had used "escort services" regularly for the past three years, although he stopped several months before reconsulting with Dr. A. He had never fallen in love with any of these women; nor had he asked for the same woman twice. Mr. G usually requested women with large breasts but reported in the consultation with me (a woman in my thirties) that he had requested for the first time an "older woman about 40 . . . to see what it was like." Mr. G also reported that when he started masturbating at age 11, he fantasized about intercourse with large-breasted women.

Although he denied feeling anxious about sex or having difficulties with potency, Mr. G admitted to occasionally ejaculating prematurely and having to fight back transient thoughts that "I was fucking my mother." He dated numerous women briefly and "platonically" and had no difficulty finding dates, but usually became "too shy and embarrassed" when the woman reciprocated his interest. Indifference and a sense of "monotony" ensued. Mr. G very much wanted to be in a long-term loving relationship with a woman, to marry, and have children. However, he felt "something is holding me back, making it impossible for me to be normal, punishing me with these anxieties and irrational fears." Mr. G denied homosexual encounters but confessed, with great anguish, that he was afraid "all this means I'm a homosexual and I don't know it."

RESULTS OF PSYCHOLOGICAL TESTING

The psychologist concluded that an interplay of psychological and organic factors produced inconsistencies in Mr. G's functioning which he regarded as evidence of mild organic pathology. He thought Mr. G's current picture was related to "minimal brain dysfunction" in childhood. He tested overall within the high end of the "Dull Normal" range of intelligence, earning a Full Scale IQ of 88 based upon a Verbal IQ of 97 and a Performance IQ of 80, a disparity approaching statistical significance. This was considered an underestimate of Mr. G's potential, which was probably within the average range. It was reported that test-taking anxiety, impaired concentration, and ambivalence disrupted Mr. G's performance and contributed to lowering the various scores.

There was wide inter- and intrasubtest scatter on verbal tests. Mr. G's fund of general information was very good, suggesting that he had profited from school and from life experience in general. His self-report of a large storehouse of "trivial facts" was posited by the examiner to serve as a compensation for his recognized intellectual limitations. Social comprehension fell within the average range. Mr. G demonstrated a good understanding of the world around him with little difficulty recognizing societal principles, operations, and standards. His retention of immediate auditory stimuli (number series) was slightly below the average range.

In contrast, verbal abstract tasks posed the most difficulty. Mr. G's thinking was concrete and relatively simplistic. He was unable to accurately state how "coat" and "suit" were alike and totally unable to indicate how "table" and "chair," "air" and "water," "poem" and "statue," were similar. More complex abstractions proved very difficult as well. On two out of three proverb tasks, he simply responded, "I don't know. I just don't know."

Mr. G's functioning on nonverbal subtests was also invaded by poor concentration and anxiety and judged to be an underestimate of his potential. He performed particularly poorly on tasks requiring analysis, synthesis and integration of parts into

wholes. Mr. G became very confused on the Block Design subtest. Even when he correctly replicated a simple item, he que-
ried, "Is this it?" unsure of himself. An exceptionally poor
performance (in the "Borderline" range, i.e., well below average) was noted on the subtest tapping Mr. G's ability to recognize details of a problem and to differentiate relevant from
irrelevant elements. Difficulties in perceptual-motor functioning were also evident on copying tasks. On the Bender-Gestalt,
Mr. G's reproductions were mildly distorted; his anxiety upon
recognizing his problems was intense. His immediate retention
of these designs was poor as well. Whether this was a function
of anxiety and/or frank weakness in immediate visual memory
was not clear. On the Trail Making Test, one which the tester
designated as quite sensitive to organicity, Mr. G performed in
the average range, despite his difficulties.

Projective testing revealed that Mr. G was preoccupied
with feelings of profound inadequacy in relationships with
women.

IMPRESSION OF ANALYZABILITY

During the consultation Mr. G, an attractive man, appeared to
be intelligent, articulate, and self-reflective. Although initially
quite anxious, he easily established rapport and freely associated. However, his use of intellectualization and isolation of
affect often gave him a stilted, humorless quality. He repeatedly
recited his list of symptoms and became bored, and boring.

As Mr. G's attention was drawn to his tendency to keep
feelings out of the sessions, he revealed glimpses of himself as
warmly humorous and affectionate and capable of insight and
introspection. His verbal abilities certainly seemed far in excess
of what had been reported in the psychological testing, although he had a tendency to misuse words. For example, he
substituted "plutonic" for "platonic" and "exasperated" for
"exacerbated."

Mr. G and I were able to establish a good working alliance.
This was in keeping with his pattern of long-lasting relationships with male friends. However, I was concerned about the

degree of anxiety he might experience in working with a female analyst. The psychological test report had pointed strongly to neuropsychological deficits that would interfere with an analysis, but my sense was that Mr. G's deficiencies had been overestimated and that psychodynamic factors had compromised his test performance. Given the long-standing and pervasive nature of Mr. G's problems, a trial of analysis seemed to offer him the best hope of treatment.

COURSE OF THE ANALYSIS

First Three Years of Analysis

Central to Mr. G's experience of analysis was his deep sense of inferiority and confusion as a patient "learning" to talk and understand in a different kind of way. This process touched upon his sense of inadequacy both intellectually and as a man. Mr. G had a deep mistrust of and wariness about his ability to deal with things "cerebral." The analytic work felt like "a lot of mental activity" to this man who had only painful and frustrating memories of failing when he tried to use his intellect. Anxiety about "not being up to snuff" characteristically spurred him to give up, expressed in wishes to quit analysis. Historically, once he quit something, he confirmed his sense of inadequacy and added to his long list of failures.

Significantly, such feelings came up around Mr. G's difficulty in free associating and exploring transference fantasies. Over time I came to realize that this problem could not be explained solely on the basis of compromise formation and defensively motivated avoidance, although these were major determinants. The direct effects of long-standing cognitive difficulties and efforts at compensation for these were also extremely important factors.

Mr. G was stumped by the abstract "as-if" quality of the transference. For example, he would say, "That's not really how I feel about you and I know you're not really that way. . . . That's not a valid conclusion I've drawn . . . I'm thinking wrong on that one. It's an example of how I tended to confuse things in school." Mr. G issued disclaimers about transference feelings and had great difficulty understanding the validity of suspending disbelief and "playing along" with perceptions that were "wrong." The deepening of our understanding of the transference kept getting shipwrecked on his need to cling to concrete logic and to that which was rationally correct.

Much work was needed regarding Mr. G's resistance to and narcissistic vulnerability concerning free association in general, and the expression of transference fantasies in particular. Mr. G was convinced he was falling short and could not "solve the puzzle" that his associations produced. Mr. G felt greater than average discomfort with the abstract, and frank bewilderment with the irrational. It was as though accessing primary process material reflected faulty apprehension and "fuzzy" thinking.

I slowly understood that transference fantasies were snuffed out, not only because of their content, but also as a consequence of their seemingly "abstract," "hazy" form. After instances when Mr. G had been particularly successful in freely associating, with greater availability of affect and fantasy, he felt uneasy that he made no sense and had become unintelligible. He concluded he was "no good at this." Mr. G likened the diffuseness of such fantasies to the dreaded experiences of childhood crossword puzzles, connect-the-dot puzzles, and jigsaw puzzles, all of which were disorienting. Did the pencil go left or right? Should the puzzle piece be rotated clockwise or counterclockwise? Why were the block letters so hard to read if they were stacked vertically? It was dizzying. He remembered having failed to pass shop. It was noteworthy that as we explored this cognitive aspect of working with his feelings about me, Mr. G gradually became more comfortable with the "letting go" of logic that occurs in free association.

It was striking how this otherwise articulate, quite competent individual, lacked the mastery-oriented attitude toward obstacles that would have allowed him to sustain confidence, striving, and hope. Years of bitterly disappointing academic failures had bred "learned helplessness"—the sense that success is impossible regardless of increased effort, motivation, or strategy. Accusatory prods, of "poor motivation," "bad attitude," or "laziness," often invoked by his frustrated parents, merely reinforced Mr. G's negative self-image and had been used to rationalize his passivity.

There were wide discrepancies between Mr. G's actual abilities and his ego ideal. He harbored fantasies of being a great baseball star, signing autographs as a famous actor, or becoming an attorney for the diplomatic corps. His academic difficulties had made it impossible to pursue law or a diplomatic career. Because he consistently panicked when taking tests, he flunked the Graduate Record Exam and law school finals. Mr. G retreated to a career as his father's apprentice in the family business, trying to deny his sense of tragedy and defeat beneath a carapace of "stoicism" and boredom. He also experienced being an analytic patient as a "blow to the self-esteem," despite his acknowledgment of its value to him in helping him to begin to feel better.

I became convinced that the narcissistic mortifications stemming from Mr. G's learning difficulties were being reenacted in his experience of me and the analysis. I was concerned that if his past learning difficulties as they were revived in the analytic experience were not thoroughly explored, the patient was at risk for fleeing the analysis in desperation and defeat, just as he had precipitously abandoned so many other pursuits in the past. I told Mr. G I noticed he feared becoming confused and tended to present himself as "too complicated a puzzle" to figure out. Memories of his prior experiences as an elementary school student came to the fore. Schoolteachers used to force him to do math problems on his own at the blackboard. He felt humiliated in front of the other children because he could not do even simple problems, despite above average achievement in English and social studies. Mr. G eventually got "bored" and "no longer cared" anymore. Analysis felt like one more humiliating trip to the blackboard.

I interpreted that Mr. G felt frustrated and humiliated in front of me about not being able to solve the problem of himself. He agreed. The boredom was like a safety switch that turned off the painful feelings. He then vividly recalled how his mother had tried to teach him to tie his shoelaces, which

took him many months to learn. She went through the steps
with him, then untied the laces, and made him do it on his
own. We both agreed that apparently she did not realize that
he experienced visuomotor difficulties. I interpreted that Mr.
G similarly experienced me as unempathic in not directing
him, as he had also experienced his schoolteachers with math
problems. He reacted as though I required him to do the impossible, withholding help and ignoring his desperation, helplessness, and rage.

Mr. G seemed thunderstruck by this discovery. He wanted
to know more about what Dr. A had meant when he told him
in the consultation sessions about the learning disability. Mr.
G was not sure he believed it. He was intrigued by this new
piece of information but did not want to use anything as a
crutch. I, too, was concerned about the risks of fostering intellectualization, and the displacement of his internal conflicts,
onto either the learning problems or his parents. I also suspected, and later received confirmation, that Mr. G's feeling
of intellectual inferiority could become elaborated into a defensively utilized pseudoimbecility.

Grappling with how to explain, I used the analogy of a boy
born with weak hand muscles who wanted to be a baseball
pitcher. This was Mr. G's favorite sport. If the problem were
identified, the boy could receive special help to strengthen the
muscles. But if the difficulty remained undiagnosed, and was
attributed instead to the boy's lack of motivation, intelligence,
or talent in baseball, the psychological outcome would be very
different. I told Mr. G that our interest would be to understand
the impact of his learning difficulties, as well as anything else
in his life.

This somewhat concrete approach was characteristic of the
technique necessary to work effectively with Mr. G, who frequently required literal analogies in order to be able to abstract
the meaning of an interpretation or clarification. I began to
use the phrase "$1 + 1 = 3$" as an extremely helpful shorthand
for highlighting Mr. G's brittle self-image. He tended to jump
to the most self-denigrating conclusions based on doubts about
himself, thereby preempting further discussion. For example,

since math was hard for him, he must be stupid. Since he questioned his manliness, he must be homosexual. Since analysis was not easy for him, he was an inadequate patient.

I often struggled with how to titrate the right amount of support for Mr. G without jeopardizing an analytic process. We constantly clarified his impulse to give up, to spare himself feelings of failure. As a consequence, he had perfected a stance as harmless and incompetent, nestled passively on the sidelines, all the while secretly thwarting others, most notably his parents, his teachers, and me in the analysis. It was essential for this patient to have me acknowledge that there had been progress. For example, he intermittently asked, "I couldn't have understood that a year ago, could I?" By the end of the first year he took pleasure in "learning" how analysis "worked"; he was delighted when he could himself "connect the dots" between seemingly unrelated thoughts and could point out aspects of his own defensive functioning. Thus he attained in the analytic work an unprecedented sense of success in something that required the use of his intellect.

Mr. G and I began to understand that there were conflicts about achievement that were related to, but separate from, his specific learning difficulties which were inborn. (I thought the inborn disability was neuropsychological in nature but Mr. G and I did not use this term.) Mr. G felt inferior to his friends and his father who had "made it on their own." However, having described a real accomplishment at work in a timid manner, he immediately minimized it. Mr. G, who had the highest percentage in sales increases for the year, revealed that his father had given him only discount accounts to work with, which constituted a significant handicap. He recalled how his father had downplayed his achievements when he played Little League, joking that if his team won, the other team had to have been "a bunch of girls." Mr. G also vividly recounted how his father severely chastised him for seeking congratulations on hitting the championship winning ball, warning his son never to become "conceited." Success meant getting "too good" for his father which was dangerous. Failure was safer, although his father's disappointment in him was tragic.

Mr. G approached the task of understanding his own fantasies with dread that he was setting himself up for one more
inevitable failure, by participating in their ambiguity. Mr. G
complained bitterly that I did not help him "get started." He
needed someone to "light a fire under" him, to get him going.
He often talked about leaving the analysis. He feared becoming
"a prisoner of psychotherapy," unable to come up with solutions, incapable of making the connections necessary to escape
one more claustrophobic situation.

Mr. G's inability to comfortably travel limited his business
opportunities, heightening his misery, and sense of failure as
a man. He said that there had always been a discrepancy between his nickname, "Big Guy," and his inner feelings. Although he was tall, he avoided the "hoop action" in basketball,
the most aggressive place in the game. In softball no one was
more shocked than he when he hit the ball hard and far. "I
feel more like [a short man] than someone tall." The lack of
structure in the analysis at times compounded the feeling of
"going nowhere." Woven throughout were conflicts concerning anality and passivity, with fears of being penetrated by interpretations or made to "eat another man's shit" by swallowing
my words.

At this point in the analysis I frequently found myself having to repeat interpretations and clarifications. Impatience and
an overwhelming sense of tedium invaded Mr. G's curiosity
and motivation to understand himself. He claimed that these
"lessons" were too difficult, as insoluble as math. It was difficult
to know when these moments resulted from resistance, and
when they were an expression of the negative transference
(e.g., obstructing my interpretive powers, making me submit
to his will), or of conflicts over success, or the result of neuropsychologically based difficulties with abstract thinking. I suspect it was a combination of all of these factors.

Mr. G and I increasingly came to see how he feared letting
me know of his competition with me, lest I "cut him down" like
his father. He likened his highly successful father to a baseball
manager who treated all his players the same without regard
for their individual sensitivities. Such a manager also expected
results from yelling, humiliating, intimidating, and "ranting

and raving." Mr. G found it painful that his father, a great admirer of Dale Carnegie, had regarded Mr. G's school difficulties as a failure of "P.I.A.T.," the acronym he employed for the family slogan "Putting It All Together" through hard work and positive thinking. Mr. G's father had hoped to spur his son on by goading him, accusing him of having a lazy mind. In fact it was Mr. G's "lazy mind" that led to the transfer from his beloved public school to a private school. Mr. G was repeating this with me regarding his analytic "prowess." He felt like he must defeat me (by coming to his own interpretations first) or be defeated by me (by agreeing to my interpretations or acknowledging he had feelings about me).

This posed an impossible bind, an insoluble puzzle; the only solution was to exit. Discussion of these issues usually sparked Mr. G's desire to flee the analysis. He agreed that his anxiety about failure caused him to steer away from trying, which then confirmed his feeling of having failed. It would be far better if he could attempt difficult things, but his impatience and vulnerability made it impossible to ask for help.

The acceptance of my help contained a paradox: the satisfaction of being able to understand himself was undermined by self-condemnation about needing assistance. He said that the weekends were like being stranded on the road with a flat tire and no mechanic or instruction manual. Mr. G was quite appreciative when I pointed out that there was a precedent for his being able to successfully learn. When he started analysis he was convinced that he was "too complicated a puzzle" to ever figure out and yet over the months we saw how he "got the hang of it" and could do a great deal on his own without my help.

I worried about the inhibiting effect of such gratifying clarifications on the analytic process. However, for this demoralized man who was so convinced of his inability to "figure things out," they seemed to propel the process forward. Although we sacrificed the clarity wrought by classical technique, I was convinced there would be no treatment at all without these parameters.

Following these explorations, Mr. G's sexual wishes in the transference began to become manifest. At first this was evident to me in the displacement of having sexual relations with a psychologist who was "a slightly older woman who worked with the problems of teenagers." Mr. G could directly articulate only the concomitant feelings of claustrophobia about being in the consulting room with me. He found Fridays particularly diffi-cult. At first we explored his feelings of loneliness on the week-ends. He suggested, cloaked in humor, that the only way to avoid this was for me to see him on Saturdays and Sundays.

We also came to see that unconsciously our verbal ex-changes had become equated with a sexual relationship. Many sessions began with brief, climaxlike bursts of material designed to impress and please me, after which he felt "spent," "emp-tied," wanting to know my reaction, at a loss as to what to do or say next. There were sessions where Mr. G experienced erections which he was unable to bring himself to talk about, with frank negations that lying on the couch had any sexual meaning to him at all. He felt constantly frustrated by my rela-tive inactivity in the sessions—I aroused his curiosity and feel-ings, yet did not respond with my own.

At this point in the analysis, Mr. G's resistance to the aware-ness of transference had additional meanings. My efforts to clarify even obvious transference material were often yawningly denied or passionately negated with accusations that I tried to manipulate him. He insisted that our separations were "vaca-tions" to be celebrated.

School was out. I often found myself feeling like a school-teacher exasperated by her student's refusal to cooperate. In analyzing my own countertransference, I realized that Mr. G's protestations of "this is too hard for me to do" contained sig-nificant elements of passive aggression and obstructionism. I interpreted that he presented himself as a harmless, incompe-tent "student" as a way of foiling me and expressing his rage. He agreed.

Helping Mr. G tolerate the transference in order to analyze it was an ongoing technical challenge. One specific aspect of this problem was finding a way of working with transference feelings without repeating Mr. G's mother's (and schoolteach-ers') intrusiveness. More generally there was the problem of

making them accessible without priming Mr. G to defensively
bat them away as analytic caricatures.

As Mr. G's unspoken sexual longings for me intensified,
he sought displacements. For example, he decided to go to a
male massage therapist although he recognized that this man
was "more an alchemist than a doctor." Nevertheless Mr. G
imagined he would offer immediate results for his anxieties
and phobias. Mr. G eventually acknowledged that he regretted
my not being more personally involved with him, my not taking
the "hands on" approach, although that would be "too
erotic."

It was the culmination of many months of painstaking work
when Mr. G himself became aware of how "flattened" in intensity his feelings and fantasies could become. He concluded with
conviction that this was part of the "antibody effect" that his
"subconscious mind" generated to avoid pain and further insight. Boredom was a defensive device, which followed intervals
where feelings were more accessible. He feared being overwhelmed if he did not "switch off" and brake their intensity.

He came to see that his impatience, pervasive boredom,
and emotional dullness with me predated both the analysis and
the onset of his phobic symptoms. Indeed he wondered if the
phobic symptoms were recent expressions of long-standing difficulties. With slowly expanding self-awareness Mr. G defined
how the claustrophobic feeling he came to recognize with me
also occurred with other women. He noted a paradox which
puzzled him. Despite his claustrophobia, which was associated
with wishes to flee, he sometimes felt he could sit on the stair-
well leading to my office all day long.

In one particularly difficult session, we analyzed his suddenly resumed resolve to decrease the number of weekly analytic meetings. Mr. G revealed that his mother had insisted he
give her my phone number so that she could arrange to meet
with me to voice her objections to the frequency of sessions
and the cost. In the same conversation she conveyed to Mr. G
her feeling that he was "shutting her out." Despite a heated
argument in which he strongly voiced his feelings that there
could be no price placed on having a person work out his life
and that analysis was not "open school week," his mother was

adamant. Ultimately Mr. G capitulated, feeling humiliated. When his mother relented, he felt too defeated to be relieved.

Mr. G subsequently reported confusing feelings of anxiety and rage when his mother wore only her underwear and his sister swam nude at the family summer house during a weekend he spent with them. Many allusions emerged to his discomfort with his mother's being "overly warm and physically affectionate" with him. At the same time, he denied that these experiences had significance. Similarly, he disavowed his fury after having reported incidents in which his mother and/or father undercut him by expressing disappointment in his social and academic success. It was clearly too frightening to accept his parents' lack of empathy. It was better to "play dumb."

Mr. G's threats to leave the analysis continued. He seemed unable to grasp my translation of this as a disguised expression of his wish to avoid painful and confusing feelings about me and his mother and father. Needing my help magnified his feelings of vulnerability and diminished masculinity. When he was eager to talk to me about his problems, he became concerned that he was becoming too dependent, like a child or a student on a teacher. Being in analysis was a confirmation of his defectiveness exposed so long ago in the classroom. His father was a model of the "superhero," a standard Mr. G could not match.

He wished that I were more active and aggressive with him. There followed fleeting sexual fantasies about his mother and then frightening violent thoughts. During periods of silence horrifying "alien thoughts" would pop to mind, such as of his parents performing "an unnatural sexual act" or himself fellating another man. He would respond by invoking Dale Carnegie's "power of positive thinking" in an effort to shut out the scary and unpleasant.

As Mr. G voiced his now familiar refusals to "go out on a limb" in speculating about me because he might be wrong, he began to realize by the third year of analysis that the quashing of his curiosity, while reminiscent of what happened in school, served another important purpose. If he allowed himself to be curious about me, he might have sexual thoughts which felt forbidden. Mr. G associated to stripping in front of me, feeling naked on the couch, as if he were submitting to me. The arousal of these feelings was often followed by tedious boredom. We appreciated a new dimension of his wishes for me to "push him harder," give him a "kick in the pants," and "light a fire under him," as his mother had done with his schoolwork.

Scattered throughout Mr. G's associations was the wish that I react to him "personally," yet the conviction that even if he were to lie down on the couch nude, I would not respond to him as a woman would to a naked man. I pointed out that he saw himself as still a "kid" who had no sexual feelings and who could not be the object of sexual feelings by a grown woman. Curiosity about me as a "flesh and blood woman" was once again followed by heightened claustrophobic feelings and then boredom. Mr. G was impressed by how this sequence repeated itself over and over again, but also felt bewildered by it. It was important to help him understand that the "mystery" lingered because of the workings of the unconscious, rather than merely because of his failure to understand what was obvious. Memories of his classroom experience, where he had failed to "get it" while everyone else seemed to understand, were omnipresent.

In keeping with Mr. G's characterological mode of mitigating anxiety through flight, his resolves to end treatment continued to be sporadic and sudden, often following periods when we had been working well together. He noted, however, that he was slowly able to drive through tunnels, eat in restaurants, and attend stadium sporting events. After a period when Mr. G had been thoroughly engaged in the analytic work concerning passive wishes and fears, he again announced that he had set a date for ending treatment. He recognized his pleasure in taking an aggressive stance toward me, which would have been impossible several months before. This was accompanied by analysis of several dreams expressing his excitement about feeling like a sexual slave, as though dominated by a teacher "laying down the rules." Announcements about leaving the analysis involved both turning the tables by making me submit to his will for a change and efforts to flee feelings of "heating up" and suffocating, stuck in the "traffic" of the analysis.

What ultimately emerged was Mr. G's struggle with two aspects of himself: the "higher" more exalted version of "pure" love (for me in the transference) pitted against the more "human" side of himself including the "universal need" for sexual fulfillment which had propelled him toward call girls. Mr. G divided women into those for whom he could have sexual feelings like the prostitutes and those for whom he cared, like his mother, sister, or me.

This was explored in the transference. Reporting a conscious transient sexual fantasy about me while masturbating, Mr. G spoke briefly of fears of being trapped, and then was bored. As we observed this sequence, Mr. G expressed his feeling that having sexual fantasies about me made him feel like he was prostituting me. I pointed out that he experienced his sexual desire for me as degrading me, rather than as the natural outcome of his attraction to me. Similarly he had recently managed to have a brief relationship with a young woman whom he considered his first girl friend, which ended when it was invaded by his defensive boredom, isolation of affect, and desire to flee.

Mr. G could see that "the tender loving care, the hugging, the kissing, are more passionate and intimate than actual sex . . . Those are the real problems for me." He subsequently revealed thoughts of making love to a male friend while they were watching football on television. He could tentatively focus on these thoughts by reminding himself that "thinking it is not the same as acting." I pointed out that the physical contact between men in football games, which he had phobically avoided, stirred up anxiety. Mr. G's initial response was one of incredulity. He then remarked that the intensity of his disbelief may well indicate a "sensitive point." Following this he became intermittently bored and upset at the idea that he was "turned on" by watching football players. I commented, "You are doing another '1 + 1 = 3' number on yourself, concluding that because you are at times interested in watching other men, you are therefore homosexual. In fact, it may be that their power attracts you." Mr. G felt freer to confess that he liked admiring their bodies, imagined watching them having sex with their partners, and fantasized about the "size of their manliness." However, he began to feel "off keel," as if he were on "shaky ground," as images tumbled to mind about homosexuality, murder, or sex with friends or strangers on the street. He had recently read that murderers had "repressed feelings about their mothers and sexuality."

Mr. G's reluctance to further explore these fantasies stemmed from mistaking thoughts for actions and reflexively flattening his fantasies in the face of anxiety. He referred to his typical reaction to challenges: "I get scared when there is a challenge. When something is not easily done, I back off out of fear of failure, I guess." This again reminded him of school. Mr. G was pained by the discrepancy between his inner state and what would be expected behavior at his chronological age: marriage, fatherhood. We spoke of his idealization of the sports figures and his vulnerability in comparing himself to them. In associating to their prowess in attracting women, he often shifted between identifying with the male athlete and the aroused woman who was attracted to him.

Fourth Year of the Analysis

Mr. G's sense of defect was a central axis around which the first three years of his analysis turned. Having begun to appreciate his phobic responses to romantic interactions with women, and his tendency to defensively "switch off" and flee, Mr. G became determined to confront the phobic situations more directly so that we could explore them. However, he did nothing other than attend his appointments with me. Mr. G spent weekends in a burst of passivity, alone in his apartment having food, rented movies, and occasionally call girls, delivered. He complained bitterly that analysis was worthless and there was no hope for change.

I repeated interpretations about Mr. G's dissatisfaction that I did not "make it all happen" and "hand him a cure on a silver platter." His wealthy mother had intervened for him throughout his childhood, encouraging the expectation that his problems would be solved by "waves of the magic wand" without his having to tackle them himself. Unconsciously these strategies had exacerbated his feeling of helplessness and inadequacy, especially in relation to other males, which were already highlighted by his learning difficulties.

Mr. G usually submitted to people he regarded as more adequate, such as me with my powerful doctor's intellect. He often felt that things were being shoved down his throat, especially by his verbally aggressive father. Mr. G associated to his tongue symptom (feeling he was choking or swallowing his tongue) as a feeling of being intruded upon and helpless—a rape. The revival of memories of adolescence became especially prominent. He felt enormously inferior to other men, even in his prized athletics. Up until puberty he was able to dodge the effects of some of these difficulties, although it was excruciating to fail at shop, where he could not manipulate the instruments or figure out the prospective shape of the finished product. He would often cry in front of the other boys, intensifying his shame. Analysis felt like shop. He feared crying in front of me. Once Mr. G became interested in girls in high school, his sense of inadequacy was heightened. In college he had no dates or sexual encounters despite being tall and handsome. Mr. G recalled watching with great shame and helplessness as fraternity brothers enjoyed experiences with girls while he remained on the sidelines.

I persistently interpreted that for Mr. G, allowing my words to affect him felt like being violated by me and confirmed as inferior. He agreed, adding his fear that if he permitted himself to change, he would be unable to leave me. In boyhood he had yearned to stay at his mother's side where things were safe and effortless. He similarly wished that I would "do" analysis for him. The prostitutes were hired to take the initiative to do things to him sexually. I was to do the same analytically, servicing him with my words, making him potent, and causing the phobias to vanish.

We highlighted the defensive aims of his character traits of passivity and entitlement. He elaborated how he allowed dates to behave inconsiderately and condescendingly, paralleled by contemptuous male colleagues at work. He feared his aggressive retaliative fantasies of becoming a killer or rapist. Inactivity seemed a safer haven. He would express his anger by covert obstructionism. In this way he could get back at women who wielded their powerful attractiveness, as well as foil the potent men who have "forced me to eat shit." Mr. G's assertion that he was "not reacting to the analysis" was reframed as a very powerful "silent reaction" which contained passive rebellion and hostility. Mr. G acknowledged that he wished to thwart and outwit me, to retaliate against my adequacy by rendering me as impotent as he felt himself to be.

Mr. G felt these clarifications had enormous relevance to other aspects of his life and were very helpful to understand. I gradually realized that I had been reacting to my own counter-aggression and his vulnerability by protecting us both from this aspect of the work. During this period Mr. G more directly confronted his anger at his mother's intrusiveness without fearing his own violent retaliation. For example, he resented how she set him up on dates, canvassed her friends for available girls, and even made dinner reservations at restaurants of her own choosing for the blind dates, all unbidden.

Less accessible to Mr. G was how he invited his mother's involvement. For him unconsciously she was his madam procuring his whores. I interpreted that despite his conscious wish to be independent, the phobias prevented him from effectively traveling or dating. Thus he could avoid separating from his mother and from me. We observed that thoughts about being away from his mother were associated with being injured in some way, alone and frightened. We explored his fantasy that women were less dangerous if they were detoxified by his mother's involvement first, although they then became inextricably associated with her. There were many associations to having me take him by the hand into the phobic situations.

Mr. G began to see how relationships with women were unconsciously the core phobic dilemma. Slowly he began to set limits on his mother's involvement, arranging for dates and weekend activities on his own. He spoke of how he "watered down" his features which were attractive to women. For example, a pretty woman was enthusiastic about the fact that he had played college baseball and was a good athlete. Mr. G proceeded to demean his athletic efforts and gave her so intellectualized a rendition of those experiences that the woman gave up asking about them. I pointed out how he did the same with me. Anything distinctive about himself was diluted and made bland. The anxiety stimulated by a woman's excitement caused him to douse her interest by becoming boring. There was something about a woman's attention that seemed very frightening.

I told Mr. G that the fantasy of "being in a woman," as a man, was connected to feeling he would suffocate and be unable to leave her body. There was both the fear and the wish to be in mother and in me in the analysis. He was able to say that his sexual encounters, while pleasurable, were marred by a sense of distancing himself from the experience; "it isn't really me." I interpreted this as a defensive maneuver related to fantasies that being "in" a woman meant to be trapped within her, with no way out. Mr. G attempted to diminish this anxiety by dousing the woman's interest and excitement in him, becoming himself boring and bored, to distance himself from the experience of being in her body during intercourse.

Anxiety-provoking fantasies about dangerous aggression toward significant males began to emerge. Mr. G associated to a dream at age 10 or 12 of his father being stabbed, leaving the patient in control, like a "power play," since he would become the man of the house. Mr. G then associated to his grandfather, a big powerful man, dying a few months before. This sequence was followed by a series of associations about several powerful men dying, including sports figures and several friends. I interpreted to Mr. G that there seemed to be a connection between being a potent, powerful male, and being killed or dying, especially if one also became involved with a woman. Mr. G felt confused and upset about the irrationality of these thoughts.

In this context, he announced that his mother was "frightened and bothered" that he continued analysis. In her view he was too dependent upon me, "like an addiction." He was upset by her comments, in part because he felt there was some truth in them. He needed to try things on his own, even though he knew there were a lot of issues yet to be discussed and that we were examining more and more issues of which he had been totally unaware. He had begun to pay special attention to his tendency to "water down" the intensity of his feelings toward women and their interest in him.

At the same time he felt his mother was right because he had seen me for years and nothing was changing. (In fact, Mr.

G had begun to change radically, especially in his independence from his mother.) He could not "in good conscience" continue the analysis any longer. He suspended all appointments for the month of August effective the next day. Mr. G knew that I would be working straight through the summer, with plans to be away in early October.

Upon his return a month later, we met only twice a week because he had released his regular appointment times. We explored more closely some of the reasons why he had needed to interrupt the analysis. Mr. G found himself beginning to change in relation to his mother, which jeopardized their relationship; this experience was quite upsetting to him. He also feared his very powerful emotional connection to me. Since he was never going to make any real progress, and I was never going to make any kind of difference to him in the long run, what was the point?

I reiterated that although he consciously wished to change, he unconsciously sought to remain at age 12. As long as he could preserve me as the teacher and himself as the recalcitrant schoolboy, bent on proving that nothing I did mattered, he could remain fixed in time forever. This way he would never have to grow into adulthood or deal with the pain of separating from his mother or from me. This last interpretation really seemed to reach Mr. G. He acknowledged that moving ahead was very frightening for him and "growing up" was agonizing. He added, "*That* for me is more of a glaring difficulty than the situation with my mother. Deep down I don't think there is that much difficulty [with her], but that might be my denial."

While trying to decide whether he wanted to continue, quit, or see another doctor, Mr. G confided that the analysis *had* been very effective for him. He decided to continue with me but only on the condition that we meet less frequently. In retrospect, I thought that he felt so confused and powerless during the summer that his mother's comment offered him an excuse to stop. We explored how getting back into analysis was like going through a tunnel again, which was associated with disturbing claustrophobic feelings.

I considered that the interruption was Mr. G's unconscious response to those aspects of the analytic situation that overlapped with his mother's attitude toward him. For example, I required his continued presence; visits to me had become part of his life. Feeling nurtured and helped by me led to feelings of never wanting to leave and to fears of being trapped. My continued interest in and involvement with him were perceived unconsciously as my being sexually excited by him. We had been discussing how a woman's excitement imperiled the man, if he did not prophylactically degrade her first through sexual intercourse.

We were able to understand that Mr. G's "defeatist" attitude served another important defensive function. An optimistic attitude was associated in his mind with "cockiness," which could lead to "bad things happening," such as castration. One form of protection was to see his manliness as defective, and thus not a threat to anyone. In this way Mr. G could preserve his penis intact. This was a key interpretation for him with which we worked extensively.

I also understood Mr. G's need to interrupt the analysis as an expression of and defense against the intensification of his wishes to have me in a different way, as he continued the developmental progress of becoming independent and confident as a man. There was the fantasy that he could treat me like a woman he hired for an hour, and fired when I did not "come across." Mr. G had been unable to tolerate the pressure of his fantasies about me and, characteristically, fled. His mother actively interfered in the analysis, as well as being the spokesperson for his resistance. It was a battle between the women over him, which was both gratifying and frightening. My interpretation about his wish never to grow up helped him mitigate his experience of out-of-control wishes for me. He was able to feel that I sided with his ego; this facilitated the reengagement of his observing identification with me which allowed him to resume the analysis, although in attenuated form.

In addition, I saw Mr. G's insistence on reducing the number of weekly sessions as an expression of progress as he attempted to "hold the line" with me. He was taking an active stance, rather than passively complying with what I had determined for him. I felt that a twice weekly treatment was better than no treatment at all, or one that repeated for Mr. G the very conflict with his mother that he was attempting to solve and which interpretation alone had been unable to mitigate.

When I agreed to meet with him twice a week for a period of time, he was both shocked and quite appreciative that I took a request of his seriously and trusted his judgment. It felt like a validation—a rare commodity in his life—and confirmed that his expectations of being castrated by me for his potency were fantasied, not real. He added that he was quite willing to consider increasing the number of sessions later on, but that for the time being it was really important to him that I allow him to "take some control."

Mr. G noticed continued improvement in his phobic symptoms. He was able to take short plane flights. For the first time in years he was not tempted to scream during religious services. He began to more actively plan business trips and could now attend theatrical events and football games without becoming anxious. He dated a woman, D, whom he both liked as a friend and found sexually attractive. He allowed himself to explore the friendship with her without having to "jump the gun" by either abandoning the relationship or diving into sexual activity with her. Mr. G remarked on "subtle changes" in the way he related to her compared to previous experiences. He found D "classy" and attractive and was jealous about the idea of her dating another man. He commented with wonderment that it was really nice to begin a relationship with a woman by becoming good friends first.

These events represented unprecedented developmental gains. I pointed out that Mr. G sounded apologetic about his sexual interest in D. He felt guilty because, in his view, "nice women" were damsels who become the degraded victims of men's animal lusts. I explained that in growing up he learned to edit out the sexual aspect of love for women that began with his natural feelings for his mother. There evolved a mental circuit breaker between sexuality and love. He was finding it difficult as an adult man to reconnect the two. This made a lot of sense to Mr. G. He reported that after masturbating to climax with a sexual fantasy about D, he noticed that he suddenly felt indifferent toward her. I interpreted he was able to temporarily reconnect the two "wires" of sexuality and affection in fantasy, but that the circuit breaker had again disconnected the two. There resulted the conscious experience of indifference. Mr. G gained increasing conviction that this process was indeed operating.

As we explored this dynamic, Mr. G and I also observed his fear that if he talked about sexual matters with me, he might begin to have sexual feelings for me which he regarded as wrong and forbidden. We began to understand that his use of polite language with me was a way to keep sexual feelings at bay and not degrade me with his dirty words.

It was troubling to Mr. G that there was something about him which made women uncomfortable. We understood that his tendency to intellectualize and dampen his spontaneity was probably discomfiting. He waited for the women to "take the lead" and thaw him out. Perhaps she responded to his lack of emotionality and took her cue from him. This tendency was, in part, also a manifestation of his identification with his father, who was not openly affectionate. Although I felt it most useful to interpret the transference in the displacement, I was guided by my counterreactions to the way Mr. G treated me.

It was hard for Mr. G to imagine that the woman might have sexual wishes of her own and might welcome sexuality as an expression of mutual caring and affection, rather than of her degradation as a whore. We were able to approach the idea that the woman who was excited or interested in him was very threatening. His penis was at risk for becoming swallowed up in her, trapped, and ultimately destroyed by her. Women who responded to him were either aggressively attacking him or making themselves vulnerable to his degradation of them through sexual intercourse. Mr. G felt that the only way to safely have a woman respond to him was to pay her to "fake it." It was hard to fathom that sexual intercourse could be an act of mutual enjoyment and caring. Either the woman had to get sullied or he would be castrated. For Mr. G, mutuality resulted in a never-ending Catch-22 of degradation and violence.

I continued to interpret to Mr. G that the decreased number of sessions were, like the August interruption he had created, a way of distancing himself from his very confusing feelings about me. Once again, it was difficult for him to tolerate not only the content of his fantasies, but also their ambiguous form. I believe this difficulty was one of the ways Mr. G's history of learning problems continued to have an impact on the progress of his analysis. We often returned to the "connect-the-dot" puzzle analogy for working with free association, replete with anxieties of becoming disoriented. "Not knowing which way to turn" had literal, as well as figurative, meaning for this analysand.

By the end of the fourth year Mr. G relied significantly less on me to "do it" for him and was instead taking more responsibility for his own treatment. He felt growing self-confidence about his ability to handle things effectively on his own. We gradually resumed a regular schedule of four meetings per week.

Fifth Year of Analysis

There was a marked diminution in Mr. G's sense of defect and deficiency, which was for years the predominant theme of his analysis. We continued to work extensively on his sexual interaction with women as his core phobic situation. He became better able to tolerate the confusion and ambiguity of his fantasies without defensively "switching off" and fleeing. He was gradually able to identify a precise moment, a "panic point," arising when he sexually approached a woman of emotional importance to him. It was at this pivotal point that he was grabbed by claustrophobic feelings and a sense of having to flee.

Unconsciously he felt rage toward attractive women whom he believed aroused him only to reject him, and whose attractiveness beckoned him to compete with other men. This predicament exacerbated his feeling of helplessness and impotence, already magnified by his lifelong difficulties with mastery and competence, especially relative to other males.

The "panic point" with women was inextricably intertwined with feelings about being engulfed and trapped, thereby losing his autonomy, his identity, his penis and his pride. This symptom also encompassed Mr. G's anxiety about identifying and competing with other men. He both feared defeating and being defeated by other men. It felt like castrating them or being castrated by them. Violence was in all of it. It was easier to sit on the sidelines, the innocuous Mr. Nice Guy who never offended or entered the fray. Safety, however, was emotionally empty.

During this period there was a significant loosening of Mr. G's passive defensive reactions, related to expanding insight about how he had co-opted the analysis in the service of passivity and entitlement. Mr. G was able to connect these wishes of me to the expectation that "if only" he could find a woman who could turn him on at first sight, his problem would be solved. I persisted in interpreting to Mr. G how allowing my words to affect him would feel like my sexual victory. I became a castrating competitor, as well as the victorious Siren who had lured and engulfed him. Passivity was the safe haven, even with me in the analysis, where secret rebellion and hostility were smuggled undercover by a stance of reasonableness and superficial compliance. Mr. G reported many episodes of romancelessly dating attractive women for weeks. They were given no hint of his sexual interest, yet were expected to surmise his "true feelings." When they eventually signaled their unwillingness to continue the relationship, they confirmed his conviction that they existed only to reject him. For Mr. G, the woman had to be deprived of a "self" in order to feel safe to him.

This dilemma was difficult for him to apprehend because consciously he treated women with consideration and courtesy. He began to understand how his assiduous avoidance of what might be anxiety-provoking with a woman (e.g., a romantic gesture) had blocked his empathy for her experience of his apparent indifference. He wanted the woman to make sexual overtures, to magically divine that he was "just shy," and then, clueless, wait until he was ready to make his move. To Mr. G's disappointment, it never worked. It was incomprehensible that a woman could also be fearful of rejection, share doubts about her body, worry about her femininity, and was not a powerful victor poised to reject him. We worked extensively on Mr. G's fantasy that the woman who was truly excited or interested in him was dangerous; he was at risk for becoming swallowed up in her, trapped, and ultimately destroyed by her, especially if she were attractive enough to require competition with other men.

We defined that, for Mr. G, the action of buying was the only safe excursion from passivity. Money was the psychological currency of his childhood that bypassed humiliation, solved problems, and maintained an oasis of passivity; thus the painful journey for mastery need never be entered. For this man, "safe sex" meant an encounter that was purchased (like the analysis), time-limited (like our sessions) and where the woman's sexual passion was "fake." He felt protected by my "not really" having sexual feelings toward him; in the analysis we were entering something "theoretically possible" in order to explore his feelings. The emotional risk he took was minimal; neither of us would actually act out anything with each other. It was hard to fathom that sexual intercourse could be something other than an act of degradation, destruction, and revenge.

Mr. G had for years avoided approaching these fears directly in a relationship with a woman. He had rationalized this avoidance with countless criticisms of dates' appearance or style. He began to realize that his adaptation was perhaps the most profoundly dysfunctional aspect of his entitled passivity and narcissism, and that it was being repeated in the analysis. "Action" could be limited to psychological discussions with me where he never had to actually "do" something. The open-endedness of analysis had become a haven for passivity, the recumbent position a metaphor for avoiding reality outside the office, free association a filibuster and attendance at appointments a substitute for real action. The narcissistic preoccupation with himself at the expense of empathically engaging with another person in an active way, promulgated by his deeply ingrained passivity and avoidance, was costing him emotional fulfillment. He was stunned and finally grieved.

Several significant changes in Mr. G's functioning evolved. Gradually, responsive women seemed less like aggressive attackers needing to be neutralized through sexuality. Instead Mr. G began to feel pleasure in being sexually desired. He became more confrontational with me, pointing out instances in which I had interrupted him or was off the mark. He worked successfully to become the head of a department at his office, to limit his mother's intrusiveness, and rebuff his father's put-downs.

Complaints about how the analysis was not working were replaced by difficult confrontations with himself regarding skirted opportunities to brave what was anxiety-provoking. He incrementally exposed himself to elevators or subways and impelled himself to risk affectionate gestures with dates. Mr. G formed at first an affectionate friendship, and then a sexual relationship, with P who refused to be treated as a purely sexual object. She was insistent on his emotional involvement with her and would not tolerate his tuning her out. This was the first time he was able to effect a loving, emotionally mutual relationship with someone who was also a sexual partner. Mr. G rejoiced in being able to persist with her without "zoning out," becoming bored, or defensively switching off, despite the ambiguities and complexities of the relationship. He felt that while he might not permanently remain with P because of several significant incompatibilities, this relationship represented a major turning point.

Mr. G decided that it was time to talk about ending his analysis. He felt that he had benefited enormously and that his ability to explore the kind of relationship he had with P was why he entered analysis to begin with. He realized that I could not "do it" for him, that the mandate for action was with him. I explored the likelihood that his involvement with P was producing heightened claustrophobia with me and the wish to leave. He thought that was possible, since at times he *was* aware of transient "trapped" feelings with me. However, he had come to realize that he had used analysis to "hide out" from actively dealing with life on his own. The regular meetings and the recumbent position, while helpful in many respects, had allowed him to perpetuate a "lackadaisical, laissez-faire" approach to life. The next step was to continue independently.

Mr. G's resolve persisted even when the relationship with P ended by mutual agreement. She wished to date others, while he was looking to settle down with someone. Mr. G felt that his newfound confidence and drive for independence, as scary as it was, had to be respected by me. He had made his decision to end. Leaving me at this point was qualitatively different from the previous avoidance and need to flee. Mr. G acknowledged that it was scary to separate from me, as it had been from his mother, but he was no longer so afraid of "really growing up." He was finally, adamantly, ready to "leave home." In other words, staying in analysis at this point felt too regressive for him at a time when he needed to make the next developmental spurt on his own.

There were several other aspects to Mr. G's desire to leave and I struggled with what I thought would be most appropriate at this point. I felt he wanted to maintain intact an only partially analyzed transference to me, which had empowered him to effect the relationship with P. This relationship contained many unanalyzed transference displacements. Feeling there was much more to explore, I was reluctant to agree to a termination.

This assessment, however, was mitigated by knowledge of Mr. G's limitations in working analytically. Although there had been enormous clinical improvements and defensive realignments over the course of his analysis, the depth of the analytic process had remained limited by his inability to fully work with the "as-if" nature of the transference, while still maintaining its affective immediacy. That transference feelings have a genetic history had been difficult for Mr. G to apprehend, limiting his ability to simultaneously explore his repressed past as currently revived in our relationship. That feelings for P contained displacements from feelings about me, and in turn were connected to multiple childhood experiences with his mother and sister, seemed too great a cognitive journey of abstraction for Mr. G to make without losing his associated affect along the way.

I was convinced that this limitation was more than defensively motivated resistance alone. It also devolved from the cognitive limitations which had been so amply objectified in the psychological testing several years before. The fact that Mr. G's preexisting cognitive deficits became even more pronounced in areas of conflict and anxiety constituted yet another neuropsychological conundrum. I was pleased with Mr. G's clinical

progress, yet felt sobered by these limitations. I had often imagined that we had progressed over the years through early childhood, to latency, preadolescence, then adolescence proper; he
had finally arrived somewhere in late young adulthood, where
paramount issues were firming independence from the primary parental objects, consolidating earlier gains, and forging
enduring relationships with new objects. I considered that we
had reached the limit of what he was able to accomplish analytically with me.

With these many factors in mind, Mr. G and I set a termination period of six months. During this phase we worked on
many memories about childhood separations, ranging from
leaving his mother for summer camp to the more recent deaths
of his grandparents. Interwoven were attempts to synthesize his
understanding of all that he had learned over the years.
Themes of personal deficiency, feelings of having been deprived of empathic feminine involvement and realistic male
models, his need to avoid anxiety-engendering situations
rather than striving to master them, adapting through passivity,
expecting special treatment and reparations, and fears about
the enigma "Woman" reappeared like a coda for additional
working through and integration.

Mr. G noted more phobic anxiety concerning airplanes,
subways, and the like, but with the resolve that he would either
"do something about it" (e.g., systematically desensitize himself through gradual exposure—a metaphor for the mandate
of personal autonomy) or "learn to live with it." It was hard
for him to recognize that the reappearance of symptoms resulted from a desire to remain in analysis or were an expression
of feelings about termination. It was painful for Mr. G to connect these events to feelings about leaving me and to directly
access feelings about our ending. At his request, he sat up
briefly in an effort to confront his feelings for me more easily
by facing me. Although this was an example of the somewhat
concrete cognitive style that plagued him, it was also an important symbolic action of assertion for Mr. G.

In the final weeks of the analysis, Mr. G and I flagged those
moments when he defensively "switched off" how important I
had become to him and how he grieved losing me. Our last

task seemed to us both to involve circling back to where we had started: Mr. G had gained the conviction that a "real man" could cry without transforming back into a helpless little boy.

DISCUSSION

As has been described in adults with childhood cognitive impairment, Mr. G had an overwhelming sense of defect that made him particularly vulnerable to anxiety about castration, separation, and dependent wishes. In addition, I believe that Mr. G's dyscalculia "dragged" along with it anxiety about his competency with verbal abstract tasks in particular, and produced inhibitions about other types of learning in general. In some ways my patient reminded me of a child with an Attention Deficit/Hyperactivity Disorder who frequently demonstrates sensory hypersensitivity, "catastrophic reactions" such as crying, problems with separation, and phobic concerns. Boredom and restlessness are the typical "shut down" reactions of such children when they feel overwhelmed. Mr. G showed many of these traits as an adult. I did not feel, however, that he warranted a diagnosis of ADHD because inattention was not his primary problem. He could concentrate, but not integrate specific types of nonverbal tasks. While he developed compensatory capacities (such as athletics and expertise in sports trivia) he continued to feel overwhelmingly defective, especially in relation to other men. A rigidity of character and a constriction in dream and fantasy life seemed to me the residua of these early childhood traumata.

Gains were made slowly in this analysis, after months of painstaking effort involving much repetition. It was not dazzling to work with Mr. G. I was often reminded of how children with learning difficulties are experienced as "disappointing." It was necessary to keep clearly in focus my countertransference reactions and expectations of this patient. At times I found myself responding to manifestations of his intelligence and unrealized potential with rescue fantasies, imagining "all he could be if only...." Interpretations had to be repeated multiple

times, more patiently and tactfully than with many other patients. Mr. G needed literal, concrete examples and analogies
to convey the meaning intended in an interpretation. Sometimes he required more of a psychotherapeutic approach,
which offered encouragement and support.

An ongoing technical dilemma involved the limits of his
ability to work directly with the transference. Most of the time
Mr. G required working in transference displacements. In wres-
tling for years with this phenomenon, I have come to understand several elements. First, dealing directly with his feelings
about me heightened his overwhelming claustrophobic panic,
and characterologically led to retreat which jeopardized the
treatment. Working with the transference displacements allowed useful analytic work to continue, but limited the extent
to which the neurosis could be consciously experienced as revived with me. Second, there were intellectual limitations in
Mr. G's ability to abstract the "as-if" nature of transference.
He could only partially grasp how feelings about one person
could contain aspects of feelings about another person. Although markedly improved, Mr. G tended to remain concretely
stimulus bound in his ability to reflect on, experience, and
comprehend transference interpretations. This, too, limited
the immediacy of his conscious experience of the revived infantile neurosis with me. Interestingly, while Mr. G's neuropsychological limitations were not solely the consequence of psychic
conflict, they were generously co-opted to serve defensive and
wish-gratifying aims.

Although Mr. G was highly motivated to change, the analytic work was often hampered by the brittleness of his self-
image. I have wondered if the exquisite vulnerability to self-
observation, which is narcissistically wounding for all analysands, becomes particularly problematic for learning disabled
patients. Like many learning disabled people, Mr. G grew into
adulthood without the clarity of a diagnosis and the promise
offered by therapeutic intervention. His parents trumpeted
their disappointment in his failure to achieve. They blamed
him and prodded him with insults. Unfortunately, this is not a
unique parental reaction to academically disappointing children. I wonder if this predisposes to a kind of sadomasochistic

adaptation in object relationships, hints of which occurred in Mr. G.

Mr. G's parents' obliviousness to their son's undiagnosed cognitive dysfunction led to many empathic failures; they could not mirror their child appropriately. Similarly there were times when I failed to empathize with Mr. G and he with me. It has been said that learning disabled children have as much trouble reading people as they have reading books, and that the "Three R's" of responsiveness, respect for self, and relationships involve perpetual struggle.

Certain aspects of the analytic process were particularly difficult for Mr. G and probably for most learning disabled adult analysands. The inherent deprivations, the tolerance for the unknown, and the "inappropriateness" of the transference caused him difficulty and dismay. We were continually working through his experience of the analysis as "confirmation" of his "defectiveness," replete with memories of "faulty thinking," bad report cards, and disappointed parents and teachers.

Chapter 20

Discussion of Mr. G's Analysis

Dr. Wyszynski's analysis of Mr. G convincingly demonstrates numerous influences upon development that a neuropsychologically based learning disability may have. It also highlights a number of technical considerations concerning diagnostic evaluation, analyzability, and indications for termination. First we will discuss the diagnostic findings and then turn to the ways in which Dr. Wyszynski worked with her learning disabled patient.

In the case of Mr. G the patient already had a diagnostic testing evaluation prior to the referral for analysis. The referring analyst, Dr. A regretted that he had failed to obtain the information (including testing results) required to establish the diagnosis when he originally treated Mr. G at age 14. Dr. A established the presence of a learning disability when Mr. G consulted with him at 27 years of age and referred him to Dr. Wyszynski for analysis.

A history of academic and other problems had alerted Dr. A to the possibility of neuropsychological features. Mr. G had been unable to tie his shoelaces at the usual age, had failed to pass shop, and suffered chronically poor performance in mathematics. This culminated in his failing algebra and receiving poor scores on the quantitative portion of the Graduate Record Examinations. Early assessment would certainly have helped Mr. G, his family, and his therapist to clarify the nature of his academic history and work experience, as well as the manner in which he elaborated upon them psychologically.

Unfortunately when Mr. G had diagnostic testing at the age of 27, the psychologist did not fully mine this opportunity to explore the existence and character of Mr. G's functioning. The presence of a neuropsychologically based learning disability was correctly diagnosed. However, its nature and extent were not carefully detailed.

There were several problems with this evaluation. The terminology used was somewhat misleading. The diagnostic impression reported was of a "positive focus for organic pathology which extended within the mild chronic range." Furthermore, the tester concluded that Mr. G "probably [had] the aftermath of minimal brain dysfunction syndrome from childhood," for which he had learned to compensate in many ways. We would prefer the term "neuropsychological dysfunction" to "organic," since in this case (as in many others, the only exception in this volume being Dr. Miller's patient Julia) there is insufficient evidence of actual organic (i.e., anatomical) change in brain structure. Although the report stated that Mr. G was highly anxious, the clinical picture, including the interrelationships between anxiety and his cognitive deficits, was not clearly delineated. The scope of the evaluation was not sufficiently comprehensive to permit such a study (Rothstein, Benjamin, Crosby, and Eisenstadt, 1988).

The diagnostic assessment also reflects several misconceptions sometimes seen in the literature. One is that "organicity" always accompanies dysfunction. Another is that "organicity" presents in a standard and consistent manner. The psychologist who tested Mr. G regarded his test results as "unusual" for an "organic" patient in that there were "signs of inconsistency." He was surprised that the patient performed one test of visuomotor functioning adequately, while he received low scores on tests of other functions. This reflects a misconception that every test which could reveal neuropsychological dysfunction ought to indicate pathology. Actually inconsistency is quite frequent and even expectable. Patients with neuropsychological dysfunction possess varied patterns of difficulty. For example, a patient may manifest impairment of immediate visual memory and sequencing without difficulties in perceiving or organizing geometric figures or reversing letters, while another will display a different constellation.

Several features of Mr. G's cognitive and emotional functioning *were* reported. He manifested a limitation in verbal concept formation and spatial concept formation (as seen in his weakness in replicating block designs). The psychologist considered his "concrete" and "relatively simplistic" thinking as inherent limitations rather than manifestations of conflict. There were suggestions of weakness in visual memory (based on the relatively few Bender-Gestalt figures Mr. G recalled) although specific tests of visual memory were not administered. In addition, the psychologist attributed a significant discrepancy between the patient's Verbal IQ of 97 and his Performance IQ of 80 (giving him a Full Scale IQ of 88) to the presence of "organicity." At the same time he felt Mr. G's performance scores underestimated his optimal abilities, given the high degree of anxiety and intratest scatter. It is unclear whether the diagnostician thought Mr. G's projective productions suggested a higher than average level of verbal intelligence in general, and in conceptual capacities in particular. Unless the material is extremely constricted, it should be possible to make such a determination, which is of great significance in determining analyzability (Rubovits-Seitz, 1988).

A diagnostic evaluation of Mr. G offered an opportunity to refine our understanding of the components of his neuropsychological and psychodynamic constellation. We ought to have been better able to understand the reasons for his problems with mathematics. Were they related to conceptual limitations, problems in spatial reasoning, and/or other specific cognitive weaknesses? Were they instead a manifestation of his intense performance anxiety due to central conflicts over competitive and sexual wishes, or some combination of these factors? Mr. G was administered one test of mathematics, the Arithmetic subtest of the Wechsler IQ test, but the psychologist did not comment on specific elements of his performance.

Finally, because the data reported were scanty, one cannot evaluate important issues, such as whether Mr. G was realistic in thinking he could not become a lawyer or a diplomat. To determine Mr. G's capabilities, a psychologist would have to study in detail an array of tests of academic skills, as well as more specialized tests of neuropsychological functions. Examinations of academic skills would include tests of various types of reading, mathematics, and written expression and conceptualization. Studies of neuropsychological functions would include different aspects of memory, language, visuomotor skills, and perceptual processing.

With the completion of the testing, the analyst has to consider how to share the findings. Dr. A decided to give Mr. G a general impression, omitting specifics. He told his patient that "everything was normal" except for evidence of a "mild learning difficulty" as a child. Although we do not know why he phrased it as he did, we may surmise that he feared abruptly traumatizing and discouraging Mr. G. Dr. A provided sufficient information so that the patient could decide on an optimal therapeutic journey. As the analysis proceeded, the patient gradually discovered many cognitive difficulties of which he was originally unaware. Dr. Wyzsynski used her knowledge, derived from the test reports and her observation of her patient, to help her patient gain insight, and to make accurate reconstructions about the impact of these cognitive problems.

Now we will turn to Dr. Wyzszynski's fascinating material on the understandings she and Mr. G gained of the interrelationship of his neuropsychological problems and his dynamic conflicts.

Mr. G agreed to the recommendation of analysis. Alert to her patient's cognitive difficulties, Dr. Wyszynski lost no time in using her knowledge to understand her patient's psychopathology and recognizing specific dangers to the analysis. She realized that he would perceive the analysis as similar to childhood situations in which he was required to learn. Indeed he felt as though his analyst, like his parents and teachers, pressed him to learn his lessons and to perform tasks of which he felt incapable. He experienced panic about these anticipated expectations and, using a defensive maneuver he had employed in childhood and still used, he felt like fleeing the situation. Dr. Wyszynski interpreted this transference configuration, with gratifying results. Her patient recognized the patterns of his behavior and discussed his desires to escape, but avoided actual flight. The insights preserved the analysis and furthered it.

In addition, the analyst recognized that she must adapt her style to fit her patient's capabilities. She had to avoid abstract terms and concepts, and had to be concrete in her confrontations and interpretations. Because his parents had often pointed out his deficiencies in a discouraging way and even attacked him for them, she had to be aware that she might inadvertently be misunderstood to imply dire consequences of the difficulties they were uncovering. She had to be alert to interpret his misinterpretations and avoid statements that Mr. G might find devastating. At times she even employed an optimistic tone while recognizing that excessive reassurance could torpedo the analysis. Dr. Wyszynski's concrete explanation that the patient was like a baseball player who could overcome his muscular weakness by exercise and thus become a good pitcher was simple, explanatory, optimistic and uncritical. She was at once able to help Mr. G understand some of the problems he was coping with and encourage his analytic participation without his feeling criticized excessively. A feeling that his analyst maligned him could not be avoided. In fact its appearance in the transference provided a valuable entry into Mr. G's inner world. But a delicate balance had to be achieved in which the fantasy of being criticized, while present, did not exceed the patient's tolerance.

As the analysis proceeded, further insights emerged that clarified the role Mr. G's learning disability played in his psychodynamic constellations. While there was no evidence that it affected him before he entered school, this does not preclude the possibility that it influenced every developmental stage. Certainly limitations in Mr. G's thinking affected his relationships with his parents who may have been sensitive to this even before his school difficulties became manifest. And he must have had difficulty interpreting their behavior even when it was benign.

During the analysis Dr. Wyszynski observed that Mr. G had a serious problem communicating with others. He used words incorrectly; for example, he said "plutonic" when he meant "platonic" and substituted "exasperated" for "exacerbated." We can imagine that when others experienced his errors in linguistic usage they responded with confusion, and perhaps with denigration of him. Quite likely, since Mr. G was unaware of his errors, and may have possessed a receptive as well as an expressive disorder, there was a potential for mutual failures of understanding and empathy during his childhood and later.

As Mr. G grew older a pervasive sense of inferiority developed. Once he was able to compare himself with others, he himself noticed his relative deficiency. This was accentuated by his parents actually berating him, calling him lazy and unwilling to overcome his troubles. His teachers too remarked on his ineptitude and underlined it in black and white on his report cards. Even when his marks were reasonably adequate, his parents remained dissatisfied; they transferred him to a more competitive school, simultaneously depriving him of his friends and camaraderie.

Mr. G's feelings of deficiency because of his learning disability magnified other normal developmental fantasies and conflicts. A preoedipal sense of incompleteness may have been accentuated in retrospect, especially as Mr. G felt he needed a powerful parent to complete him and make him feel whole. Normal castration anxiety was certainly intensified by his feeling inferior and vulnerable.

Positive and negative oedipal wishes appeared in exaggerated and even distorted form. Mr. G's parents' actual behavior influenced his oedipal urges, but so too did his own inner propensities which influenced his perception of his parents. His mother repeatedly urged him to work and be independent, so much so that his feelings of being nagged became an essential element in his psyche; he developed a desire to please his mother and obtain her love through getting her to pressure him. Furthermore, Mr. G felt he could not achieve the goals she set. This was, in part, an expression of his realistic evaluation but also of his need to avoid success, particularly oedipal success.

He had strong feelings for his father as a man. He admired powerful men like football players and hoped to acquire their strength through contact with them, sometimes with a masochistic coloring. This we assume derived from Mr. G's wishes to obtain power from his capable, successful, but dissatisfied father. Sexualization of his wishes to acquire power led to the very homosexual wishes Mr. G feared.

Mr. G's antagonistic feelings toward his parents appeared not only as a reflection of rivalry, but also as an expression of irritation that they both demanded too much of him, and were constantly unhappy about his performance. We assume that Mr. G also became unhappy as a result of frustration when he was unable to achieve his own goals or live up to his own ideals; he not only attacked himself, but also directed his anger at his parents. The common dynamic of fury on the part of learning disabled children toward adults whom they believe to have failed them in not recognizing their condition was not apparent during Mr. G's analysis.

In any case, the presence of intense rage from these sources, as well as strong positive and negative oedipal wishes, require defenses to keep impulses under control. Mr. G used a variety of defenses, many of which derived from the way he dealt with his learning disability and the family interactions that emerged. Some of his defenses were determined in part by the characteristics of his learning disabilities; that is, he could use his learning difficulties for defensive purposes. Mr. G felt defective and harmless, a stance which provided a "safe haven" from violent, competitive wishes toward those he loved and needed, while at the same time expressing these very wishes.

Dr. Wyszynski attempts to differentiate between a primary cognitive disorder and one based on conflict. At the same time she implies that it is impossible for totally nonconflictual manifestations to appear. We agree with her in assuming that the existence of a nonconflictually based failure to comprehend or to become confused is a myth. Rather the patient's primary cognitive disturbance soon becomes immersed in conflict and is used defensively. Nevertheless it may sometimes be valuable for patient and analyst to distinguish primary and secondary aspects of his or her difficulties. For example, Dr. Wyszynski attempted to show Mr. G when he was confused and bewildered because of his neuropsychological disturbance and when the confusion was employed as a defense. However, such differentiations were sometimes difficult to make.

Dr. Wyszynski noted that Mr. G had "difficulty expanding on transference fantasies, in addition to . . . [a] tendency to discount reactions to" Dr. Wyszynski. On the one hand the learning disability involved failure to understand the meaning of words and sentences, especially if they were abstract, and to appreciate the abstract and "as if" aspects of the transference. At times Mr. G could not understand the analyst's interpretations or develop a feel for the irrational aspects of the transference. On the other hand, he could become confused or fail to comprehend as a means of averting anxiety or other noxious affects; he would in effect utilize his cognitive difficulties defensively to avoid disturbing emotions.

Because of cognitive difficulties, Mr. G was especially upset about being illogical. He and Dr. Wyszynski referred to his reaching incorrect conclusions as "1 + 1 = 3." Mr. G's logical failures did not occur randomly. Analyst and patient observed his tendentious quality; he would reach the most devastating conclusions. For instance, he would say that "since math was hard for him, therefore he must be stupid." Or "since he questioned his manliness, therefore he must be a homosexual." Mr. G thus used his learning disability to attack himself. In this way he not only satisfied superego demands for punishment but also identified with his parents, especially his father, who attacked him. After all his parents too used non sequiturs, such as, "if you have trouble studying, you must be lazy and procrastinating."

Mr. G's learning disability made it very difficult to accomplish tasks that others achieve relatively easily. As a result his self-esteem suffered. In addition, as Dr. Wyszynski succinctly states, he "lacked the mastery-oriented attitude toward obstacles that would have allowed him to sustain confidence, striving, and hope." This predicament could be used defensively. Mr. G could thwart fearful oedipal accomplishments through a conviction that he could not succeed. If he did accomplish forbidden goals, he could mobilize his sense of inevitable failure to defensively deprecate his victory, and at the same time punish himself for his wishes. Through analysis and the successful attainment of insight and improvement, Mr. G began to feel he could achieve mastery. Dr. Wyzsynski would sometimes underline Mr. G's achievements to fortify his recognition of his capabilities. However, she recognized that it was best to be careful not to be excessively supportive.

Difficulties learning and understanding can produce boredom because the work is highly frustrating and/or uninteresting. The boredom can then be used defensively, as occurred with Mr. G. When he became anxious at being pressed to do schoolwork that was too much for him, he reacted with a boredom that tended to dispel anxiety. Boredom could then be used to protect himself in other situations, as when painful emotions appeared in the analysis.

Failures could be used aggressively. As a child Mr. G recognized the pain his parents suffered when he bungled. He could thus hurt them through his cognitive failures with their untoward consequences. Similarly in the transference he could frustrate his analyst by not understanding her and not profiting from her interventions. He could attempt to produce a sadomasochistic interaction in which his foiled analyst would become angry and even sadistic. Or he could try to evoke an affectionate desire to save the patient from his emotional bankruptcy. In that way he could create a parent who was different from his own deficient father and mother, mitigating the need to be angry at his parents or analyst. Dr. Wyszynski was impressed with the fact that, at times, she did desire to rescue Mr. G.

We may surmise from Mr. G's reported memories and his transferences that his parents reacted to their son's pathology in a variety of ways. They appeared narcissistically wounded by their son's deficiencies, as if his failure made them deficient. They became angry at his putting them in that position, and attacked him for it. They criticized him, but tried to rescue him. At the same time his father may have denigrated Mr. G even if he had no learning disability, because he considered him an oedipal rival. Mr. G's parents' behavior served to facilitate particular defensive maneuvers: denial, stoicism, escape, intellectualization, and isolation.

We will discuss each of these.

Mr. G's cognitive disabilities caused his parents great pain which they attempted to minimize through defenses, including denial. Narcissistically disturbed by their son's deficiency and his subsequent school difficulties, they attempted to turn away

from what caused this. Rather than recognize his basic incapac-
ity, they attributed his failures to laziness and blamed the
school. Instead of realizing that his school had failed to diagnose his disorder, they sent him to another school in which his
difficulties remained unrecognized. Nor did Mr. G's parents
appreciate that they were further taxing their son by interfering
with his friendships.

Mr. G identified with them in utilizing denial. He too did
not perceive the causes of his trouble. Denial is basically a failure
in perception of the world about one. The patient's denial may
have been facilitated by specific aspects of his neuropsychological disorder, such as the suggestion of weakness in visual memory, which would affect the accuracy with which he discerned the
world about him. In the absence of a detailed diagnostic evaluation, the relationships between the neuropsychological contribution and central defenses cannot be determined. Mr. G used
denial not only as a defense against recognizing the nature of his
troubles, but in other areas as well.

Mr. G's defensive use of stoicism and flight was catalyzed
by his mother's encouragement of her son to "bite the bullet"
and press on when he faced adversity. She forced him to isolate
himself and study, even when the odds were against success
because he did not have appropriate tutoring or other educational help for his learning difficulties. She also insisted that
he be impassive, forcing him to "tough it out" at sleep-away
camp when he was miserable and wanted to go home. This
defensive maneuver, which he called "stoical" and which involved denial as well, was not effective. Although at times Mr.
G could master his anxiety through a stoical determination,
often enough the anxiety snowballed until he had to attempt
to flee from the distressing situation. This defense formed a
basis for his phobic symptoms and behavior.

Mr. G's mother encouraged certain phobic symptoms by
promoting the feeling that he must try to both remain in and
escape from a claustrum and that being away from home was
dangerous. He also feared being in enclosures as well as out in
the unprotecting and threatening world. He feared examinations so much that he, at times, ran out of the room in which
they were given. No doubt Mr. G's anxiety interfered with his

cognitive capacities and thus with his ability to succeed on tests as well. Mr. G also used flight as a defense in other situations. He feared and then avoided attendance at ball games for complicated reasons. For example, the aggression and disguised homosexuality at the games frightened him, prompting his wish to escape.

It may seem paradoxical that Mr. G, who had such great difficulty using his mind well, should have employed intellectualization as a defense. In fact one of the things that made analysis interesting to Mr. G was that he liked to figure things out, even though he was often convinced that he could not succeed in doing so. His mother was a former college administrator who admired hard work and achievement. His family ideals, which he adopted, included the use of the brain. Mr. G's parents wanted so much for him to be an intellectual person that they sent him to a private school they thought would be helpful to him in this regard. The patient, being basically intelligent, sought friends who were bright and wanted to succeed.

We have not yet focused on the appearance of sexual feelings toward Dr. Wyszynski and the ways in which these became intermeshed with the transferences related to his learning disabilities. At first Mr. G expressed his erotic transferences by engaging in intercourse with a female psychotherapist who was somewhat older than he, and seeking treatment by a male massage therapist who he said was "more an alchemist than a doctor." Mr. G came to recognize that he wanted Dr. Wyszynski to be more personally involved with him, but feared that a "hands on" approach would be "too erotic." He responded to the intensifying transference with fantasies of leaving the analysis. Wanting the analyst, he felt dependent, vulnerable, and less masculine. The analyst appeared to be a sexual threat (like his mother who walked about the house wearing only a bra and slip), as well as a source of pressure to work in the analysis (as his mother had tried to force him to do schoolwork and now urged him to quit the analysis). Sadomasochistic fantasies started to appear.

Before long Mr. G began to have actual sexual feelings on the couch. The analysis was experienced as foreplay, but without the gratification of completing the sex act. Talk of sexuality in the transference appeared in conjunction with wishing the analyst would "push him harder" as his mother had. Flight and boredom and then homosexual fears appeared as defenses. Mr. G began to recognize that sexual feelings were associated with being trapped and forced to do things. On the one hand he was being mistreated. On the other hand, he felt that his amorous feelings toward his analyst demeaned and degraded her, making her a prostitute.

As Mr. G talked about his sexual wishes, his symptoms started to fade. Interpretation of the effects of his learning disability became a less prominent focus, although Dr. Wyszynski remained alert to its persistent influence. Central at this point was the way in which Mr. G experienced women as embodiments of the core phobic situation. This was related to his feelings and fantasies about his mother, as well as the analyst in the transference. Mr. G's mother pressured him to depend on her, trying to make herself the center of his universe and arranging for blind dates. As he became more independent of her, she encouraged him to quit the analysis. He temporarily interrupted the treatment, which he ultimately resumed, because he needed to satisfy his mother and because getting close to Dr. Wyszynski frightened him. He feared being engulfed, being inside a woman, and more specifically having his penis inside a woman's body. His fear of losing his genitals to his mother appeared more prominently in the analysis than his anxiety about being castrated by his father. However, Mr. G did express wishes and fears of castrating his father and being castrated by him.

A month after quitting the analysis Mr. G returned. He and Dr. Wyszynski discussed his motives for leaving, including his need to be in control. He was pleased that Dr. Wyszynski let him take charge by attending sessions less than four times a week until he was ready to resume a full schedule. His symptoms diminished markedly as a result of the analytic work in the context of his being able to exert control and feel potent. Less phobic, he could take short plane trips and attend the theater and football games without anxiety.

The learning disability, although not the center of attention of the analysis at this point, was still important. One reason

Mr. G ended the analysis was his anger about Dr. Wyszynski's inability to wave a magic wand to cure him; she could not do the analysis *for* him. His mother had tried to intervene and magically set things right; she had hired people to correct his difficulties and Mr. G had the fantasy he was doing the same when he engaged Dr. Wyszynski to analyze him.

Dr. Wyszynski kept her eye on her patient's difficulties with abstraction. Her use of metaphor in her interpretations contained a careful balance of the concrete and the general. Mr. G better understood when she said that he used a "circuit breaker" between sexuality and love. Later she showed him that he was able to temporarily reconnect the two wires. He himself talked of the analyst's "handing him a cure on a silver platter."

In the fifth year of analysis Mr. G decided to talk about ending his analysis. He had achieved the kind of relationship with a woman, P, for which he had entered analysis. During the termination phase, a series of problems directly related to the learning disability arose. As the treatment comes to a close it is optimal for patient and analyst to evaluate the results of their work together. Mr. G had done rather well. He had overcome many of his symptoms, had achieved insight into the role of his learning disability, and learned to cope with it effectively in many ways. He was able to accomplish previously forbidden goals. But, of course, some problems remained.

Despite this Mr. G was eager to end treatment and escape the trap he felt analysis could be. In her report Dr. Wyszynski describes little of the usual disappointment and antagonism that erupts at termination, perhaps because of the defenses Mr. G erected that prevented their appearance.

Reading between the lines of Dr. Wyszynski's discussion of Mr. G's termination, one can see her concern about the outcome of the treatment as she gauged how close to the ideal the analysis had come. She describes her attempts to decide whether she had done right by her patient. Reluctantly, she reached the conclusion that, although a great deal was achieved in their analytic work together, Mr. G's learning disability limited what he could accomplish. His conceptual limitations in grasping the "as if" nature of the transference, while experiencing its affective immediacy, seriously interfered with the achievement of insight.

At the same time Dr. Wyszynski recognized that opposing Mr. G's desire to end treatment would interfere with his attempts at independence. It seems inevitable that a man such as Mr. G with a complex of preoedipal and oedipally based conflicts, as well as cognitive difficulties, would require a lengthy analysis. We feel that, although perhaps more could have been achieved in a more prolonged analysis, the analytic gains were impressive.

Conclusion

This book is intended both to sensitize analysts to the presence of learning disabilities in selected cases in which they might not consider this possibility, and to elaborate diagnostic and therapeutic considerations in working with such patients. We have stressed the importance of attending to the specific features of a patient's neuropsychological dysfunction and the individual ways in which this dysfunction contributes to development and psychic conflict. The process of analytic discovery is enriched by an exploration of the interrelationships between the patient's particular cognitive difficulties (e.g., disturbances in perception, memory, and receptive or expressive language) and his or her wishes, defenses, moral concerns, and affects, as well as the shaping influences of the environment. Thus the neuropsychological becomes interwoven with and shapes the distinctive configuration of an individual's psychic conflicts in general, and his unconscious fantasies in particular (Rothstein, 1992, 1998). We have also described the nature of the comprehensive diagnostic evaluation which facilitates such an understanding.

While maintaining an emphasis on the specific features of individual patients in this regard, some of the trends which emerged in the nine cases in this book may be useful to bear in mind. Our study revealed some commonalities in the patients' vulnerabilities, dynamics, transference configurations, and issues relevant to successful analytic collaboration. These are offered as potential (but by no means invariant) considerations in psychoanalytic work with patients with learning disabilities.

INTENSIFICATION OF CONFLICT

Although the specific clinical features of the nine patients' learning disabilities varied, the presence of a learning disability appeared to heighten neurotic conflict. There were a number of reasons for this which we could identify. The presence of the disability frequently compromised patients' abilities to achieve satisfaction, since they were subject to repeated experiences of frustration and poor performance, when compared with their peers, even when they exerted great effort. This contributed to anger at their parents and teachers who did not recognize their difficulties or, when they did, were unable to prevent such experiences. Feeling neglected and abandoned, these analysands frequently blamed their parents for their defects.

In addition many experienced an intensification of sexual desires. In part this served as a defense against their rage. It also arose from the greater than usual need of such patients to depend on their parents to help them learn, control their impulses, and adapt in a world that was particularly difficult for them in some respects. In only one case (Leah/Barrett)[1] was difficulty traversing separation-individuation and intensified rapprochement substage conflict a clear-cut feature; however, we imagine that more subtle preoedipal disturbances were even more common, but often difficult to analyze (Julia/ Miller, for instance). Oedipal conflict can be exaggerated by the necessity of greater than ordinary parental involvement with a child with neuropsychologically based difficulties. In extreme cases (for example, Dr. Gilmore's patient's experience of being tutored and given medication by her father), it is particularly likely that the competitive and sexual urges of this phase of development will be even more accentuated.

Similarly parental demands regarding learning may accentuate the impact of persisting anal stage conflicts. The child may rebel against his mother's or teacher's pressing him to do schoolwork, as if he were still being urged to participate in toilet training. Conversely an especially intense early toileting experience may make later academic achievement difficult (Leah/Barrett).

In addition, distractibility and impulsivity of neuropsychological etiology (e.g., in patients with ADHD) may result in a

---

[1] Throughout this chapter we refer to specific cases by placing the patient's pseudonym and the name of the analyst in parentheses. The examples given are not all inclusive.

heightened proclivity for conflict with parents and others in the patient's environment. Lack of verbal facility may also contribute to a penchant for expression through activity. Another neuropsychologically determined condition we noted was a perceptual hypersensitivity that may have contributed to the prominence of anxiety in some patients (Leah/Barrett, Rebecca/Gilmore).

In many of our cases pronounced conflicts surrounded achievement and standards of right and wrong. This was sometimes related to a discordance between the patient's capabilities and his or her own aspirations, as well as with parental demands for a high level of performance. Parents frequently set high standards which their children internalized but could not achieve. A number of the parents were characterologically perfectionistic and found it difficult to bear their sons' or daughters' weaknesses or failures. Some of our patients reacted to such desires (their own and those of their parents) for a more perfect state with anger and projection as seen, for example, in their berating others for failing to attain perfection. The existence of a learning disability can also influence the superego in other respects (Julia/Miller, Frank/Waldron). In Dr. Waldron's case the patient's misunderstanding of adults due to his receptive language disorder contributed to his thinking they were untruthful; he identified with them and became untruthful himself. The fact that Frank's parents encouraged dishonesty solidified these identifications. His sense of defect further promoted his desire to cheat, as in the psychology of the exception. There were times when patients who carried out their wishes for gratification, experienced as forbidden, sought to assuage a sense of guilt by inviting punishment.

The patients studied typically regarded themselves as defective and suffered from self-esteem problems. This laid the foundation for an even more intense experience of depressive affect, when other determinants of depression (e.g., guilt or self-directed rage) appeared. It was also common for feelings of deficiency and intense shame to be associatively linked with fantasies of being inferior as a female or a castrated male.

The brain was frequently selected as the organ of inferiority. Some patients felt their brains were damaged; others thought they were lacking a brain. At times they expressed greater concern for some other part of the body, the genitals for instance. But patients generally focused on the brain because the experience of neuropsychological dysfunction potentiated a focus on this part of the body. In some cases, a patient remembered a past experience in which there was a brain injury. Past or current bodily sensations associated with brain damage could also be recalled, as was the case with Julia, Dr. Miller's patient. She had cerebral bleeding in infancy and suffered from repeated petit mal seizures, during which she lost consciousness and, with that, contact with those she loved. It is also possible for a patient to have been told of past episodes in which brain damage occurred, or to have heard (after a psychiatric consultation or psychological testing) that he or she is cognitively disabled or suffered from some type of "brain damage." Other patients may deduce that something is wrong with their brains from experiences of lack of control or impulsive behavior.

SHAPING OF DEFENSIVE PROCLIVITIES

We found that many of our learning disabled patients had a propensity for particular defenses which was potentiated by their neuropsychological dysfunction. Denial, reversal, and employment of the learning disability or Attention Deficit/Hyperactivity Disorder for defensive purposes were common. So too was the appearance of a configuration of defenses, superego demands, and drive derivatives to produce a sadomasochistic picture.

Denial is defined as a "primitive or early defense mechanism by which an individual unconsciously repudiates some or all of the meanings of an event. . . . The ego thus avoids awareness of some painful aspect of reality and so diminishes anxiety or other unpleasurable affects" (Moore and Fine, 1990, p. 50). Since denial involves problems in the perception of reality, it is not surprising that people with learning disabilities which involve poor or distorted perception were prone to utilize this defense (Leah/Barrett, Frank/Waldron, Rebecca/Gilmore, Mr. Young/Green). Combined with this neuropsychological foundation was the contribution of the frequent denial by parents of their children's disabilities. They did so in the service of overcoming their sense of narcissistic insult, their shame, their humiliation, and their anger at their learning disabled offspring. The patient, identifying with his father or mother, had a penchant for denial as well.

We thought it was likely that patients who had difficulties with visual or auditory memory would be predisposed to rely upon repression, a phenomenon we have observed in other patients. However, this was not a prominent feature of the population studied in this book, although there was some mention of it in the case of Ms. Ames; she displayed an amalgam of intense psychic conflict and visual memory weakness, i.e., difficulty in retrieving visually registered memories.

Reversal in the form of turning from a passive state, in which one is the victim, to an active position occurred frequently, but did not seem to be directly facilitated by a neuropsychological disturbance. Rather many of the patients described felt like victims, or *were* actual victims, as others attacked and criticized them. In an attempt to avoid feeling defective and inferior, they identified with the aggressor and treated others as deficient (Eric/Yanof, Leah/Barrett, Rebecca/Gilmore). (Barrett's patient also made defensive use of reversal in a different sense. Her sequencing problems which were probably of neuropsychological origin, manifested in reversing letters and word sounds, were also a channel for expression of disguised aggressive and sexual wishes.) Defensive grandiosity was another common way of dealing with their deep sense of inferiority.

Many of our patients employed their neuropsychological difficulties for defensive purposes. By failing they could regressively avoid the fantasied consequences of a forbidden oedipal victory and/or remain in an infantile relationship with their parents, or their analysts in the transference (Frank/Waldron, Rebecca/Gilmore). In a similar way patients who believed that they could not succeed, even if they tried (Frank/Waldron, Mr. G/Wyszynski, Rebecca/Gilmore), often relinquished their efforts. Unconsciously they felt, why exert the effort when you will inevitably fail at school or at work? Development of a defensive stance of not caring was thus invoked to avoid disappointment and shame. This sometimes took an overdetermined sadomasochistic form (Glenn and Bernstein, 1995). Disabilities (e.g., motor coordination problems which affected the tying of shoelaces) could be used to taunt and provoke parents, who themselves harbored unconscious wishes to engage in relationships of this sort (Frank/Waldron, Rebecca/Gilmore, Mr. Young/Green). Some patients unconsciously failed or sought attack as punishment for superego violations. Sexual pleasure could be derived from such self-destructive or self-punitive tendencies.

TECHNICAL ISSUES

While there is nothing unique about the psychoanalysis of patients with learning disabilities, or other manifestations of neuropsychological dysfunction, a number of specific technical issues arose in our nine cases.

The patient's suspicions or fantasies of "brain damage" may create a dilemma for the analyst. He will not want to support a patient's denial of this possibility, but rather to interpret such defensive activity. However, excessively abrupt confrontation or even interpretation of the patient's denial of a disability may be so upsetting that he becomes unable to face the truth of his condition. By contrast, in some instances the analysand may turn to the neuropsychological explanation of his difficulties to the exclusion of the psychodynamic determinants.

A great deal of tact and conceptual scope is required to maintain a proper balance. Optimally the analyst will be able to focus first on one area, then on another, and eventually to integrate the various aspects interpretively. In the case of a child patient, his cognition may not be sufficiently mature to permit him to fully understand the relationship between brain and behavior. However, such a failure of understanding is probably also attributable to the emotional impact of such connections. This is certainly true as well for adult patients with learning disabilities or other neuropsychological difficulties. Some patients cannot fully face the possibility of neuropsychological dysfunction and its effect on cognition; thus interpretation of this aspect of their personalities remains incomplete. At other times the analysis of frightening unconscious fears of damage, from which the anxiety about brain functioning has been displaced, permits a marked diminution of worries about the brain.

Other technical issues were highlighted by our cases. When the need for psychological testing arises during the course of the analysis, the analyst may have to prepare the patient for this consultation which he may resist taking or may even find traumatic (Julia/Miller). Once this evaluation is completed, the analyst has to decide whether and how much to tell his patient, and how to integrate the test findings into the ongoing analytic exploration of the patient's conflicts and unconscious fantasies. The analyst may rely on the psychologist to report the results to the patient, the patient may read the test report, or the analyst may explain the results himself; a combination of methods of conveying this information is also possible. The analyst has simultaneously to analyze with the patient his fantasies about the testing process and the role of the learning disability in his development and current life.

Since the analyst may only appreciate the importance of his patient's cognitive difficulties for the first time following the diagnostic evaluation, his understanding of the patient and/or aspects of technique may require modification. Previous suspicions may be confirmed and details of neuropsychological aspects of the patients' conflicts may be clarified as well. In some instances the analyst may alter his way of speaking to his patient. For example, he may become more concrete in his interpretations, avoiding abstractions the patient may not understand (Mr. G/Wyszynski) and explaining what he means in greater detail (Frank/Waldron, Mr. G/Wyszynski). This is not to say that abstractions will be avoided. What may sometimes be mistaken for concreteness can in fact be a manifestation of the efforts of analyst and patient to create a shorthand way of communicating an issue. An example was Dr. Wyszynski and her patient's use of the phrase, "1 + 1 = 3," to signify that he reached incorrect conclusions (as when he decided that he was a homosexual because he thought of men).

The knowledge gained from a diagnostic evaluation may also enable the analyst to broaden his interpretations. To illustrate, the patient may be helped to see that difficulties with spatial concepts and sequencing contribute to obsessive symptoms and slowness, as well as being a product of identification with the family's characteristics of perfectionism, order, and cleanliness (Ms. Ames/Green).

Awareness of the patient's neuropsychological (or frankly neurological) problems may alert the analyst to hitherto unrecognized, but important features of the patient's bodily experiences. For example, Dr. Miller helped Julia identify bodily feelings connected with petit mal seizures and periods of confusion resulting from her neurological state, and attempted to differentiate this from confusion due to conflict and fear of object loss. This set the stage for the analysis of Julia's terrifying unconscious fantasies of abandonment and injury. Dr. Yanof's analysis of Eric included an awareness of his somatic feelings of lack of control, which he experienced as "crazy" and explosive. He expressed and identified these through drawings which he produced with his analyst. In this manner they proceeded beyond the surface to discover the unconscious conflictual fantasies he harbored.

Generally child analyses involve action to a greater degree than adult analyses. The impulsive behavior of child patients, which may be an especially great problem in cases of ADHD, may require the analyst's verbal or even physical restraint. In learning disabled children (including those without ADHD) who have difficulties with expressive language, expression through action rather than words may be fostered. To illustrate, as her patient Eric's impulsiveness dominated the sessions, Dr. Yanof skillfully verbalized what he was doing and how he felt, bringing his behavior into the analytic arena. Eventually she could interpret the significance of this behavior. As his verbalization provided another channel for expression of his emotions, it served to control his impulsiveness.

OUTCOME

We cannot gauge the degree and frequency of success analysis affords patients with learning disabilities from the reports of a mere nine cases. This is especially true since the nature of the disabilities treated varied so greatly. Nevertheless, we are impressed with the fine results in the six patients who started analysis when children or adolescents, as well as the three adult patients. Some of these patients did well, even though the tutoring or medication recommended by the analyst or other professionals who became involved with these patients were not instituted, sometimes because the families did not accept them.

Despite the presence of serious learning difficulties, most of the child and adolescent patients fared well academically. One patient entered law school after scoring in the 98.4 percentile on an untimed LSAT (Frank/Waldron). He also did well socially. A second patient had a rocky postanalytic course. After the analysis she entered college but, with her parents' encouragement, dropped out rather than seek further cognitive evaluation and psychotherapeutic help. However, after a period of time she returned to psychotherapy with her analyst, completed college, and entered graduate school (Rebecca/Gilmore). Another patient changed from a restless, active child who could not achieve academically to a normally quiet and social child who could concentrate and earn A's and B's (Eric/Yanof). (Despite this, his parents believed he did not perform up to his potential.) One child became well adapted socially and academically, but continued to require tutoring after the analysis (Leah/Barrett). Another child did well academically and socially without the remedial help which had been recommended (Andy/Peltz). The analyses of Dr. Green's two adult patients were also remarkable for their results. These two patients came to understand and adapt to their learning disabilities which, although persistent, had a significantly less compromising effect on their overall functioning personally and in work.

Still another patient, Julia (Miller), had persistent neurological problems but made remarkable improvements academically and socially, especially in light of her frank brain damage

as an infant. Although her physicians had deemed her progno-
sis dim, her parents demonstrated extraordinary persistence
in pursuing many types of treatments. While her neurological
condition remained and she required anticonvulsants, she did
remarkably well in school and in her family. That treatment is
still ongoing.

There were limits in other cases as well. Dr. Wyszynski decided not to oppose her adult patient's desire to end the analysis, in part because she thought his cognitive limitations
compromised the degree of insight he could acquire, and
hence the extent of symptom relief possible. This was despite
the fact that his symptoms receded significantly and his ability
to function independently, which included having a satisfying
romantic life, was greatly enhanced.

THE ANALYST'S EMOTIONAL REACTIONS

The analyst of learning disabled patients may grapple with a
desire to achieve a perfect result in which even a neuropsychologically based learning disability disappears. We believe in
those cases in which there is such an etiology, the disability will
remain after the analysis, although the patient may learn to
cope with it, and find means of compensating for or navigating
around his deficiency. Unfortunately, in all but one of our cases
we do not have the benefit of diagnostic testing both before
and after the analysis. Thus we could not assess the degree to
which cognitive disabilities were diminished or analysands better coped with these disabilities as a result of analysis. In the one
case in which an evaluation was done years after the treatment
(during a follow-up), a learning disability remained (Frank/
Waldron).

Although we have not had the experience of analyzing
analysts who have treated patients with learning disabilities, we
have speculated about potential unconscious fantasies. The fact
that analysts work with their brains, and value their intelligence
and insight, may affect their work with the learning disabled.
Their intense investment in thinking may result in a blind spot,

a reluctance to recognize neuropsychological disorders in patients with whom they identify. Awareness of one's own heightened investment in thinking will, one hopes, help the analyst understand his or her patients' struggles with cognitive difficulties.

Certainly the analysts who contributed to this volume have demonstrated their emerging awareness of the inevitable intertwining of the neuropsychological with wishes, defenses, superego elements, affects and environmental influences in their patients' psychic development: the major emphasis of this book. As we worked together to develop their cases and our discussions for publication, we experienced a rich process of discovery of unexpected interrelationships, making this an enriching collaboration for all involved.

References

Abend, S. M., Porder, M. S., & Willick, M. S. (1983), *Borderline Patients.* New York: International Universities Press.

Abraham, K. (1924), The influence of oral eroticism in character formation and contributions to the theory of the anal character. In: *Selected Papers.* London: Hogarth Press, 1965, pp. 393–406.

Abrams, J. C., & Kaslow, V. (1976), Learning disability and family dynamics: A mutual interaction. *J. Clin. Child Psychol.,* 5:35–40.

Aleksandrowicz, D., & Aleksandrowicz, M. (1987), Psychodynamic approach to low self-esteem related to developmental deviations: Growing up incompetent. *J. Amer. Acad. Child Adol. Psychiatry,* 26:583–595.

Allen, J. G., Lewis, L., Peebles, M. J., & Pruyser, P. W. (1986), Neuropsychological assessment in a psychoanalytic setting: The mind–body problems in clinical practice. *Bull. Menninger Clin.,* 50:5–21.

American Psychiatric Association (1980), *Diagnostic and Statistical Manual of Mental Disorders,* 3rd ed. (DSM-III). Washington, DC: American Psychiatric Press.

——— (1987), *Diagnostic and Statistical Manual of Mental Disorders,* 3rd ed. rev. (DSM-III-R). Washington, DC: American Psychiatric Press.

——— (1991), *DSM-IV Options Book: Work in Progress.* Washington, DC: American Psychiatric Press.

——— (1994), *Diagnostic and Statistical Manual of Mental Disorders,* 4th ed. (DSM-IV). Washington, DC: American Psychiatric Press.

Andersen, H. C. (1981), The little mermaid. In: *Michael Hague's Favorite Hans Christian Andersen Fairy Tales.* New York: Henry Holt.

Anthony, E. J. (1973), A psychodynamic model of minimal brain dysfunction. *Ann. NY Acad. Sci.,* 205:52–60.

Arlow, J. A. (1969), Unconscious fantasy and disturbances of conscious experience. *Psychoanal. Quart.,* 38:1–27.

Athey, G. I. (1986), Implications of memory impairment for hospital treatment. *Bull. Menninger Clin.,* 50:99–110.

Barkley, R. A. (1990), *Attention Deficit Hyperactivity Disorder: A Handbook for Diagnosis and Treatment.* New York: Guilford.

473

Baumgardner, T., & Reiss, A. L. (1994), Fragile x syndrome. In: *Learning Disorder Spectrum: ADD, ADHD and LD,* ed. A. J. Capute, P. J. Accardo, & B. K. Shapiro. Baltimore: York Press, pp. 67–84.

Beitchman, J. H., & Young, A. R. (1997), Learning disorders with special emphasis on reading disorders: A review of the last 10 years. *J. Amer. Acad. Child Adol. Psychiatry,* 36:1020–1032.

Benson, D. F. (1993), Aphasia. In: *Clinical Neuropsychology,* 3rd ed., ed. K. M. Heilman & E. Valenstein. New York: Oxford University Press, pp. 17–36.

Beres, D., & Brenner, C. (1950), Mental reactions in patients with neurological disease. *Psychoanal. Quart.,* 19:170–191.

Berger, M., & Kennedy, H. (1975), Pseudobackwardness in children; maternal attitudes as an etiological factor. *The Psychoanalytic Study of the Child,* 30:279–306. New Haven, CT: Yale University Press.

Black, W. F. (1974), The word explosion in learning disabilities: A notation of literature trends, 1962–1972. *J. Learn. Dis.,* 7:323–325.

Blanchard, P. (1946), Psychoanalytic contributions to the problems of reading disabilities. *The Psychoanalytic Study of the Child,* 2:163–187. New York: International Universities Press.

Bornstein, B. (1930), Zur Psychogenese der Pseudodebilitat. *Internat. J. Psycho-Anal.,* 16:378–399.

Brenner, C. (1976), *Psychoanalytic Technique and Psychic Conflict.* New York: International Universities Press.

——— (1982), *The Mind in Conflict.* New York: International Universities Press.

Breuer, J., & Freud, S. (1893–1895), Studies on Hysteria. *Standard Edition,* 2. London: Hogarth Press, 1955.

Buchholz, E. S. (1987), The legacy from childhood: Considerations for treatment of the adult with learning disabilities. *Psychoanal. Inq.,* 7:431–452.

Burka, A. A. (1983), The emotional reality of a learning disability. *Annals of Dyslexia,* 33:289–302.

Burland, J. A. (1984), Dysfunctional parenthood in a deprived population. In: *Parenthood: A Psychodynamic Perspective,* ed. R. Cohen, B. Cohler, & S. Weisman. New York: Guilford, pp. 148–163.

——— (1986), The vicissitudes of maternal deprivation. In: *Self and Object Constancy,* ed. R. Lax, A. Black, & J. A. Burland. New York: Guilford, pp. 324–348.

Buskirk, J. R. (1992), Headlock: Psychotherapy of a patient with multiple neurological and psychiatric problems. *Bull. Menninger Clin.,* 56:361–378.

Buxbaum, E. (1964), The parents' role in the etiology of learning disabilities. *The Psychoanalytic Study of the Child,* 19:421–447. New York: International Universities Press.

Casey, J. E., Rourke, B. P., & Picard, E. M. (1991), Syndrome of nonverbal learning disabilities: Age differences in neuropsychological, academic and socioemotional functioning. *Dev. Psychopathol.,* 3:329–345.

Chelune, G. J., Ferguson, W., Koon, R., & Dickey, T. O. (1986), Frontal lobe disinhibition in attention deficit disorder. *Child Psychiat. Hum. Dev.,* 16:221–232.

Chernow, B. A., & Valassi, G. A. (1993), *The Columbia Encyclopedia,* 5th ed. New York: Columbia University Press.

Chomsky, N. (1965), *Aspects of the Theory of Syntax.* Cambridge, MA: MIT Press.

Coen, S. (1986), The sense of defect. *J. Amer. Psychoanal. Assn.,* 34:47–67.

Cohen, D. J. (1998), Marianne Kris memorial lecture. Meeting of the Association for Child Psychoanalysis, April 5.

Cohen, J. (1985), Learning disabilities and adolescence: Developmental considerations. *Adol. Psychiatry,* 12:177–196.

———— (1993), Attentional disorders in adolescence: Integrating psychoanalytic and neuropsychological diagnostic and developmental considerations. *Adol. Psychiatry,* 19:301–342.

———— Cohler, B. (In preparation), *The Psychoanalytic Study of Lives Over Time: Clinical and Research Perspectives on Children Who Return to Treatment in Adulthood.*

Coulmas, F. (1989), *The Writing Systems of the World.* Oxford: Basic Blackwell.

De Hirsch, K. (1975), Language deficits in children with developmental lags. *The Psychoanalytic Study of the Child,* 30:95–126. New Haven, CT: Yale University Press.

Dement, W., & Kleitman, N. (1957), Cyclic variations in EEG during sleep and their relation to eye movements, bodily mobility and dreaming. *Electroencephal. & Clin. Neurophysiol.,* 9:673–690.

Denckla, M. B. (1972), Clinical syndromes in learning disabilities: The case for "splitting" versus "lumping." *J. Learn. Dis.,* 5:401–406.

Doris, J., & Solnit, A. (1963), Treatment of children with brain damage and associated school problems. *J. Amer. Acad. Child Psychiatry,* 2:618–635.

Edgcumbe, R. (1993), Developmental disturbances in adolescence and their implications for transference and technique. *Bull. Anna Freud Centre,* 16:107–120.

Fenichel, O. (1937), The scoptophilic instinct and identification. *Internat. J. Psycho-Anal.*, 18:6–34.

Fisher, C. (1954), Dreams and perception. *J. Amer. Psychoanal. Assn.*, 2:389–445.

Fonagy, P., Moran, G., Edgcumbe, R., Kennedy, H., & Target, M. (1993), The roles of mental representations and mental processes in therapeutic action. *The Psychoanalytic Study of the Child*, 48:9–48. New Haven, CT: Yale University Press.

——— Target, M. (1996), Predictors of outcome in child psychoanalysis: A retrospective of 763 cases at The Anna Freud Center. *J. Amer. Psychoanal. Assn.*, 44:27–77.

Freud, A. (1962), Assessment of childhood disturbances. *The Psychoanalytic Study of the Child*, 17:149–158. New York: International Universities Press.

——— (1963), The concept of developmental lines. *The Psychoanalytic Study of the Child*, 18:245–265. New York: International Universities Press.

——— (1965), *Normality and Pathology in Childhood*. London: Hogarth Press, 1980.

——— (1974), A psychoanalytic view of developmental psychopathology. In: *The Writings*, Vol. 8. New York: International Universities Press, 1981, pp. 57–74.

Freud, S. (1891), *On Aphasia*. New York: International Universities Press, 1953.

——— (1895), Project for a scientific psychology. *Standard Edition*, 1:281–391. London: Hogarth Press, 1966.

——— (1905), Three Essays on the Theory of Sexuality. *Standard Edition*, 7:123–243. London: Hogarth Press, 1953.

——— (1909), Family romances. *Standard Edition*, 9:235–241. London: Hogarth Press, 1959.

——— (1912), The dynamics of transference. *Standard Edition*, 12:97–108. London: Hogarth Press, 1958.

——— (1919), "A child is being beaten." *Standard Edition*, 17:179–204. London: Hogarth Press, 1955.

——— (1923), The Ego and the Id. *Standard Edition*, 19:1–66. London: Hogarth Press, 1961.

——— (1926), Inhibitions, Symptoms and Anxiety. *Standard Edition*, 20:75–172. London: Hogarth Press, 1959.

——— (1937), Moses and Monotheism. *Standard Edition*, 23:1–137. London: Hogarth Press, 1964.

Fries, M., & Lewi, B. (1938), Interrelated factors in development. *Amer. J. Orthopsychiatry*, 8:726–752.

Furman, E. (1974), *A Child's Parent Dies.* New Haven, CT: Yale University Press.

—— (1985), On fusion, integration and feeling good. *The Psychoanalytic Study of the Child,* 40:81 110. New Haven, CT: Yale University Press.

—— (1991), Early latency—Normal and pathological aspects. In: *The Course of Life: Psychoanalytic Contributions toward Understanding Personality Development,* Vol. 3, ed. S. I. Greenspan & G. H. Pollock. Madison, CT: International Universities Press, pp. 161–203.

Furman, R. A. (1996), Methylphenidate and "ADHD" in Europe and the U.S.A. *Child Analysis,* 7:132–145.

Gabbard, G. (1990), *Psychodynamic Psychiatry in Clinical Practice.* Washington, DC: American Psychiatric Press.

Galin, D. (1977), Lateral specialization and psychiatric issues: Speculation on the development and evolution of consciousness. *Ann. NY Acad. Sci.,* 6:396–410.

Garber, B. (1988), The emotional implications of learning disabilities: A theoretical integration. *The Annual of Psychoanalysis,* 16:111–128. Madison, CT: International Universities Press.

—— (1989), Deficits in empathy in the learning disabled child. In: *Learning and Education: Psychoanalytic Perspectives,* ed. K. Field, B. Cohler, & G. Wool. Madison, CT: International Universities Press, pp. 617–635.

—— (1991), The analysis of a learning-disabled child. *Annual of Psychoanalysis,* 19:127–149. Hillsdale, NJ: Analytic Press.

—— (1992), The learning disabled adolescent: A clinical perspective. *Adol. Psychiatry,* 18:322–347.

Geleerd, E., Ed. (1967), *The Child Analyst at Work.* New York: International Universities Press.

Gensler, D. (1993), Learning disability in adulthood: Psychoanalytic considerations. *Contemp. Psychoanal.,* 29:673–692.

Gilberg, C., Melander, H., von Knorring, A. L., Janos, O. L., Thernlund, G., Hagglof, B., Eidevall-Wallin, L., Gustafsson, P., & Kopp, S. (1997), Long-term stimulant treatment of children with attention deficit hyperactivity disorder symptoms: A randomized double blind placebo control trial. *Arch. Gen. Psychiatry,* 54:857–964.

Gilbert, S. (1997), Study supports use of stimulants for children with hyperactivity. *New York Times,* F10. September 16.

Glenn, J., & Bernstein, I. (1995), Sadomasochism. In: *Psychoanalysis. The Major Concepts,* ed. B. E. Moore & B. D. Fine. New Haven, CT: Yale University Press, pp. 252–265.

Glover, E. (1925), Notes on oral character formation. *Internat. J. Psycho-Anal.*, 6:131–154.

Grigorenko, E. L., Wood, F. B., Meyer, M. S., Hart, L. A., Speed, W. C., Shuster, A., & Pauls, D. L. (1997), Susceptibility loci for distinct components of developmental dyslexia on chromosomes 6 and 15. *Amer. J. Hum. Genet.*, 6:27–39.

Gross-Glenn, K., Duara, R., Barker, W. W., Lowenstein, D., Chang, J. Y., Yoshii, F., Apicella, A. M., Pascal, S., Boothe, T., Savush, S., Jallad, B. J., Novoa, L., & Lubs, H. A. (1991), Positive emission tomographic studies during serial word-reading by normal and dyslexic adults. *J. Clin. Exper. Neuropsych.*, 13:531–544.

Hallowell, E. M., & Ratey, J. J. (1994), *Driven to Distraction*. New York: Pantheon Books.

Halperin, J. M., Gittelman, R., Klein, D. F., & Ruddel, R. G. (1984), Reading disabled hyperactive children: A distinct subgroup of attention deficit disorder with hyperactivity? *J. Abnorm. Child Psychology*, 12:1–14.

Harley, M., Ed. (1974), *The Analyst and the Adolescent at Work*. New York: Quadrangle.

Harris, J. C. (1995), *Developmental Neurology*, Vol. 2. New York: Oxford University Press.

Hartmann, H. (1950), Comments on the psychoanalytic theory of the ego. In: *Essays on Ego Psychology: Selected Problems in Psychoanalytic Theory*. New York: International Universities Press, 1964, pp. 113–141.

Hartocollis, P. (1968), The syndrome of minimal brain dysfunction in young adult patients. *Bull. Menninger Clin.*, 32:102–114.

Heinicke, C. M. (1972), Learning disturbances in childhood. In: *Manual of Child Psychopathology*, ed. B. B. Wolman. New York: McGraw-Hill, pp. 662–705.

Heisler, A. B. (1983), Psychosocial issues in learning disabilities. *Ann. of Dyslexia*, 33:303–310.

Hellman, I. (1954), Some observations on mothers of children with intellectual inhibitions. *The Psychoanalytic Study of the Child*, 9:259–273. New York: International Universities Press.

Herman, J. L., & Lane, R. C. (1995), Cognitive ego psychology and the psychotherapy of learning disorders. *J. Contemp. Psychother.*, 25:15–34.

Hoffman, D., Stockdale, S., Hicks, L., & Schwaninger, J. (1995), Diagnosis and treatment of head injury. *J. Neurother.*, 1:14–21.

Hoope, J. (1977), Split brains and psychoanalysis. *Psychoanal. Quart.*, 46:220–244.

Hooper, S. R., & Swartz, C. (1994), Learning disability subtypes: Splitting versus lumping revisited. In: *Learning Disabilities Spectrum: ADD, ADHD, & LD*, ed. A. J. Capute, P. J. Accardo, & B. K. Shapiro. Baltimore: York Press, pp. 37–66.

Hughes, J. R. (1985), Evaluation of electrophysiological studies of dyslexia. In: *Behavioral Measures of Dyslexia*, ed. D. Gray & J. K. Parkton. Baltimore: York Press.

Interagency Committee on Learning Disabilities (1987), *Learning Disabilities: A report to the U.S. Congress.* Washington, DC: U.S. Government Printing Office.

Janzen, T., Graap, K., Stephanson, S., Marshall, W., & Fitzsimmons, G. (1995), Differences in baseline EEG measures for ADD and normally achieving preadolescent males. *Biofeedback Self Reg.*, 20:65–82.

Jarvis, V. (1958), Clinical observations on the visual problem in reading disability. *The Psychoanalytic Study of the Child*, 13:451–470. New York: International Universities Press.

Jones, E. (1953), *The Life and Work of Sigmund Freud*, Vol. 1. New York: Basic Books.

Kafka, E. (1984), Cognitive difficulties in psychoanalysis. *Psychoanal. Quart.*, 53:533–550.

Kagan, J. (1981), *The Second Year: The Emergence of Self-Awareness.* Cambridge, MA: Harvard University Press.

Kanzer, M., Ed. (1971), *The Unconscious Today.* New York: International Universities Press.

Katan, A. (1961), Some thoughts about the role of verbalization in early childhood. *The Psychoanalytic Study of the Child*, 16:184–188. New York: International Universities Press.

Kaye, S. (1982), Psychoanalytic perspectives on learning disability. *J. Contemp. Psychother.*, 13:83–93.

Kennard, M. A. (1960), Value of equivocal signs in neurological diagnosis. *Neurology*, 10:753–764.

Keogh, B. K. (1971), Hyperactivity and learning disorders: Review and speculation. *Exceptional Children*, 38:101–109.

Kernberg, O. (1975), *Borderline Conditions and Pathological Narcissism.* New York: Jason Aronson.

Kestenberg, J. (1975), Outside and inside, male and female. In: *Children and Parents: Psychoanalytic Studies in Development.* New York: Aronson, pp. 101–154.

Klein, E. (1949), Psychoanalytic aspects of school problems. *The Psychoanalytic Study of the Child*, 3/4:369–390. New York: International Universities Press.

Klein, M. (1931), A contribution to the theory of intellectual inhibitions. *Internat. J. Psycho-Anal.*, 12:206–218.

Kohut, H. (1977), *The Restoration of the Self.* New York: International Universities Press.

Kris, E. (1956), The recovery of childhood memories in psychoanalysis. *The Psychoanalytic Study of the Child,* 11:54–88. New York: International Universities Press.

Kuperman, S., Johnson, B., Arndt, S., Lindgren, S., & Wolraich, M. (1996), Quantitative EEG differences in a nonclinical sample of children with ADHD and undifferentiated ADD. *J. Amer. Acad. Child Adol. Psychiatry,* 35:1009–1017.

Landwehrmeyer, B., Gerling, J., & Wallesch, C. W. (1990), Patterns of task-related slow brain potential in dyslexia. *Arch. Neurol.,* 47:791–797.

Leichtman, M. (1992), Psychotherapeutic interventions with brain-injured children and their families: II. Psychotherapy. *Bull. Menninger Clin.,* 56:338–360.

Levin, F. M. (1991), *Mapping the Mind: The Intersection of Psychoanalysis and Neuroscience.* Hillsdale, NJ: Analytic Press.

——— (1995a), Psychoanalysis and the brain. In: *Psychoanalysis: The Major Concepts,* ed. B. E. Moore & B. D. Fine. New Haven, CT: Yale University Press, pp. 537–552.

——— (1995b), Psychoanalysis and knowledge. Part 1. *Annual of Psychoanalysis,* 23:95–115. Hillsdale, NJ: Analytic Press.

——— Kent, E. (1995), Psychoanalysis and knowledge. Part 2. *Annual of Psychoanalysis,* 23:117–130. Hillsdale, NJ: Analytic Press.

——— Vuckovich, D. M. (1983), Psychoanalysis and the two cerebral hemispheres. *Annual of Psychoanalysis,* 10:171–197. New York: International Universities Press.

Levy, F., Hay, D. A., McStephen, M., Wood, C., & Waldman, I. (1997), Attention-deficit hyperactivity disorder: A category or a continuum? Genetic analysis of a large-scale twin study. *J. Amer. Acad. Child Adol. Psychiatry,* 36:737–744.

Levy, J. (1974), Psychobiological implications of bilateral asymmetry. In: *Hemisphere Functions in the Human Brain,* ed. S. J. Dimond & J. G. Beaumont. New York: Halstead Press, pp. 121–183.

Lewis, L. (1986), Individual psychotherapy with patients having combined psychological and neurological disorders. *Bull. Menninger Clin.,* 50:75–87.

——— (1992), Two neuropsychological models and their psychotherapeutic implications. *Bull. Menninger Clin.,* 56:20–32.

Lou, H. C., Henricksen, L. E., & Bruhn, P. (1964), Focal cerebral hypoprofusion in children with dysphasia and/or attention deficit disorder. *Arch. Neurol.*, 41:825–829.

Lubar, J., & Shouse, M. (1976), Use of biofeedback in the treatment of seizure disorders and hyperactivity. *Adv. in Clin. Child Psychology*, 1:203–265.

Lubs, H., Gross-Glenn, K., Duara, R., Feldman, E., Stottun, B., Jallad, B., Kushch, A., & Rabin, M. (1994), Familial dyslexia. In: *Learning Disorder Spectrum: ADD, ADHD and LD*, ed. A. J. Capute, P. J. Accardo, & B. K. Shapiro. Baltimore: York Press, pp. 85–105.

Mahler, M. S. (1942), Pseudoimbecility; a magic cap of invincibility. *Psychoanal. Quart.*, 11:149–164.

—— Pine, F., & Bergman, A. (1975), *The Psychological Birth of the Human Infant*. New York: Basic Books.

Mann, C. A., Lubar, J. F., Zimmerman, A. W., Miller, C. A., & Muenchen, R. A. (1992), Quantitative analysis of EEG in boys with attention-deficit-hyperactivity-disorder. *Ped. Neurol.*, 8:30–36.

Mattis, S., French, J. H., & Rapin, I. (1975), Dyslexia in children and young adults: Three independent neuropsychological syndromes. *Development. Med. & Child Neurol.*, 17:150–163.

McDevitt, J. B. (1975), Learning disturbances. In: *Personality Development and Deviation*, ed. G. H. Wiedeman & M. Summer. New York: International Universities Press, pp. 148–160.

McGee, R., & Share, D. L. (1988), Attention deficit disorder-hyperactivity and academic failure: Which comes first and what should be treated? *J. Amer. Acad. Child Adol. Psychiatry*, 27:318–325.

Meers, D. R. (1970), Contributions of a ghetto culture to symptom formation. Psychoanalytic studies of ego anomalies in childhood. *The Psychoanalytic Study of the Child*, 25:209–230. New York: International Universities Press.

—— (1973), Psychoanalytic research and intellectual functioning of ghetto-reared black children. *The Psychoanalytic Study of the Child*, 28:395–417. New Haven, CT: Yale University Press.

Migden, S. D. (1983), Issues in concurrent psychotherapy-remediation. *Annals of Dyslexia*, 33:275–288.

—— (1990), Dyslexia and psychodynamics: A case study of a dyslexic adult. *Annals of Dyslexia*, 40:107–116.

—— (1996), Dyslexia and self control: An ego psychoanalytic perspective. Typescript.

Miller, J. (1996), Anna Freud: A historical look at her theory and technique of child psychoanalysis. *The Psychoanalytic Study of the Child*, 51:142–171. New Haven, CT: Yale University Press.

Miller, L. (1991), *Freud's Brain: Neuropsychodynamic Foundations of Psychoanalysis.* New York: Guilford.

—— (1993), Freud's brain: Toward a unified neuropsychodynamic model of personality and psychotherapy. *J. Amer. Acad. Psychoanal.*, 21:183–212.

Moore, B. E. (1995), Narcissism. In: *Psychoanalysis. The Major Concepts,* ed. B. E. Moore & B. D. Fine. New Haven, CT: Yale University Press, pp. 229–251.

—— Fine, B. D. (1990), *Psychoanalytic Terms and Concepts.* New Haven, CT: Yale University Press/American Psychoanalytic Association.

Moran, G. (1984), Psychoanalytic treatment of diabetic children. *The Psychoanalytic Study of the Child,* 39:407–447. New Haven, CT: Yale University Press.

Myers, W. A. (1989), Cognitive style in dreams: A clue to recovery of historical data. *Psychoanal. Quart.,* 58:241–244.

—— (1994), Addictive sexual behavior. *J. Amer. Psychoanal. Assn.,* 42:1159–1183.

Nathan, W. A. (1992), Integrated multimodal therapy of children with attention-deficit hyperactivity disorder. *Bull. Menninger Clin.,* 56:283–312.

Newman, C. J., Dember, C. F., & Krug, O. (1973), He can but he won't: A psychodynamic study of so-called gifted underachievers. *The Psychoanalytic Study of the Child,* 28:83–129. New Haven, CT: Yale University Press.

Palombo, J. (1985a), The treatment of neurocognitively impaired children. *Clin. Soc. Work J.,* 13:117–128.

—— (1985b), The treatment of borderline neurocognitively impaired children: A perspective from self psychology. *Clin. Soc. Work,* 13:114–125.

—— (1987), Selfobject transferences in the treatment of borderline neurocognitively impaired children. *Child & Adol. Soc. Work,* 1:18–33.

—— (1991), Neurocognitive differences, self cohesion, and incoherent self narratives. *Child Adol. Soc. Work,* 8:449–472.

—— (1994), Incoherent self-narratives and disorders of the self in children with learning disabilities. *Smith College Studies in Soc. Work,* 64:129–152.

—— (1995), Psychodynamic and relational problems of children with nonverbal learning disabilities. In: *The Handbook of Infant, Child and Adolescent Psychotherapy: A Guide to Diagnosis and Treatment,* Vol. 1, ed. J. A. Incorvia & B. Mark. Northvale, NJ: Jason Aronson, pp. 147–178.

———— Berenberg, A. H. (1997), The psychotherapy of children with nonverbal learning disabilities. In: *The Handbook of Infant, Child and Adolescent Psychotherapy: New Directions in Integrative Treatment*, Vol. 2, ed. J. A. Incorvia & B. Mark. Northvale, NJ: Jason Aronson, pp. 25–67.

———— Feigon, J. (1984), Borderline personality development in childhood and its relationship to neurocognitive deficits. *Child Adol. Soc. Work*, 13:114–125.

Pearson, G. H. J. (1952), A survey of learning difficulties in children. *The Psychoanalytic Study of the Child*, 7:322–386. New York: International Universities Press.

Peltz, M. L. (1992), The wish to be soothed as a resistance. *Psychoanal. Quart.*, 61:370–399.

Pennington, B. F. (1991a), *Diagnosing Learning Disorders: A Neuropsychological Framework*. New York: Guilford.

———— (1991b), Annotation: The genetics of dyslexia. In: *Annual Progress in Child Psychiatry and Child Development*. New York: Brunner/Mazel, pp. 193–201.

Piaget, J. (1923), *The Language and Thought of the Child*, 2nd ed. London: Routledge, 1932.

Pine, F. (1980), On phase-characteristic pathology of the school-age child: Disturbances of personality development and organization (borderline conditions) of learning and of behavior. In: *The Course of Life: Psychoanalytic Considerations Toward Understanding Personality Development*, Vol. 2, ed. S. I. Greenspan & G. H. Pollock. Washington, DC: U.S. Government Printing Office, pp. 165–203.

———— (1991), Interrelations of specific cognitive deficits and broader psychological functioning. In: *The Course of Life*, Vol. 3, ed. S. I. Greenspan & G. H. Pollock. Madison, CT: International Universities Press, pp. 421–425.

———— (1994), Some impressions regarding conflict, defect, and deficit. *The Psychoanalytic Study of the Child*, 49:222–240. New Haven, CT: Yale University Press.

Pinker, S. (1994), *The Language Instinct*. New York: Morrow.

Plank, E. N., & Plank, R. (1954), Emotional components in arithmetical learning as seen through autobiographies. *The Psychoanalytic Study of the Child*, 9:274–293. New York: International Universities Press.

Rappaport, S. R. (1961), Behavior disorder and ego development in a brain-injured child. *The Psychoanalytic Study of the Child*, 16:423–450. New York: International Universities Press.

Reiser, M. F. (1984), *Mind, Brain, Body: Toward a Convergence of Psychoanalysis and Neurobiology.* New York: Basic Books.

———— (1991), *Memory in Mind and Brain.* New York: Basic Books.

Richters, J. E., Arnold, L. E., Jensen, P. S., Abikoff, H., Conners, C. K., Greenhill, L. L., Hechtman, L., Hinshaw, S. P., Pelham, W. E., & Swanson, J. M. (1995), NIMH collaborative multisite multimodal treatment study of children with ADHD: I. Background and rationale. *J. Amer. Acad. Child Adol. Psychiat.,* 34:987–1000.

Roiphe, H., & Galenson, E. (1981), *Infantile Origins of Sexual Identity.* New York: International Universities Press.

Roth, N. (1990), Does neurology inform psychoanalysis? A case report. *J. Amer. Acad. Psychoanal.,* 18:512–518.

Rothstein, A. (1992), Neuropsychological "deficit" and psychological conflict. Presented at the Seminar for Clinicians sponsored by the American Psychoanalytic Association, New York, October.

———— (1998), Neuropsychological dysfunction and psychological conflict. *Psychoanal. Quart.,* 67:218–239.

———— Benjamin, L., Crosby, M., & Eisenstadt, K. (1988), *Learning Disorders: An Integration of Neuropsychological and Psychoanalytic Considerations.* Madison, CT: International Universities Press.

Rubenstein, B. O., Fallick, M. L., Levitt, M., & Eckstein, R. (1959), Learning problems; learning impotence, a suggested diagnostic category. *Amer. J. Orthopsychiatry,* 29:315–323.

Rubovits-Seitz, P. (1988), Intelligence and analyzability. *Annual of Psychoanalysis,* 16:171–216. Madison, CT: International Universities Press.

Rumsey, J. M., Andreason, P., Aquino, T., Hamburger, S. D., Picus, A., Rapaport, J. I., & Cohen, R. M. (1992), Failure to activate the left temporoparietal cortex in dyslexia: An oxygen 15 positron emission tomographic study. *Arch. Neurol.,* 49:527–534.

———— Dorwart, R., Vermes, M., Denckla, M. G., Krues, M. J. P., & Rapoport, J. L. (1986), Magnetic resonance imaging of brain anatomy in severe developmental dyslexia. *Arch. Neurol.,* 43:1045–1046.

Sandler, J., Kennedy, H., & Tyson, R. (1980), *The Technique of Child Psychoanalysis: Discussions with Anna Freud.* Cambridge, MA: Harvard University Press.

Sarvis, M. A. (1960), Psychiatric implications of temporal lobe damage. *The Psychoanalytic Study of the Child,* 15:454–481. New York: International Universities Press.

Satterfield, J. H., Schell, A. M., Backs, L. W., & Hidaka, K. C. (1984), A cross-sectional and longitudinal study of age effects of electrophysiological measures in hyperactive and normal children. *Biol. Psychiatry*, 19:973–990.

Schmukler, A., Ed. (1991), *Saying Goodbye. A Casebook of Termination in Child and Adolescent Analysis.* Hillsdale, NJ: Analytic Press.

Schore, A. N. (1994), *Affect Regulation and the Origins of the Self.* Hillsdale, NJ: Lawrence Erlbaum.

Schwaber, E. A. (1992), Countertransference: The analyst's retreat from the patient's vantage point. *Internat. J. Psycho-Anal.*, 73:349–361.

Shane, E. (1984), Self-psychology: A new conceptualization for the understanding of learning disabled children. In: *Kohut's Legacy: Contributions to Self-Psychology*, ed. P. Stepansky & A. Goldberg. Hillsdale, NJ: Analytic Press, pp. 191–203.

Shapiro, B. K. (1994), Early detection of learning disability. In: *Learning Disabilities Spectrum: ADD, ADHD, & LD*, ed. A. J. Capute, P. J. Acardo, & B. K. Shapiro. Baltimore: York Press, pp. 121–131.

Shapiro, D. (1965), *Neurotic Styles.* New York: Basic Books.

Shaywitz, S. E., Fletcher, J. M., & Shaywitz, B. A. (1994), A new conceptual model for dyslexia. In: *Learning Disabilities Spectrum: ADD, ADHD, & LD*, ed. A. J. Capute, P. J. Accardo, & B. K. Shapiro. Baltimore: York Press, pp. 1–15.

————— Shaywitz, B. A., Pugh, K. R., Fulbright, R. K., Constable, R. T., Mencl, W. E., Shankweiler, D. P., Leberman, A. M., Skudlarski, P., Fletcher, J. M., Katz, L., Marchione, K. E., Lacadie, C., Gatenby, C., & Gore, J. C. (1998), Functional disruption in the organization of the brain for reading in dyslexia. *Proc. Nat. Acad. Sci.*, 95:2636–2641.

Sholevar, G. P., & Glenn, J., Eds. (1991), *Psychoanalytic Case Studies.* Madison, CT: International Universities Press.

Silbar, S., & Palombo, J. (1991), A discordant consolidation of the self in a late adolescent male. *Child Adol. Soc. Work*, 8:17–31.

Silver, L. (1981), The relationship between learning disabilities, hyperactivity, distractibility, and behavioral problems. *J. Amer. Acad. Child Adol. Psychiatry*, 20:385–397.

————— (1989), Psychological and family problems associated with learning disabilities: Assessment and intervention. *J. Amer. Acad. Child Adol. Psychiatry*, 29:219–325.

————— (1992), *Attention-Deficit Hyperactivity Disorder: A Clinical Guide to Diagnosis and Treatment.* Washington, DC: American Psychiatric Press.

Silverman, M. A. (1971), The growth of logical thinking. Piaget's contribution to ego psychology. *Psychoanal. Quart.*, 40:317–341.

——— (1976), The diagnosis of minimal brain dysfunction in the preschool child. In: *Mental Health in Children*, Vol. 2, ed. D. V. Siva Sankar. Westbury, NY: PJD Publications, pp. 221–301.

Silverstein, S. (1981), *The Missing Piece Meets the Big O.* New York: HarperCollins.

Smith, H. F. (1986), The elephant on the fence: Approaches to the psychotherapy of Attention Deficit Disorder. *Amer. J. Psychother.*, 40:252–264.

Smokler, I. A., & Shevrin, H. (1979), Cerebral lateralization and personality style. *Arch. Gen. Psychiatry*, 36:949–954.

Solms, M. (1995), New findings in the neurological organization of dreaming. *Psychoanal. Quart.*, 64:43–67.

——— (1997), *The Neuropsychology of Dreams.* Hillsdale, NJ: Lawrence Erlbaum.

Sprince, M. P. (1967), The psychoanalytic handling of pseudo-stupidity and grossly abnormal behavior in a highly intelligent boy. In: *The Child Analyst at Work*, ed. E. R. Geleerd. New York: International Universities Press, pp. 85–114.

Squire, L. R. (1987), *Memory and Brain.* New York: Oxford University Press.

——— (1995), Contribution to panel on memory. Fall Meetings of the American Psychoanalytic Association. New York, December 16.

Staver, N. (1953), The child's learning difficulty as related to the emotional problems of the mother. *Amer. J. Orthopsychiatry*, 23:131–141.

Sterman, M., & Macdonald, L. (1978), Effects of central EEG feedback training on incidences of poorly controlled seizures. *Epilepsia*, 19:207–222.

Stone, L. (1954), The widening scope of indications for psychoanalysis. *J. Amer. Psychoanal. Assn.*, 2:567–594.

Strachey, J. (1930), Some unconscious factors in reading. *Internat. J. Psycho-Anal.*, 11:322–331.

Vereecken, P. (1965), Inhibition of ego functions and the psychoanalytic theory of acalculia. *The Psychoanalytic Study of the Child*, 20:535–566. New York: International Universities Press.

Waldhorn, H. F. (1960), Assessment of analyzability: Technical and theoretical observations. *Psychoanal. Quart.*, 29:478–506.

Watt, D. F. (1990), Higher cortical functions and the ego: Explorations of the boundary between behavioral neurology, neuropsychology, and psychoanalysis. *Psychoanal. Psychol.*, 7:487–527.

Weil, A. P. (1961), Psychopathic personality and organic behavior disorders—different diagnostic and prognostic considerations. *Comp. Psychiatry,* 2:83–95.

——— (1970), The basic core. *The Psychoanalytic Study of the Child,* 25:422–460. New York: International Universities Press.

——— (1971), Children with minimal brain dysfunction. *Psychosoc. Process,* 1:80–97.

——— (1977), Learning disturbances with special consideration of dyslexia. *Issues Child Ment. Hlth.,* 5:52–66.

——— (1978), Maturational variations and genetic-dynamic issues. *J. Amer. Psychoanal. Assn.,* 26:461–491.

Weinberg, W. A., & Brumback, R. A. (1992), The myth of attention deficit hyperactivity disorder: Symptoms resulting from many causes. *J. Child Neurol.,* 7:431–445.

Wender, P. H. (1971), *Minimal Brain Dysfunction in Children.* New York: John Wiley.

Willick, M. (1991), Working with conflict and deficit in borderline and narcissistic patients. In: *Conflict and Compromise: Therapeutic Implications,* ed. S. Dowling. Madison, CT: International Universities Press, pp. 77–94.

Wolff, P. (1960), The Developmental Psychologies of Jean Piaget and Psychoanalysis. *Psychological Issues,* Monogr. 5. New York: International Universities Press.

Zametkin, A. J., Liebenauer, L. L., Fitzgerald, J. A., King, A. C., Minkunas, E. V., Herscovitch, P., Yamada, E. M., & Cohen, R. M. (1990), Brain metabolism in teenagers with attention-deficit hyperactivity disorder. *Arch. Gen. Psychiatry,* 50:333–340.

Name Index

Subject Index